**Current
Respiratory
Care**

given out
Boston, April, 1978

'

Current Respiratory Care

Edited by

Kenneth F. MacDonnell, M.D.

Associate Professor of Medicine,
Tufts University School of Medicine, Boston;
Director, Pulmonary Unit,
St. Elizabeth's Hospital of Boston

Maurice S. Segal, M.D.

Professor (Emeritus) of Medicine,
Tufts University School of Medicine, Boston;
Director, Foundation for
Research in Bronchial Asthma
and Related Diseases, Cambridge

Little, Brown and Company
Boston

To Ann and the children and to Sylvia, who
should be glad to find us at home now that
the book is completed.

Library of Congress Catalog Card No. 76-42687

ISBN 0-316-54191-5

Printed in the United States of America

Preface

An annual inhalation and respiratory therapy postgraduate course, founded by Maurice S. Segal, M.D., serves as the model for this textbook. The goal of both is to bridge the "knowledge gap" and update recent technical and medical advances for the various members of the respiratory care team (physician, therapist, nurse). The physician charged with respiratory care must have an understanding of the operational mechanics and construction of those instruments so necessary for modern respiratory therapy. So too, the respiratory therapist must have an understanding of the basic pathophysiologic mechanisms of pulmonary disease. The expanding role of the nurse in the clinical care of patients is well known to all. Thus, each member can most effectively discharge his or her responsibilities only with an understanding of the total process of respiratory care. Such a format requires the presentation of current and proposed technical innovations as well as therapeutic and diagnostic trends in respiratory therapy.

Whenever a team approach is employed in respiratory care, there are areas (ventilators, monitors, therapeutic agents) that are more familiar to some members of the team than to others. Nonetheless, it remains true that the most effective patient care is rendered when all members of the team have at least a modest understanding of the basic concepts and present state of the art of the entire field of pulmonary medicine. With this goal in mind, we have divided this textbook into sections dealing first with instrumentation, then the latest diagnostic techniques, then topics of special clinical importance and interest. Following these discussions are sections dealing with therapeutic agents and nursing care and nursing responsibilities to the respiratory patient, and the final section, which is concerned with glimpses into the future of respiratory care as a discipline. Thus, a cross-section of respiratory care topics, not intended to be encyclopedic or exhaustive, is presented and discussed within the framework of the respiratory team concept.

K. F. M.
M. S. S.

Acknowledgments

We wish to thank Richard Johnston for his many sketches and artistic contributions. Mrs. Pat Filley spent many hours typing and retyping the manuscript; her expert performance facilitated its completion. Many others readily volunteered their help; they include Linda Healy, Susan Dalton, Judy Pierce, Judy Yarosz, and Tom Bartosek.

We gratefully acknowledge the help of our colleagues: David McGoldrick, M.D., for his review of pathologic specimens, R. E. Langevin, M.D., for his review of the radiographic material, and a special thanks to Francis Donovan, M.D., for his assistance.

Little, Brown and Company and its staff, especially Sarah Boardman and Diane Faissler, were invaluable in their advice and assistance.

In conclusion, there are many we have deprived of much during the past year, and we have gained much more. They will recognize their influence.

K. F. M.
M. S. S.

Contents

Preface　　*v*

Acknowledgments　　*vii*

Contributing Authors　　*xiii*

Section 1　Instrumentation
1　Mechanical Ventilators　　3
Daniel J. Donovan
Richard P. Johnston
Kenneth F. MacDonnell

2　Respiratory Monitoring: Systems and Devices　　25
Daniel J. Donovan
Richard P. Johnston
Kenneth F. MacDonnell

3　Gas Delivery Systems　　59
Daniel J. Donovan
Richard P. Johnston
Kenneth F. MacDonnell

Section 2　New Diagnostic Techniques
4　Pulmonary Function Testing: New and Old　　69
Doraswamy Saroja Moorthi

ix

5 Sputum and the Respiratory Therapist 113
Mauricio J. Dulfano
Don E. Davis

6 Bronchoscopy 129
Kenneth F. MacDonnell
Doraswamy Saroja Moorthi

Section 3 Clinical Topics
7 Hemodynamic Aspects of Respiratory Care 137
Bernard D. Kosowsky

8 Immunologic Processes in Respiratory Disease 151
Bernard A. Berman
John M. O'Loughlin

9 Microbiology: Epidemiology, Diagnosis, and Therapeutics as Applied 169
to Respiratory Therapy
Terrence Murphy

10 Oxygen: Therapeutics, Toxicity, Advances 191
Grace R. Baldwin

11 Positive Pressure Breathing: Physiologic Effects and Consequences 229
Kenneth F. MacDonnell
Bijan Sadrnoori

12 Weaning: Criteria; Intermittent Mandatory Ventilation 245
Kenneth F. MacDonnell

13 Tracheal Stenosis 253
Armand A. Lefemine

14 Controlled Ventilation: Neuromuscular Blocking Agents 277
Robert E. Flynn

15 Chronic Obstructive Pulmonary Disease 291
Kenneth F. MacDonnell

16   Bronchial Asthma: Nature and Management   307
Maurice S. Segal
Kenneth F. MacDonnell

17   Adult Respiratory Distress Syndrome   321
Kenneth F. MacDonnell

18   Recent Advances in the Care of Neonatal Respiratory Disorders   339
Marguerite J. Herschel
Joseph L. Kennedy, Jr.

Section 4   Therapeutic Agents
19   Therapeutic Aerosols   357
Maurice S. Segal

20   Methylxanthines   373
Maurice S. Segal

Section 5   Nursing Care
21   Nursing Care of the Patient with Respiratory Disease   389
Marsha Goodwin
Ellen Moloney Bergeron

Section 6   On the Horizon
22   Lung Transplantation   417
Armand A. Lefemine

23   Respiratory Assistance Using the Artificial Lung   427
Armand A. Lefemine

24   Glossary of Therapeutics   447
Maurice S. Segal

Index   465

Contributing Authors

GRACE R. BALDWIN, M.D.
Assistant Instructor of Medicine, Tufts University
School of Medicine; Maurice S. Segal Pulmonary Fellow,
St. Elizabeth's Hospital of Boston

ELLEN MOLONEY BERGERON, R.N.
Head Nurse, Respiratory Intensive Care Unit,
St. Elizabeth's Hospital of Boston

BERNARD A. BERMAN, M.D.
Assistant Clinical Professor of Pediatrics, Tufts
University School of Medicine; Chief, Pediatric
Allergy Department, St. Elizabeth's Hospital of
Boston

DON E. DAVIS, A.A., A.R.R.T.
Supervisor, Respiratory Therapy Technicians, Brooklyn
Veterans Administration Hospital, Brooklyn, New York

DANIEL J. DONOVAN, A.B.
Chief, Respiratory Therapy Department, St. Elizabeth's
Hospital of Boston

MAURICIO J. DULFANO, M.D.

Associate Professor of Medicine, State University of New York Downstate Medical Center College of Medicine, Brooklyn; Chief, Respiratory Care Center, Brooklyn Veterans Administration Hospital, Brooklyn, New York

ROBERT E. FLYNN, M.D.

Associate Professor of Medicine, Tufts University School of Medicine; Director, Department of Medicine, and Chief of Neurology, St. Elizabeth's Hospital of Boston

MARSHA GOODWIN, R.N., B.A.

Chairman, Nursing Level I, St. Elizabeth's Hospital of Boston

MARGUERITE J. HERSCHEL, M.D.

Assistant Professor of Pediatrics, Tufts University School of Medicine; Assistant Clinical Professor of Pediatrics, Boston University School of Medicine, Boston; Neonatologist, St. Margaret's Hospital, Dorchester, Massachusetts

RICHARD P. JOHNSTON

Chief Pulmonary Function Technician, St. Elizabeth's Hospital of Boston

JOSEPH L. KENNEDY, Jr., M.D.

Associate Professor of Pediatrics, Tufts University School of Medicine, Boston; Director of Nurseries, St. Margaret's Hospital, Dorchester, Massachusetts

BERNARD D. KOSOWSKY, M.D.

Associate Professor of Medicine, Tufts University School of Medicine; Chief of Cardiology, St. Elizabeth's Hospital of Boston

ARMAND A. LEFEMINE, M.D.

Associate Professor of Surgery, Tufts University School of Medicine; Chief of Cardiovascular Surgery, St. Elizabeth's Hospital of Boston

KENNETH F. MACDONNELL, M.D.

Associate Professor of Medicine, Tufts University School of Medicine; Director, Pulmonary Unit, St. Elizabeth's Hospital of Boston

DORASWAMY SAROJA MOORTHI, M.D.

Instructor of Medicine, Tufts University School of
Medicine; Director, Pulmonary Physiology Laboratory,
St. Elizabeth's Hospital of Boston

TERRENCE MURPHY, M.D.

Instructor of Medicine, Tufts University School of
Medicine; Staff Physician, St. Elizabeth's Hospital
of Boston

JOHN M. O'LOUGHLIN, M.D.

Instructor in Medicine, Harvard Medical School;
Senior Staff Allergist, Department of Allergy and
Dermatology, Lahey Clinic Foundation, Boston

BIJAN SADRNOORI, M.D.

Pulmonary Fellow, St. Elizabeth's Hospital of Boston

MAURICE S. SEGAL, M.D.

Professor (Emeritus) of Medicine, Tufts University
School of Medicine, Boston; Director, Foundation for
Research in Bronchial Asthma and Related Diseases,
Cambridge

Notice

The indications and amounts of all solutions in this book have been recommended in the literature and conform to
the practices of the general medical
community in which the various authors
practice. The solutions described do not
necessarily have specific approval by the
Food and Drug Administration for use
in the situations and the amounts for
which they are recommended. The
package insert or label for each solution
should be consulted for use and dosage
as approved by the FDA. Because standards for usage change, it is advisable to
keep abreast of *all* recommendations,
particularly those concerning new
solutions.

Current
Respiratory
Care

Instrumentation

1

Daniel J. Donovan
Richard P. Johnston
Kenneth F. MacDonnell

Mechanical Ventilators

1

Mechanical ventilators are clinically useful in a variety of applications ranging from intermittent positive pressure breathing (IPPB) therapy to the complex task of continuous controlled ventilatory support. It follows that the design and character of the respirator should fit its clinical assignment; it seems wasteful to utilize an expensive, sophisticated machine for routine IPPB treatment. Those responsible for the assignment and use of mechanical ventilators should be thoroughly acquainted with the capabilities and limitations of each type.

A number of classifications have been prepared, categorizing ventilators according to such criteria as flow, volume, and pressure. For our purpose, we have divided ventilators into three major categories: pressure-cycled (Bird Mark 7; PR 1,2), volume-cycled (Ohio; Bennett MA–1; see below), and time-cycled (Air Shield; Engstron), the reference source in each device remaining constant.

The pressure-cycled ventilator depends on the creation of a pressure gradient from the mouth to the pleural space (and generally has no volume control on the machine) to deliver a volume of gas. This volume may be quite variable from breath to breath, depending on any changes that might occur in the mechanical characteristics of the patient's lung. This necessitates scrupulous attention to tidal volume and minute volume.

One of the advantages of a volume-cycled apparatus is its relative independence of changes in patient mechanics, although this is not to say that careful observation is unnecessary.

Both inspiratory and expiratory time are preset in the classic time-cycled ventilator. Variations in flow, pressure, and volume are possible. The constant reference source is time, and cycling of the device is not affected by alterations in lung dynamics.

For any change in lung compliance, a thorough diagnostic search should be instituted to be sure that the patient has not suffered a pneumothorax or atelectasis.

Only those ventilators that are new or of special interest are considered in this chapter: Bennett MA-1; Ohio Critical Care; Siemens Servo Ventilator 900; Searle VVA; Chemetron Gill 1; Emerson 3MV; Foregger 210; Monaghan 225; Cavitron PV-10 Pediatric Ventilator; Amsterdam Infant Ventilator. Modifications that we have found useful are also described (see also Chapter 11).

Humidifiers and nebulizers, once thought of as accessories to ventilators, are now recognized as integral components. For this reason, they are discussed separately in this chapter.

THE BENNETT MA-1 VENTILATOR

Classified as volume-cycled, the Bennett MA-1 ventilator is electronically controlled with a double gas circuit that isolates the patient's inspired gas from the machine compressor and pneumatic circuitry (Figure 1-1). The obvious advantage of this type of system is to ensure a relatively "clean" air supply for the patient. Ambient air is drawn into the ventilator through a coarse filter 2½ inches in diameter (A). Oxygen is stored in the oxygen reservoir (B). These gases are mixed to obtain the desired FI_{O_2} in the oxygen-proportioning valve (C). Gas is then delivered to the main bellows (D). Desired tidal volumes are controlled by a pair of potentiometers. The volume knob on the control panel adjusts one potentiometer; movement of the main bellows adjusts another. When the resistances of the potentiometers are equal, the machine cycles to expiration. Movement of the bellows is controlled by pressure changes initiated from the main compressor (E), via line (F) through solenoid valve (O) to flow control (G). The flow control manipulates the speed of the gas as it passes from the compressor (E) to the bellows chamber (H). Diaphragm valve (J) opens and closes, providing for expiration and inspiration. Gas passes through outlet valve (K) to the patient circuit.

There is a separate compressor (L) for the nebulizer, which derives its gas supply from the main bellows, thus assuring uniform FI_{O_2}. Once activated, the compressor (L) stays on. Nebulization occurs only during inspiration because of the action of the nebulizer solenoid valve (M), which alternately opens and closes according to the inspiratory-expiratory pattern. The inspiration-control solenoid valve (O) connects the main compressor and the exhalation valve during inspiration. During expiration it powers the positive end expiratory pressure (PEEP) regulator and outlet valve (K).

The maximum pressure generated by the main compressor is 7.5 PSI; however, through a series of reductions, a maximum of 80 cm H_2O is effectively generated. The pressure control knob regulates the pressure exerted upon a microswitch against a diaphragm, which in turn communicates with the patient circuitry. If the preset

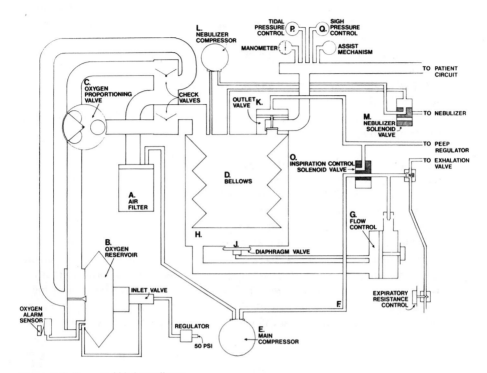

Figure 1-1. Bennett MA-1 ventilator.

pressure is exceeded, the machine cycles to expiration. There are separate pressure alarms for tidal pressure controls (P) and sigh pressure controls (Q), as well as separate pressure limit knobs.

The sensitivity device consists of a metal diaphragm that makes electrical contact as long as the pressure within is at or above the preset sensitivity level; once pressure drops below this level, then contact is broken, and the inspiratory phase of respiration is activated. This mechanism is involved in assist positive end expiratory pressure (PEEP) (see Chapter 11). The rate-controlling knob is a timing device that automatically starts an inspiratory phase. A slow-rate circuit card is offered as an option that allows for a minimum respiratory rate of one breath every 150 seconds (±50 sec); this option is valuable if intermittent mandatory ventilation (IMV) is to be employed.

Oxygen percentage may be adjusted to deliver concentrations varying from ambient to 100%. It should be noted that the oxygen alarm system is sensitive to pressure change and not to oxygen concentration. A device similar to the pressure limit control is used as a sensor, measuring the pressure in the oxygen reservoir.

The sigh volume mechanism employs a volume-determining device that is similar to that used to set tidal volume. A timing device activates the sigh volume system at the desired frequency.

The amount of PEEP is determined by a variable-pressure regulator that is powered by the main compressor.

MA-1 ventilator alarms are tidal and sigh volume pressures, I:E ratio, and O_2 pressure.

The cascade humidifier is a heated bubble-through type with a heating range from room temperature to $140°F$.

OHIO CRITICAL CARE VENTILATOR

Ohio Critical Care Ventilator (Figure 1–2) is a volume-cycled apparatus that is electronically controlled and that has a double gas circuit. Ambient air is drawn in through a coarse air filter (A) and travels past the oxygen-mixing valve (B) to the bellows (C). Oxygen enters at 50 PSI, is reduced to 12 PSI by regulator (D), then passes the pressure sensor (E) and enters reservoir (F), from which it passes to the oxygen-mixing valve (B). The prescribed FI_{O_2} may then be delivered to the patient. The volume adjustment knob (G) turns a spool (H) attached to a cord (I) in turn attached to the base of the bellows (C). The height of the bellows determines the volume of gas delivered to the patient. Power is provided by the turbine (J). Either sigh volume actuator (K) or tidal volume actuator (L) opens diaphragm (M), allow-

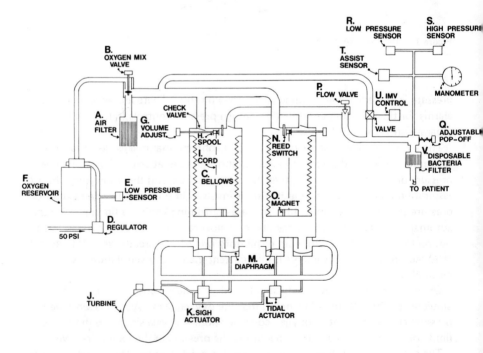

Figure 1–2. Ohio Critical Care Ventilator.

ing air into the bellows housing and forcing the bellows upward, delivering the preset tidal volume and oxygen concentration to the patient. At the end of inspiration a reed switch (N) responds to a field from a magnet (O) located in the base of both bellows and cycles to expiration. Gas flow is regulated by needle valve (P). Pressure limitation is adjusted by pop-off valve (Q).

The controls for two pressure-sensing devices that activate alarms in the event that preset high or low pressure limits are exceeded are located on the main panel. The low-pressure sensor (R) consists of a diaphragm with a preset force exerted on it. If during inspiration 8 cm H_2O pressure is not attained, then activation of an audiovisual alarm ensues. A variable, spring-loaded, pressure-regulated diaphragm (S) is the basic device employed in the high-pressure alarm system. Movement of the diaphragm, which activates a microswitch, triggers an audiovisual alarm and cycles the respirator to exhalation should airway pressure exceed two times in a row the upper limit set by the operator. There is a maximum pressure limit available to the patient circuitry of 100 cm H_2O. Sensitivity is photoelectrically regulated via a diaphragm connected to a shutter that gates the light source and photodiode sensor. Adjustment of the sensitivity knob alters the responsiveness of the photodiode receptor. Output from the photodiode is amplified and transmitted to the tidal volume and sigh volume activators.

The PEEP mechanism employs a needle valve to bleed gas from the turbine outlet and directs this gas to the exhalation valve line. This serves to maintain pressure on the exhalation balloon, producing PEEP.

Variable oxygen concentrations are obtained via the oxygen-mixing valve (B). However, the audiovisual oxygen fail alarm is not a concentration but a pressure sensor, and inspiratory gas must be checked if specific concentrations of oxygen are required; excess oxygen is vented.

Inflation hold is accomplished by a timing circuit with a range from 0 to 2 seconds. Intermittent mandatory ventilation (U) is a standard feature that, when activated, bypasses the bellows; gas is drawn through the oxygen-mixing valve, thus allowing for convenient continuation of humidified oxygen. Gas then travels to the patient via bacteria filter (V).

Alarms systems for the Ohio Critical Care Ventilator are as follows: high and low pressure, oxygen, failure to cycle, and power failure.

The humidifier is a heated bubble-through type with a heating range to 90°F.

SIEMENS SERVO VENTILATOR 900

The Siemens Servo Ventilator 900 (Figure 1-3) is a volume-cycled, electropneumatically powered ventilator. Controls on the front are used to select the required respiratory pattern. These values are converted into electrical signals and stored in the electronic control unit where they later serve as reference values. Air and oxygen may be mixed (range 21% to 100%) to prescribed concentrations in the pneumatic blender (A) before entering the ventilator through the inlet valve (B). Gas enters the bellows (C), which is under a pressure load variable from 0 to 100 cm H_2O. The bel-

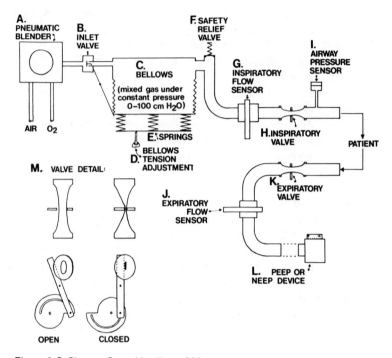

Figure 1-3. Siemens Servo Ventilator 900.

lows tension is adjusted by a turnkey (D) that adjusts the tension of springs (E) against the bellows. Maximum inspiratory pressure is also adjusted in this way. Gas then passes out of the bellows past the safety relief valve (F) to the inspiratory flow sensor (G). This sensor is integrated with the minute volume and rate controls found on the front panel. When the prescribed tidal volume is reached, flow is interrupted by the inspiratory valve (H), which closes, occluding the pliable inspiratory tubing. The airway pressure sensor (I) is a strain gauge transducer which transmits to the electronic control unit an electronic signal proportional to the actual flow. This signal is compared to the preset reference values. The servomotors are controlled so that the actual and reference values are integrated; thus, the prescribed ventilation pattern is maintained. An expiratory flow sensor (J) analyzes the expired minute volume, which is displayed on a panel meter. Upper and lower limits of minute volume can be set; if these limits are violated, then an audiovisual alarm system is activated.

Flow control allows alteration in wave form. Flow rate is a function of inspiratory time control, pressure, and tidal volume.

Sigh volume is activated every 100 breaths automatically. The options of sigh volumes are three: (1) no change in tidal volume, (2) two times the tidal volume, (3) three times the tidal volume.

The airway pressure control knobs are responsible for both sensitivity and high pressure relief. A strain gauge transducer transmits an electronic signal; the sensitivity control is regulated by a low-limit pressure knob, which either initiates or interrupts inspiratory flow.

Both inspiratory and expiratory control valves are servomotors (M) and allow metered inspiratory and expiratory control. Expiratory resistance can be adjusted from 1 liter/min to zero resistance.

Inflation hold can be varied from 0 to 20% at 5-second intervals; the PEEP mechanism (L) is a spring-loaded valve that obstructs the expiratory port; it is adjustable from 0 to 20 cm H_2O.

The negative end expiratory pressure (NEEP) device (L) bleeds gas from the blender, then utilizes a venturi on the exhalation dump port to generate negative end expiratory pressure.

The Siemens Servo Ventilator allows the operator to set high and low alarm limits for both expired tidal volume and airway pressure.

SEARLE VVA (VOLUME VENTILATOR ADULT)
The VVA (Figure 1–4) is a volume-cycled machine that is electronically controlled with a single gas circuit. Gas is drawn into the machine through a coarse filtering sys-

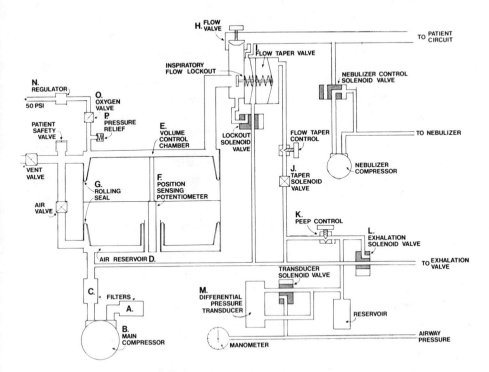

Figure 1–4. Searle VVA (Volume Ventilator Adult).

tem (A); it is then directed under pressure by a carbon vane compressor (B) to a gas reservoir consisting of two chambers, located one atop the other. The superior chamber (E) is for volume control; the amount of gas contained therein will determine the amount of gas delivered to the patient, i.e., tidal volume. The inferior chamber (D) functions as a reservoir, refilling the superior chamber following each patient inspiration. The volume of gas expelled by the piston and rolling seal (G) of the superior chamber is determined by adjustment of the tidal volume control knob, which regulates a potentiometer.

Inflow of gas into the superior chamber will continue until the resistance between the tidal volume potentiometer and the superior chamber sensing potentiometer (F) are equal, at which time all gas inlets are closed. Volume is adjustable between 250 and 2,200 ml. Two flow control valves are located on the main panel of the VVA. The main flow control knob (H) is a needle valve that can regulate flow between 2 and 200 liters/min. The taper valve (I) produces either a square wave or a tapered wave flow curve, depending on whether or not it is engaged. The sensitivity control adjusts automatically by means of the exhalation solenoid valve (L) to varying levels of end expiratory pressure. A differential pressure transducer (M) samples airway pressure proximal to the exhalation port; if line pressure falls below the predetermined values, then machine inspiration is initiated.

The concentration of oxygen in the superior chamber, which is in fact the concentration of oxygen in each tidal breath, is accomplished by a logic control system of the VVA. This control circuit receives information from the chamber potentiometer (F) and adjusts oxygen inflow to arrive at the prescribed oxygen concentration.

Pressure control of the VVA consists of two main panel knobs, one that regulates a high-pressure alarm and one that regulates a high-pressure relief cycle. The high-pressure alarm employs a differential pressure transducer that compares the signal output from the alarm potentiometer and the pressure transducer; when pressure limits are exceeded, an audiovisual alarm is initiated. The high-pressure relief control functions in a similar manner. When it samples pressures in excess of its preset limits, it automatically cycles the machine to expiration. Both controls are adjustable to pressure ranges from 0 to 100 cm H_2O. Pressure from the main carbon vane compressor is directed through a needle valve (K) (PEEP control knob) to the exhalation valve balloon.

The humidifier is a disposable bubble-through humidifier, refilled by a constant infusion setup. A heating element is provided.

A wedge spirometer with an audiovisual apnea alarm is standard equipment. As an added feature, electronic outputs for volume measurement may be connected to a remote recording device or to a visual display.

Respiratory rate is controlled by an electronic timing circuit and is displayed digitally. The inspiration-expiration ratio is also displayed digitally. If the 100% oxygen button is pressed, 3 minutes of 100% oxygen will be delivered to the patient.

An optional battery pack is available with this ventilator.

The following are the types of alarms that can be used with the Searle VVA:

1. Airway disconnect. Samples are taken during end inspiration; if the pressure of the sample is less than 1 cm H_2O, then an audiovisual alarm is activated.
2. Short exhalation. A ratio alarm; if the inspiratory time is greater than the expiratory time, then an audiovisual alarm is activated.
3. Failure to cycle. If 15 seconds pass without a machine inspiration, an audiovisual alarm is activated.
4. Low oxygen pressure. An alarm will be activated if line pressure is less than 15 PSI.

CHEMETRON GILL 1 VENTILATOR

Volume-cycled with a double gas circuit, the Gill 1 ventilator (Figure 1–5) is electronically controlled. Air is drawn in through a filtered inlet (A) and delivered to the main reservoir, which is separated into an upper control chamber (B) and a lower delivery chamber (C). A vacuum compressor pump (D) draws up a weighted piston (E) in the control chamber to a height commensurate with the preset tidal volume. Gas is then expelled from the delivery chamber by the movement of a rolling seal (F), which is gravity-powered and pneumatically controlled. The gas then travels through a high-efficiency particulate air (HEPA) filter (see Chapter 3) past an oxygen analyzer to a heated bubble-through humidifier and into the patient circuitry.

Flow control is accomplished by altering the rate at which the piston falls in the delivery chamber. A valve control (G), located on the inlet side of the piston chamber, controls the rate at which gas fills the chamber; this in turn regulates the speed at which the gravity-powered piston can fall in the delivery chamber. A square-wave flow rate of 0 to 120 liters/min is possible.

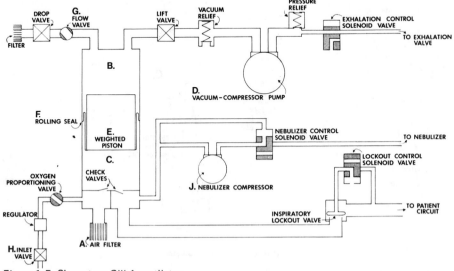

Figure 1–5. Chemetron Gill 1 ventilator.

The oxygen inlet (H) delivers the gas under pressure to the delivery chamber; mixing continues until the desired oxygen concentration is obtained. This concentration is adjusted by the operator until the desired oxygen concentration is displayed on the main panel.

A needle valve regulates a venturi positioned downstream from the exhalation port, generating NEEP during expiration if that is desired.

Alarms for the Gill 1 consist of pressure limit, improper cycle, low pressure, power failure, improper O_2 I:E ratio, and low water level in the humidifier.

EMERSON 3MV INTERMITTENT MANDATORY VENTILATION VENTILATOR

The Emerson 3MV with intermittent mandatory ventilation (Figure 1-6) is an electrically powered volume-preset ventilator. It utilizes a wheel-and-pulley mechanism to drive a cylindrical piston (F). A series of one-way valves is employed to ensure a unidirectional air flow. A mixture of air and oxygen from either a mixing valve or a blender enters through a valve (A). Relief valve (B) is set at 3 cm H_2O. One-way valves (C) provide for patient "breathe-through" should power fail. The 5-liter bag (D) provides a reservoir for intermittent mandatory ventilation. Gas at the prescribed oxygen concentration then passes through another one-way valve (E) into the piston (F). The same mixture is fed through valve (G) to the patient reservoir bag (H). Volume is regulated by adjusting the length of the piston (F) stroke, which is powered by a 115-volt motor attached to a wheel-and-pulley system. The preset volume passes through a third one-way valve (J), past the oxygen sensor (K), into the humidifier (L), which is situated on top of the heater (M). Gas passes over the heated water, and then out the patient inspiratory supply line (N) through a copper mesh filter, which has an oligodynamic effect. Pressure limits are controlled by ad-

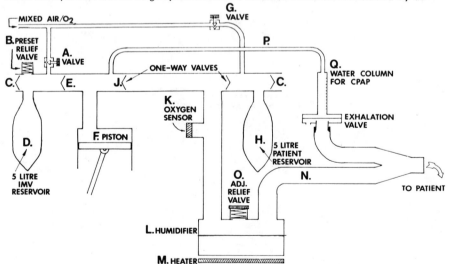

Figure 1-6. Emerson 3MV intermittent mandatory ventilation ventilator.

justing relief valve (O). Line (P) supplies pressure to the combined water PEEP and exhalation valve (Q) on the expiratory patient supply line. Flow rate is regulated by a variable-speed control on the motor.

FOREGGER 210 VENTILATOR

The Foregger 210 is an electrically powered, single-circuit volume ventilator (Figure 1–7). Air and oxygen at 50 PSI are mixed in the pneumatic blender (A) and are regulated to 33 to 35 PSI after passing the 5 μ sintered bronze filter (B) and the inlet pressure sensor (C), which is preset to signal an alarm at pressures less than 20 PSI. If piped-in compressed air is not available, the Foregger can be ordered with an optional air compressor. A portion of this mixed gas is further regulated to 2 to 3 PSI and made available to the adjustable PEEP regulator (D) and exhalation solenoid valve (E). During inspiration, the exhalation solenoid valve directs the 2 to 3 PSI mixed gas to the patient circuit exhalation valve balloon. During expiration, this flow is then directed to the exhalation solenoid valve, which connects the exhalation valve balloon with its PEEP solenoid valve (F). In this manner, PEEP pressures up to 35 cm H_2O are made available to the patient (when the PEEP solenoid valve is connected to the activated PEEP regulator). The PEEP control is uncalibrated, and PEEP pressures are set while observing the airway pressure manometer. If the PEEP regulator is not activated, the PEEP solenoid valve is opened to room air

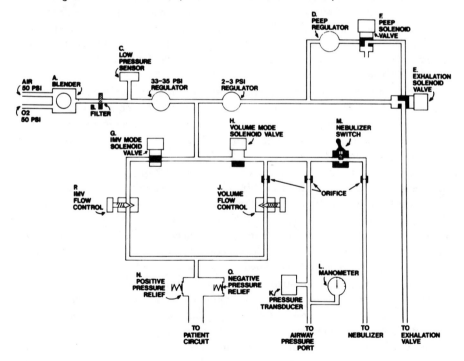

Figure 1–7. Foregger 210 ventilator.

(ambient pressure) depending upon whether the 210 is in the IMV or volume mode. The remaining portion of the 33 to 35 PSI mixed gas is directed through either the IMV mode solenoid valve (G) or the volume mode solenoid valve (H).

During inspiration a small flow of mixed gas is directed past the airway pressure transducer and manometer to prevent condensation buildup in the airway pressure line. Also during inspiration, the nebulizer switch, in its on position, directs flow through a flow-limiting precision orifice to the patient circuit nebulizer. When the nebulizer's switch is in the off position, flow is directed downstream distal to the volume mode flow control (not shown in diagram), thereby allowing the Foregger 210 to deliver the same tidal volume regardless of whether the nebulizer is activated or not. The tidal volume and respiratory rate of the Foregger 210 are regulated by a combination of three controls: the I:E control, which is continuously adjustable from a ratio of 1:1 to a ratio of 1:4; the inspiratory time control, which is continuously adjustable from 0.5 to 4.0 sec; and the volume flow control, which is adjustable from 0.2 to 2.0 liters/sec. Tidal volume and respiratory rate are computed from these parameters and are displayed digitally on the control unit.

When the ventilator is operating in the IMV mode, the 33 to 35 PSI mixed gas is directed through the IMV flow control (P) (which is adjustable from 0.2 to 0.8 liter/sec) to the patient circuit. IMV rate is adjustable from 0.5 to 15 breaths per minute. The volume of these IMV breaths is determined by the volume mode inspiratory time control and volume mode flow control, and is digitally displayed.

In the volume mode, the 33 to 35 PSI mixed gas trifurcates and is directed via a flow-limiting precision orifice to the volume flow control (J), via a flow-limiting precision orifice to the airway pressure transducer (K) and manometer (L), and to the nebulizer switch (M).

The inspiratory pause control keeps the patient's lungs inflated at end-inspiration for a period adjustable from 0.2 to 2.0 sec. The Foregger 210 considers the inspiratory pause to be part of the inspiratory period and automatically increases expiratory time in accordance with the setting of the I:E ratio control, thereby decreasing the delivered respiratory rate.

Sigh breaths are given in multiples of 1, 2, or 3, at rates of 4, 6, 8, 10, or 15 per hour. Sigh volume is adjustable from 25% to 100% above normal tidal volume.

Assist pressure sensitivity is an uncalibrated control, and the assist level must be set in conjunction with the airway pressure manometer. The assist control is self-compensating for PEEP pressures, thereby allowing assisted ventilation at all levels of PEEP. Airway pressure is limited to a maximum of 100 cm H_2O and a minimum of -10 cm H_2O by positive (N) and negative (O) safety relief valves.

The pressure alarm is an audiovisual alarm with two functions, and it is activated if line pressure drops below 20 PSI or if inspiratory pressure during a sigh or normal breath exceeds the limits preset by the pressure limit control. The ventilator automatically cycles to expiration if inspiratory pressure limits are exceeded.

The apnea alarm, a patient disconnect alarm, is activated if a computed airway pressure threshold is not reached during inspiration. For tidal volumes less than 0.2 liter, airway pressure must exceed 3 cm H_2O to prevent activation of the apnea alarm. For tidal volumes greater than 0.2 liter, the apnea alarm's minimum pressure threshold is computed from the formula [15 X TV (liters)]. The alarm threshold pressures are automatically referenced to PEEP pressure if PEEP is used.

The internal failure alarm is activated if a patient breath is not initiated within 16 seconds from the end of the last expiration. The internal failure alarm is deactivated when the ventilator is in IMV mode.

The Foregger 210 comes with a heated Bennett cascade bubble-through humidifier and, except for the addition of an airway pressure port, uses the standard MA–1 ventilator circuit. The Foregger 210 also comes with an expiratory spirometer that uses a unidirectional, vane-type sensor. The spirometer displays either tidal or minute volume and provides adjustable high and low audiovisual alarms in the minute volume mode only. The manufacturer claims an accuracy of ± 5% for its spirometer.

MONAGHAN 225 VENTILATOR

The Monaghan 225 is a pneumatically powered, fluidically controlled volume ventilator. The 225 can operate in a time-cycled, pressure-cycled, or volume-cycled mode. The source gas enters the ventilator with a pressure of 50 PSI. A sintered filter excludes all particles greater than 5 μm in size from the inlet gas. The availability of clean air is essential to the operation of a fluid device, for its flow characteristics can be adversely affected by particulate contamination. All fluidic and timing devices are pneumatically regulated (see page 16). Beyond the filter, the gas flow bifurcates. One limb is delivered under 50 PSI pressure, which serves to power (1) the minifluid amplifier valve that operates the air-oxygen bellows system; (2) the flow controller; and (3) the nebulizer system. The second limb delivers gas first to a 5 to 7 PSI-reducing regulator, after which it serves to power the remaining components of the ventilator. A bypass relief valve assures a pressure ceiling of less than 10 cm H_2O. Gas then flows to the mode-select module, which allows for selection of either assist, controlled, or assist-controlled ventilation. When in the assist or assist-controlled mode, the patient trigger module responds to a reduction in pressure in the patient tubing.

Using ambient pressure as a reference, the amount of negative pressure required to initiate inspiration may be varied from 1 cm H_2O to –10 cm H_2O. The PEEP control is connected to the patient trigger module. Sensitivity reference is automatically adjusted to the level of end expiratory pressure that allows for assisted ventilation during PEEP.

The timing module controls respiratory rate, inspiration-expiration ratio, and pressure limits. Two identical timing bellows initiate inspiration and expiration, respectively. Inspiratory time is controlled by the inspiration-expiration ratio control. Gas flows into the inspiratory timer chamber, which surrounds the inspiratory timing bellows. A signal is sent to the dual or/nor module, which allows 50 PSI to reach the air-oxygen bellows via the minifluid amplifier valve, the flow-control needle valve, and the bronze filter. The bellows is moved upward, delivering the prescribed gas volume to the patient tubing. Volume is set by adjusting the bellows height with a crank. A high-pressure signal is sent back to the timing module when the baseplate of the air-oxygen bellows touches an actuator rod. This results in the vertical movement of the inspiratory timer bellows, causing a plunger to change a pressure signal, switching the timer module to expiration. The flow of gas at 50 PSI stops. The diaphragm check valve at the patient tubing outlet closes. A high-pressure signal travels to the timing module. The expiration timing bellows cylinder fills in the same manner as the inspiratory bellows. Cycling frequency is determined by varying the distance traveled by the exhalation bellows, and hence varying the exhalation time.

During exhalation, the air-oxygen bellows falls because of the lack of pressure in the cannister. Gas is expelled from the cannister via a diaphragm valve into the air-oxygen mixing chamber; as the bellows descends, ambient air is entrained through a 120 μ filter. A valve diverts some of the gas expelled from the cannister and mixes it with the ambient air. An oxygen control governs the amount of oxygen that is mixed with ambient air. Excess oxygen is vented to the atmosphere.

Pressure limits are controlled by the positive-pressure cutoff mode. When a preset limit is exceeded, this module sends a pneumatic signal to the timing module, and exhalation is initiated.

FLUIDICS

Although the Monaghan 225 is a departure from the usual design for ventilators, its function is based on the concept of fluidics, or the technology of amplifiers, valves, and switches powered and controlled solely by the flow of liquid or gas. Fluidic technology has its basis in phenomena first recognized and described by Henri Coanda 40 years ago. The Coanda effect, as this observation has come to be known, states that when a flowing fluid stream (gas or liquid) is directed across a surface, it becomes attached to that surface until some counterforce or change in surface contour forces a separation [2]. Fluidic stream attachment forces can best be understood through the Bernoulli effect, which states that the lateral pressure of a fluid decreases as its velocity increases. Breakaway of a high-velocity fluidic stream from a surface is resisted by the low-pressure void generated between the surface and the fluidic stream by the low lateral pressure of that stream (Figure 1-8, diagram I).

Fluidic stream attachment can be manipulated through alteration of the stream-surface interface. In a bistable manifold (Figure 1-8, diagram II), where a fluidic stream has equal opportunity to flow in either of two paths (A, B), the stream's direction can be chosen by preventing the formation of a low-pressure void on one path. This acts to direct the fluidic stream to the opposite path. The low-pressure void in a bistable device can be controlled through ports (C, D) that allow pressure to be added to either path at the critical interaction region of the manifold. In the RETEC manifold (Figure 1-9), gas enters pressure inlet (A). The design of the de-

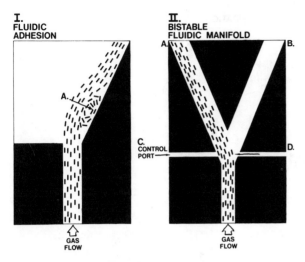

Figure 1–8. Fluidics: The Coanda effect.

vice is such that gas flows selectively past the antivortex airfoil (B) into arm (C) and hence to the patient. Back pressure created by the patient's exhalation changes flow direction from arm (D) and redirects the gas out the exhalation port (E). In the MSA IPPB manifold (Figure 1-10), a bistable fluidic valve structurally more sophisticated than the RETEC, the negative pressure of patient inspiration affects the interaction region of the fluidic valve, directing gas flow to the patient outlet (A). Feedback

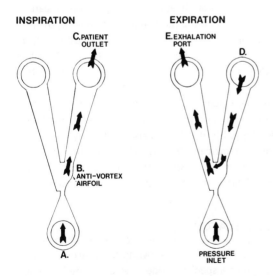

Figure 1–9. RETEC fluidic IPPB manifold.

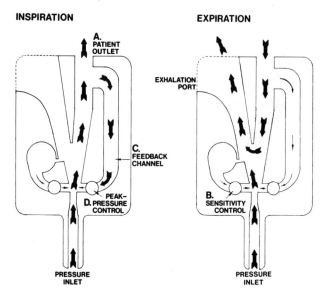

Figure 1-10. MSA fluidic IPPB manifold.

from the expiratory channel adjusted by the sensitivity control (B) determines the amount of negative pressure required to switch the valve from expiration to inspiration. Once established in the inspiratory mode, gas will continue to flow to the patient outlet until pressure in the feedback channel (C), adjusted by the peak pressure control (D), switches the valve to expiration.

Fluidic technology contains a wide range of applications in the pulmonary care field. In its simplest form, a fluidic valve can be the basis of an IPPB device, or fluidic valves can be arranged in more complex patterns that mimic those of a computer. In several pneumatic volume ventilators, i.e., the Cavitron PV-10 and Monaghan 225, fluidic logic circuitry is used to control factors and devices such as timing, flow rates, alarms, and pressures.

Fluidic devices, although sensitive to particulate matter, have high reliability, require little maintenance, and have no moving parts, thus showing many advantages over conventional gas control technology. Fluidic devices also find many applications in gas or liquid control, where an electrically powered device would introduce an undesirable hazard, or in remote or special environments, where electricity is unavailable. The following Cavitron PV-10 Pediatric Ventilator is another example of a fluidically controlled device.

CAVITRON PV-10 PEDIATRIC VENTILATOR
The Cavitron PV-10 is a pneumatically powered, fluidically controlled neonate pediatric ventilator. The PV-10 is extremely versatile, allowing for a variety of different operational modalities. Selection of a specific mode is accomplished by the use of the cycle/CPAP switch.

When the CPAP (continuous positive airway pressure) mode is selected, all timing and limit controls are bypassed, and continuous flow ventilation with or without positive pressure (CFV or CPAP) is made available to the patient. In the cycle mode, time-cycled positive pressure ventilation, either volume-limited or pressure limited, with or without PEEP, can be delivered. IMV, with an additional uncalibrated range to 30 seconds and rates as low as 2 breaths/minute, is also available. This ventilator utilizes gas as its power source. For these reasons, it may be considered useful for transporting patients who require uninterrupted mechanical ventilation.

Oxygen at 50 PSI is necessary and must be provided to operate the fluidic logic of the PV–10. Air at 50 PSI is needed if oxygen concentrations of less than 100% are to be delivered. The FI_{O_2} of inspired gas is set by adjusting the oxygen and air flow meters on the front panel, utilizing the provided slide rule nomogram. The inspiratory time control, calibrated from 0.2 to 2.0 sec, and the expiratory time control, calibrated from 0.25 to 2.5 sec, with an additional uncalibrated range to 30 sec for IMV, together set the rate for the ventilator in the time-cycled mode. Tidal volume is calculated on a slide rule nomogram using inspiratory time, expiratory time, and combined minute volume of the air and oxygen flow meters.

The PEEP/CPAP control and maximum-pressure control are uncalibrated, and their limits are determined by an airway pressure manometer. A safety relief valve located on the patient tubing connector is preset to vent the airway pressures above 70 cm H_2O and to open at airway pressures of less than 4 cm H_2O.

Because of the mode of operation of the fluidic logic, inspiratory time and expiratory time increase over their calibrated setting about 2.5% per 1,000 feet of altitude above sea level.

AMSTERDAM INFANT VENTILATOR
The Amsterdam is an electrically powered, electronically controlled, continuous-flow ventilator capable of providing tidal volumes from 20 to 300 ml. The Amsterdam operates in the time-cycled intermittent positive pressure breathing (IPPB) mode with PEEP, NEEP, or ZEEP (zero end expiratory pressure).

Oxygen concentration is determined using a nomogram and independent air and oxygen flow meters. 50 PSI of air and of oxygen must be provided to the flow meters. The mixed gas is passed through a heated humidifier to the PEEP-NEEP proportioning valve (Figure 1–11, A). Two separate inspiratory breathing circuits (B, C) exit from the proportioning valve, the gas flow through either circuit being determined by the valve setting. Both inspiratory lines run to the Ayre T-piece (D), an integral part of the Amsterdam ventilator. During inspiration, the expiratory side of the breathing circuit is occluded by a solenoid valve (E), and the inspired gas may come from either of the two inspiratory circuits. During patient inspiration, the continuous gas flow is directed, according to the PEEP-NEEP proportioning valve setting, to an expiratory venturi for NEEP, to the patient's airway for PEEP, or to both for ZEEP.

A capacitor-discharge timing circuit controls the solenoid valve. The frequency

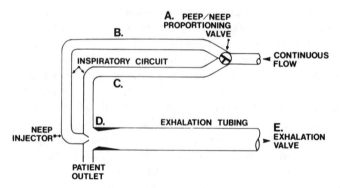

Figure 1–11. Amsterdam infant ventilator.

of the timing pulse (respiratory rate) is determined by the setting of the respira-
tions-per-minute control; pulse width (I:E ratio) is determined by the inspiration-
percent-of-cycle control. Inspiration time may also be manually controlled by the
pushing of a button located on the rear of the solenoid valve housing that mechanically closes the solenoid valve.

Peak airway pressures are limited by a spring-loaded pop-off valve located on the
front of the solenoid valve housing. Uncalibrated, this control limit is set in conjunction with the airway pressure manometer.

Tidal volumes are determined by a nomogram using the combined minute volumes
of the air and oxygen flow meters, respiratory rate, and inspiration time.

NEBULIZERS
Ventilators provide some of the drama in respiratory care. The following devices
might be described as more mundane, but they are equally necessary. Equipment
such as the Puritan and the McGaw Hydro-Sphere pneumatically powered nebulizers and the Devilbiss ultrasonic nebulizer (USN) will be described as representative
of traditional and new methods of providing safe humidification and nebulization.

Puritan Nebulizer
In pneumatically powered jet nebulizers, such as the Puritan nebulizer (Figure 1–
12), a source gas is delivered through a narrow aperture (A) and enters a water
reservoir (B). A syphon tube (C) connected to a filter (D) is placed at right angles
to the stream of gas. Water is drawn up the tube in accordance with Bernoulli's
principle, which states that where the velocity of a gas is high, its lateral pressure is
low. Thus, a reduction in pressure is realized at the top of the syphon tube. Because
atmospheric pressure exerted on the water surface is greater than the pressure at the
top of the syphon tube, a pressure gradient is formed, resulting in water being drawn
up the tube. The water is then entrained into the stream of gas at the nozzle. The
water surface (E) serves as a baffle system, with the larger particles reentering the

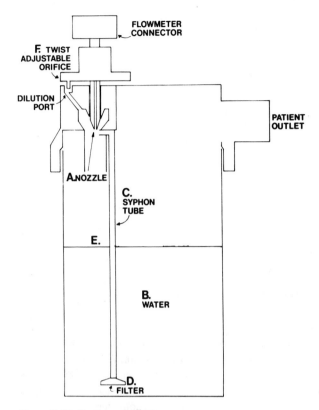

Figure 1–12. Puritan nebulizer.

reservoir. Small particles remain in aerosol form and are delivered to the patient via wide-bore tubing.

Oxygen concentrations are obtained by manipulating an adjustable orifice (F) that mixes ambient air and pure oxygen. Concentrations of 40, 70, and 100% may be obtained. Entrainment charts are provided by the manufacturer.

A 2 PSI or 40 torr pressure relief valve is used as a safeguard against excessive pressure.

An immersion heater is available to increase the humidity of the nebulized gas. The heater's thermostat is preset by the manufacturer to maintain water temperature at approximately 140°F. It is estimated that the temperature of the gas delivered to the patient will approximate normal body temperature. Newer models provide a calibrating screw to allow for temperature adjustment.

McGaw Hydro-Sphere Nebulizer

The hydro-sphere is a pneumatically powered nebulizer (Figure 1–13) that operates on the "hydronamic" (Babington) principle. Its aerosol output is comparable to that of an ultrasonic nebulizer [1]. Water from an upper reservoir (A) is continuously

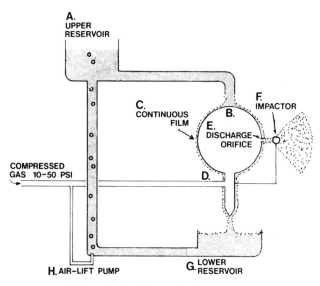

Figure 1-13. McGaw Hydro-Sphere nebulizer.

fed to the top of a nebulizer sphere (B). The effect of surface tension causes the water to form a film (C) on the surface of the nebulizer sphere. Compressed gas is delivered through an inlet port (D) to the interior of the sphere. When it exits at the outlet port (E), the gas is traveling at supersonic velocity, carrying with it a portion of the water film from the nebulizer sphere. This aerosol then strikes an impactor (F), further reducing mean particle size. Excess water is collected in a lower reservoir chamber (G) and is pumped back to the upper reservoir by a compressed air pump (H).

The Hydro-Sphere nebulizer is powered by compressed gas and will operate on inlet pressures from 10 to 50 PSI.

The Hydro-Sphere system can employ two separate nebulizer spheres simultaneously: a single-port sphere and a double-port sphere. The double-port sphere can be replaced by a plug, thus converting the system to a low-flow aerosol generator. The amount of aerosol produced is also dependent upon inlet pressure and the configuration of the nebulizer spheres.

All parts of the Hydro-Sphere can be sterilized by ethylene oxide or by chemical solutions. All parts, except the aerosol tubing, the tubing adaptors, and the aspiration dilution control valve, are autoclavable.

Ultrasonic Nebulizers

The ultrasonic nebulizer (USN) is based on the piezoelectric principle discovered in the late nineteenth century. Some crystalline substances produce electric charges when subjected to increasing pressure levels. Conversely, when an electric charge is placed across a crystal, it alters the dimensions of that crystal. This mechanical de-

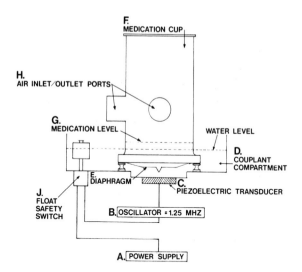

Figure 1–14. Devilbiss ultrasonic nebulizer (USN).

formation is the result of an electric potential that is formed along certain of the crystal's axes in response to the movement of the charges. The crystal changes its physical dimensions according to the applied voltage. The vibrational energy generated is utilized in aerosol production.

Power for the Devilbiss USN (Figure 1–14) is supplied by an AC power supply (A). This current is boosted in voltage, converted from AC to DC, transmitted through a capacitor resonance oscillator (B), and converted into 1.25 MHz oscillating current. The voltage of the signal, which can be controlled by the operator, will determine the number of particles produced. This extremely high energy (1 MHz = 1 million cycles/second) is transmitted to a piezoelectric transducer (C). Water is introduced into the couplant compartment (D). Vibrational energy is transmitted through the diaphragm (E). The medication cup (F) is partially immersed in the water. The substance to be aerosolized (G) is placed in the cup and is atomized into minute droplets. A small electric blower is attached to an air inlet port (H), providing the power to move the aerosol through an outlet port (H) to the patient. A float safety switch (J) guards against damage to either patient or equipment caused by lack of water in the system.

SUMMARY
There are a number of reliable and durable mechanical ventilators, humidifiers, and nebulizers commercially available. It is incumbent upon those charged with the responsibility of providing respiratory care to be thoroughly acquainted with their varying design advantages, in order to select the instrument most appropriate for a particular clinical situation.

REFERENCES

1. Calderwood, H. W., et al. Distribution of nebulized aerosols in spontaneous-breathing puppies. *Anesthesiology* 41:4, 1974.
2. Donnenfeld, R. S., and London, T. R. Fluidics: A new concept of controlled gas flow. *Exhibit at International Anesthesiology Research Society Meeting,* 1969.

Daniel J. Donovan
Richard P. Johnston
Kenneth F. MacDonnell

Respiratory Monitoring: Systems and Devices

2

The word *monitor* is derived from the Latin *monēre,* "to warn." Webster defines *monitor* as ". . . a person chosen to keep order . . . who advises, warns or cautions, . . . something that reminds or warns." Total care of the critically ill patient requires that accurate data must be gathered, stored, and presented in a logical fashion. Thus, according to the simplest definitions, physiologic monitors keep order and warn against changes in status.

It must be remembered that close observation by trained personnel is the fundamental basis for good patient care, and mechanical monitoring devices are mainly an adjunct to the keen eye of the trained observer. They should in no way be construed as an acceptable substitute. The major advantage of surveillance by an electronic device is the ability of such a device to be dedicated to a specific task for extended periods of time. Selective monitoring devices can accurately gather voluminous amounts of information and present moment-to-moment observations as a complete logical record, allowing critical care personnel to be freed from repetitive duties and enabling them to concentrate on the special tasks that people perform better than electronic equipment—decision-making and patient contact.

Mechanical monitoring is not without its disadvantages. Electrical hazards are omnipresent. Personnel must be thoroughly trained in calibration, use, and maintenance of the equipment. Despite these limitations, electronic physiologic monitoring has come of age. Unfortunately, however, respiratory monitoring has lagged behind other forms of clinical monitoring and is a relatively recent innovation. A reference as recent as the *1974 Medical Equipment Buyer's Guide* showed that most monitors do not have modules for recording respiratory function and fall short of providing meaningful indications of change in the characteristics of respiration.

Monitoring in the modern respiratory intensive care unit can be a complex procedure requiring a number of interrelated subsystems: apnea and rate detectors, devices for the detection of respiratory gas values, measurement of respiratory mechanics, and monitoring of blood gas values. Central to the ideal system is a collecting, processing, and storage capability. This is most efficiently accomplished by using a computer properly programmed to gather, process, record, and display all pertinent information.

Figure 2–1 illustrates the basic configuration of a 5-bed monitoring system employing a computer and a master module that gathers information by means of sensors attached to the patient. At each bedside is an American Optical physiologic monitor (A). Direct patient measurements are electrocardiogram (ECG); heart rate (maximum, minimum, mean); blood pressure (BP), pulmonary artery pressure (PAP), airway pressure (P_{aw}), and pulmonary capillary wedge pressure (PCWP); body temperature; and respiratory rate. These data in analog form are transmitted via the line drivers transmission cable (B) to the analog multiplexer (C). The analog signal is then

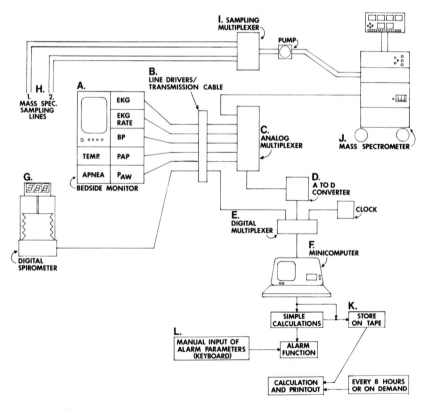

Figure 2–1. Computerized central respiratory intensive care unit monitoring system.

transformed into a digital signal in the analog to digital (A–D) converter (D), from which the signals pass through a digital multiplexer (E) to the minicomputer (F). A digital spirometer (G) measures tidal volume. This signal is sent to the minicomputer via the line drivers cable and digital multiplexer.

Two sampling lines (H) are pumped via a sampling multiplexer (I) to the mass spectrometer (J), which is then connected to the minicomputer via the same route as the physiologic monitor. PI_{O_2}, PE_{O_2}, and PE_{CO_2} are measured and stored.

In the minicomputer, data are stored on tape or disc (K) and the following calculations are made by the Fick method: O_2 uptake, CO_2 output, respiratory quotient (RQ), static compliance, alveolar-to-arterial oxygen gradient (AaP_{O_2}), dead space volume to tidal volume ratio (VD/VT), shunt fraction of flow to total pulmonary flow ratio ($\dot{Q}s/\dot{Q}T$), cardiac output ($\dot{Q}$). These data are organized and printed out every 8 hours or on demand.

A multiplexer is an electronic device capable of sorting many signals and arranging them into an order easily accepted by the computer. The minicomputer serves as a storage apparatus as well as a processing unit for calculation. The digital data enter the memory of the computer and are then processed under the direction of the central processing unit. The computation and logical data analysis needed for display and information are carried out during the time between the reading of points of data. Such programming is well within the capabilities of the minicomputer; a large, expensive computer is not required for basic monitoring procedures. An 8K memory capacity is adequate in this system.

The individual sensing and recording devices of any respiratory monitoring system may be employed singly or in combination. For this reason, each component will be presented and discussed individually: computers; magnetic mass spectrometers; direct patient measuring devices; display systems and recorders; measurement of blood gases and pH; and spirometers.

COMPUTERS

The dictionary defines a computer as a mechanical device capable of solving problems by accepting data, performing prescribed operations on the data, and supplying the results of these operations. The first computer ever used was the abacus. This was followed during the seventeenth century by the gear-driven calculator, designed by a young Frenchman named Blaise Pascal. In 1888 an American, Herman Hollerrath, devised a system that automatically counted punched holes in a card. This method, first used in 1890, is still in use today.

The computer industry as we know it today was developed and perfected in several American universities between 1937 and 1945. There have been three generations of computers since that time. The first generation was the vacuum tube computer, used from 1946 to 1959. The most widely known was the UNIVAC (Universal Automatic Computer) computer, a large, expensive apparatus necessarily restricted in use and scope. The second generation computer was a transistorized model, and the years 1959 to 1965 marked the era when computers with large memories and microsecond access time became available for general use. The transistor replaced the vacuum tube, thus shrinking the physical size of the computer without decreasing its effectiveness. A monolithic memory system is the major characteristic distinguishing the third from the second generation of computers. The third generation makes up the bulk of presently existing computers

Today's computers are made to handle large quantities of information at high rates of speed. Our modern computers work basically by counting and calculating. All work done must be reduced to mathematical terms.

The computer performs four basic operations: input, storage, processing, and output. These operations are very much like the steps in establishing a patient's treatment plan. The results of the patient's test and/or the doctor's examination is the input. The patient's medical history to date is storage. The physician, who is himself the processor, then diagnoses what is wrong with the patient, and the treatment plan is the output.

All the information needed to start computing, as well as the initial instructions, first must be gathered. The next step is to enter the data into the input unit. This may be done with a punched card, punched paper tape, or magnetic tape.

One of the indirect benefits of a computer is the discipline that it imposes upon the user. For example, to solve a problem with a computer, the user must first understand the problem and then give the computer a sequential set of instructions, or a *program,* to give the right answer. Understanding the problem to a depth of detail and insight required to program the computer is a more difficult task than one might expect.

Analog Computers

An analog signal represents the variable being measured in terms of the amplitude of an electrical signal (e.g., 150 torr in a transducer could equal 1.5 volts). The analog computer performs its calculations by manipulating these voltage amplitudes. An analog computer is programmed by interconnecting circuit components that mathematically manipulate the voltages representing the variables.

A common example of an analog computer is an integrator that calculates volume from a flow signal. If a 1-volt signal, representing a flow rate of 1 liter/sec is put into the integrator, after 5 sec the output from the integrator would be 5 volts, representing 5 liters of accumulated volume.

Analog computers are ideal for use when physical measurements are manipulated as data for arithmetic operations; when the solution of the problem needs one cycle of operation; and when a high degree of accuracy (typically limited to within 0.1 percent) is not critical. Digital computers are used when 100 percent accuracy is required, and when repetitive, routine mathematical operations are involved.

Digital Computers

People count using the decimal system, in which the position of each number is worth 10 times the one to the right. The zero in 150 represents zero ones; the five tens; the one, one one-hundred; 100 plus 50 plus 0 equals 150.

10,000	1,000	100	10	1
0	0	1	5	0

Information in a digital signal is represented in the binary number system. The binary number system uses only two digits, 1 and 0. Usually these 1s and 0s, called *bits,* are organized into "words" of specific length, most commonly consisting of 8, 16, 24, or 32 bits. In the binary system, each position is worth twice the one to the right, as opposed to being worth 10 times the one to the right in the decimal system. 150 is represented in binary notation as 10010110.

128	64	32	16	8	4	2	1
1	0	0	1	0	1	1	0

Computer components used for storage and processing work on a simple principle. Like an ordinary light bulb, they have only two possible states, on and off. In computers, "on" can represent a 1 and "off" a 0. Various combinations of on and off represent binary numbers.

On the most basic level, a modern digital computer is composed of such elements as transistors, diodes, capacitors, and resistors. With the advent of integrated circuits, these formerly discrete components have been organized into composite units. Each of these units (Figure 2-2), variously called *and gates, or gates, inverters, nand gates, nor gates, exclusive-or gates,* and *flip-flops,* performs a specific function in Boolean algebra, the algebra of the binary number system. The truth tables summarize the output states for each possible input for each device. In the central processing unit of a computer, these functional units are arranged into registers, random access memories, read-only memories, multiplexers, counters, decoders, adders, subtractors, multipliers, dividers, and other components. Although Boolean algebra performs mathematical operations with only two states, on and off or 1 and 0, its range of capabilities is as all-embracing as any arithmetic system based on the decimal system. Thus, when a program is run, the decisions and mathematical computations performed by a digital computer are limited in complexity and time only by the computer's architecture and the number of internal components.

The layman's understanding of a computer is usually limited to the fact that such a machine is able to store and retrieve large quantities of data. This capability of the digital computer is invaluable when dealing with the voluminous amounts of information that are generated from continuous monitoring of critically ill patients. With proper programming, the computer organizes the collected information in a method most convenient for the individual user. Thus it becomes possible to reference information as to date, patient's name or hospital number, disease process, type of therapy, or any other convenient method of retrieval. This capability of assimilating and organizing information can be utilized to perform tasks that normally could not be done by a person or that would require such a vast amount of time and effort that the net result would be the same: the task would not be performed.

An example of this type of task was described by Krekule and Radil-Weiss [9],

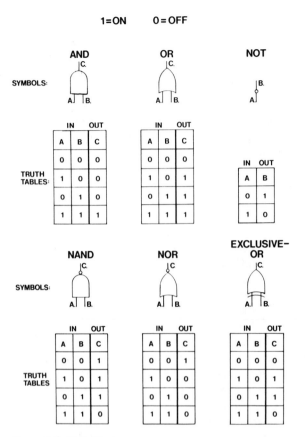

Figure 2-2. Digital logic.

using two simple computer techniques for analyzing the time relationship between cardiac activity and respiration, a nearly impossible task on a long-term basis for the human observer, but one easily completed by a computer. The computer detects the statistical time relationships between cardiac activity and respiration. This process not only makes use of the assimilation and organization capabilities of the computer but is also an example of what is known as data reduction and transformation, a sophisticated capability of the digital computer. When sending voluminous amounts of data, such as pressure and volume information from a patient on a ventilator, the analog signal obtained from the bedside monitoring device is transformed into a digital form and then must be manipulated into a display meaningful to the user. This can be accomplished by reducing it to the written word or, as Powers et al. [16] have done, a computer display of a pressure-volume curve in which pressure is on the abscissa and volume on the vertical axis for each breath. When projected side by side, a visual representation of the patient's breathing pattern enables the observer to make instantaneous note of any change in the patient's status.

The computations done by the computer in particularly difficult examples of data reduction form a highly complex subject involving higher mathematics and going beyond the scope of this discussion. Suffice it to say, however, that the capability of the digital computer to transform a vast amount of information and to provide a meaningful display of it is a particularly useful clinical tool.

Just as one need not be a mechanic to drive an automobile, one need not be a computer repair expert or programmer to operate a computerized central monitoring system. It is essential, however, to understand the basics of how a digital computer functions. There are certain principles that all computers share. Each computer must have some type of central processing unit that controls the overall operation of the device. Information must travel both into the computer and back out after processing has been completed. There must then be some method of communication between the user and the computer, or between the peripheral monitoring devices, which gather data from the patient, and the computer. Therefore, there are available a variety of devices that can either input information to the computer or output information to the user.

Memory Bank

Once information has been placed in the computer, it can be stored for future reference. Thus, each computer has some type of memory bank. The overall cost of a computer is greatly influenced by the amount of information that can be stored and manipulated by the particular device.

A digital computer can operate as the heart of any monitoring system, for certainly it satisfies the basic definition of a monitor in that it can organize data, keep them in order, and warn against changes in the status of the patient. The computer can be utilized most efficiently in postoperative recovery rooms, intensive care units, or in any other setting where the patient must be observed closely and continuously.

Analog-to-Digital Converter

When properly used in conjunction with other biomedical instruments, the computer can automatically accept and transcribe data from biologic sensing instruments. The electrical signals from most sensing devices at the patient's bedside appear in a wave (analog) form and must be translated into a numerical (digitized) form to allow for manipulation by the computer. This is a conversion process that matches analog waves to a series of numbers that describe the relative height of each portion of those waves. This is accomplished by an analog-to-digital (A–D) converter.

Hardware-Implemented Algorithms

Several investigators have used the analog computer for monitoring patients who are critically ill [13, 14, 19]. Many of the on-line continuous-measurement monitors used in intensive care units are analog devices, and as such they produce a wave form as their graphic output. The analog computer is well suited for measuring respiratory work efficiently and at reasonable cost. Such a system allows for dedicated task assignment with a rapid response time. However, the bulk of the information found in the literature concerns the digital computer. There has been interest in developing a computer combining the advantages of the analog and digital models. An interesting new approach employs special devices called *hardware-implemented algorithms* (HIA). An algorithm is any special method of solving a certain kind of problem, for example, the repetitive calculations used in finding the largest common divisor of two numbers. Such a system operates nearly independently of the central computer. The major advantage of the HIA is that the mechanics of processing information consumes only 5 μsec per second of central processing time rather than the usual 75,000 μsec required when the main computer does the entire processing. This is certainly an interesting and promising method [3] .

Any of the raw data collected through physiologic monitors can be presented to the computer's memory and used to generate calculations that give meaningful data on that particular patient. For example, the computer can be programmed to accept pertinent data, such as tidal volume and breathing pressures, from which it can calculate static compliance. Compliance is the change in pressure (in centimeters of water) that accompanies each cubic centimeter increase in lung volume, at the time of no air flow. At the point between inspiration and expiration there is, of course, no air flow. The program to perform this operation is not a difficult one to write. The computer must be programmed to know when there is no air flow and to record the airway pressure at that point. This observation is then repeated at maximum tidal volume [15] .

Alarm Systems
Alarm systems can be triggered simply by programming upper and lower limits for any given parameter. Should these limits be exceeded, the computer will then activate an alarm device.

Display of Information
When combined with the user's choice of output devices, the digital computer can provide information in many different forms. Graphs, charts, or numerical data can be shown either on paper or on a viewing screen.

Use of Data
Heretofore we have been discussing the capabilities of the computer to accept data and manipulate it in such a way that the person using it can make decisions based on information more complete than could be derived in any other fashion. However, the computer may be used to assimilate data, make a decision according to the information programmed into it by the user, and then activate another device that will in turn affect the course of the patient's treatment. A system in which a digital computer assimilates information on respiratory mechanics and then incorporates the information into a feedback system that controls the basic adjustments of minute ventilation and dead space for a patient undergoing artificial mechanical ventilation has been described [7] .

Summary

Properly programmed, a minicomputer can function as the central key to any respiratory monitoring system capable of accepting, processing, and in some instances reacting to data gathered by the various biologic sensing devices that will be discussed later in this chapter.

MAGNETIC MASS SPECTROMETER

A major aspect of our monitoring system is the use of a mass spectrometer, which is capable of reliable, continuous, and almost immediate (50 msec) gas analysis. Sampling with the mass spectrometer is sufficiently fast to allow sampling every 30 sec at each bedside.

The analysis of inspiratory and expiratory gases provides much valuable patient information, such as respiratory quotient, alveolar gas, oxygen consumption, and dead space calculation. Also, the flexibility of the system, as described earlier (Figure 2-1), allows for either full-time dedication to one patient or time-sharing with other patients.

This instrument's mechanism of operation is as follows (Figure 2-3). A sample is introduced into the device and ionized. The mass spectrometer first sorts the ions into a spectrum, according to their mass-to-charge ratios, then determines the quantity of individual ions present and displays this information in some fashion, usually a digital readout. The ion analyzer and ion detection stage of all mass spectrometers operate in a vacuum. The background pressure in the device, that is, the

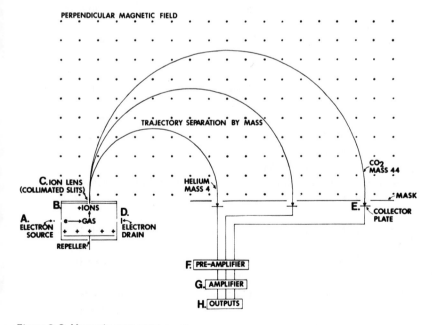

Figure 2-3. Magnetic mass spectrometer.

pressure in the vacuum without a sample having been introduced into the machine, is usually approximately 10^{-6} torr. The ion source, which is basic to the operation of the spectrometer, includes three major parts—the electron source (A), which is a hot filament; an ion chamber (B) (see also Figure 2-4); and an ion lens (C). The electron source is heated and the electrons (e) produced then travel through the ion chamber. The molecules to be analyzed are drawn into the ion chamber by vacuum. Collision between the activated stream of electrons and the vaporized sample molecule then occurs; as a result, the filament-produced electron removes one electron from the sample molecule. The positive ion (+) that is generated is then focused into a beam and accelerated out of the ion chamber by a repeller. The excess filament-produced electrons are removed from the ion chamber by the electron drain (D).

In the magnetic field, the beam of ions forms a semicircular trajectory whose radius depends upon the mass of the various sampled ions (see Figure 2-3). The mass of a particular ion determines the distance it will travel from the ion chamber to the collector plate (E). When leaving the ion chamber, there is one ion beam that contains all possible ions formed from the sample. This beam is then separated into as many beams as there are different mass ions. Each individual beam is detected by a collector upon which the ion falls. The collector then measures the ion current and sends this measurement through the preamplifier (F) and amplifier (G) to an output device (H), usually a digital meter that can display either the partial pressure or the fractional concentration of the gas involved. Because the ions of each sample are of differing masses and thus travel with different trajectories, the various ion beams will fall sequentially on the collector plate and the mass spectrum of the entire sample can be obtained.

An enlargement of the ion chamber (B) in Figure 2-3 (Figure 2-4) permits us to view the interior. A gas sample is introduced into the ion chamber via the gas inlet (A). These sample molecules collide with a stream of electrons (B) that enters at point (C) from the heated filament. The gas sample and the electron stream collide. One way the activated particle dissipates its energy is by ejecting an electron and becoming positively charged. One electron is removed from the sample. These positive ions are accelerated out of the chamber by the repeller (D) and are focused into a beam by the ion lens (E), a series of collimated slits. Excess filament-created electrons are removed at point (F) by an electron drain.

Fowler [4] lists the characteristics a mass spectrometer should possess to be of value in respiratory studies.

1. A mass range of 25 to 50 atomic mass units is regarded as essential; 15 to 50 is valuable.
2. The ability to record simultaneously the partial pressures of at least three gas components.
3. A sensitivity such that a full-scale deflection is produced by a gas component of 5 mol per 100 mol is essential, with a signal-to-noise ratio such that the accuracy of measurement is not impaired.

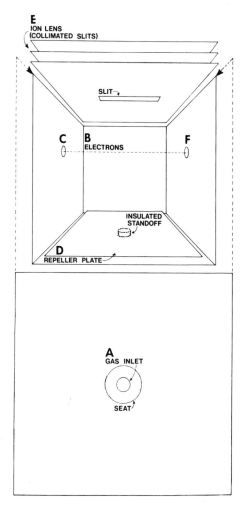

Figure 2-4. Mass spectrometer ion chamber.

4. A linear response to the partial pressure of the gas component at the sampling point with an accuracy of ±2 percent of the range in use.

5. A response time such that 90 percent of the change in gas concentration is recorded in 100 msec or less.

6. A gas sampling system that draws off less than 1 percent of the patient's turnover and maintains a constant sample chamber pressure in face of changes in gas composition, viscosity, temperature, and water vapor.

7. A vacuum system such that partial pressures in the ionizing region are proportional to those in the sample chamber, irrespective of changes in the viscosity, and can follow pressure changes in the latter within the response times specified.

8. The merits of compactness, simplicity, and reliability, with minimum requirement for high technical skill in operation and maintenance.

DIRECT PATIENT MEASURING DEVICES

The monitoring system as depicted in Figure 2-1 employs an American Optical con-
sole which receives its input from patient sensors. The patient's catheter lines are
connected to strain gauge transducers (see Figure 2-6) which are zeroed at the level
of the heart. These transducers are sensitive instruments, requiring a good deal of
care, and excessive pressure exerted on the transducer during flushing or calibration
may result in permanent damage and thus faulty determinations. Operation manuals
will define the pressure limits for each specific transducer. The transducer cable is
connected to the master module and transmits a signal to a differential amplifier. (A
single-ended amplifier is one that receives input from one input signal, amplifies it,
and uses ground as its zero. A differential amplifier receives two input signals, and
the difference between the two is the signal that is amplified.) The zero setting on
the master module is obtained by depressing the zero button or turning a zero screw,
thus programming the differential amplifier. Subsequent changes in voltage input
will be compared to this zero and displayed on the module panel. The calibration
procedure involves first adjusting the transducer to the proper height, then opening
the transducer stopcock to sample atmospheric pressure and adjusting the zero
point. A known pressure load is then delivered to the transducer (via mercury manometer, etc.) and the appropriate gain calibration is made. At this point, the stopcock
may be opened to the patient sampling line and the desired pressure determinations
obtained. The output signal is displayed as systolic (peak), diastolic (ebb), and mean
(a filtered signal). These values are either transmitted to be displayed on panel
meters or as an analog output to an oscilloscope or computer system.

As with any physiologic event measured by electrodes, movement causes a variation in impedance and produces unwanted signals.

The temperature module employs a thermistor that varies its output according to
temperature; this signal can be displayed or recorded.

Differential Transformer Transducer

The transducer is a central piece of equipment in nearly all pressure and flow measurements in both the clinic and the research laboratory. Simply stated, a transducer
is a device that serves to convert one form of energy to another. The determinants
of blood pressure and gas flow are converted to electrical energy and are displayed
on an appropriate recording device.

Two types of transducers are generally employed in common medical practice —
the differential transformer transducer (Figure 2-5) and the strain gauge transducer.
The latter is the more popular. In the differential transformer transducer, a magnetic
field is generated by passing a low-voltage alternating current through the primary
windings (A), composed of coiled wire, across to the secondary windings (B, C).
When the transformer core (D) is symmetrically placed between the two secondary
windings, then the differential output (between the two secondary windings) is zero.

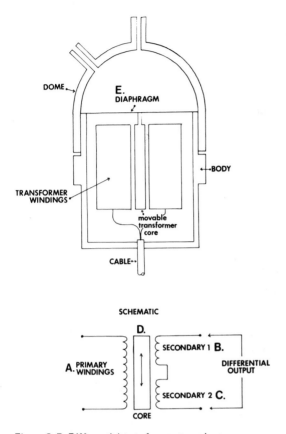

Figure 2–5. Differential transformer transducer.

If pressure is exerted on the transducer's diaphragm (E), this results in an asymmetric core-to-secondary-coil relationship, thus changing the transducer's output voltage, which must be amplified and then recorded. This transducer is linear in its output within its rated range.

Unbonded Strain Gauge Transducer
The resistance of an electrical conductor is determined by its cross-sectional area as well as its electrical properties. This principle serves to explain the operation of the unbonded strain gauge transducer (Figure 2–6). A sampling catheter attached to the dome (A) transmits pressure (either gas or liquid) to a diaphragm (B), which is attached to an armature (C), which in turn is connected to the strain gauge wire (D). With movement, the wire stretches, with a resultant decrease in its cross-sectional area. Electrical resistance is increased, and the electrical signal that passes through the wire is reduced. This signal is amplified and recorded. The output of the strain gauge transducer is also linear over its rated range.

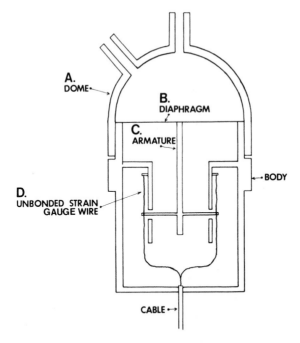

Figure 2–6. Unbonded strain gauge transducer.

Electrocardiograph

The electrocardiograph (ECG) measures bioelectric potentials that are generated by ionic flow in the heart. The ionic flow is converted to electronic by electrodes and the electrode paste. Electrodes are attached to the patient and connected to an amplifier. Once amplified, the signal may be displayed or recorded. The ECG tachometer samples the ECG signal; voltage change per unit time is analyzed, computed, and displayed as rate per minute.

Apnea Alarm

Impedance pneumography is a noninvasive method used to measure the volume and rate of respirations. The changes in impedance (electrical resistance) across the thorax during respiration were first noted in 1944. An impedance system for recording respiration was subsequently developed in 1949. Later, the transthoracic impedance changes were shown to be directly related to the volume of respiration.

The changes in impedance are measured by passing a high-frequency (50 to 600 kHz) signal through two electrodes placed on either side of a patient's thorax (right and left). The signal is then filtered and amplified, with the frequency of the change in the impedance wave form being displayed as respiratory rate.

Typically, the changes in impedance are relatively linear and range from 1 ohm/liter for subjects of heavy build to 6 ohms/liter for subjects of slight build. Because of the linearity of the impedance measurement, it is possible to calibrate and use the ohm signal as a volume measurement.

Two electrodes of the three used to record ECG can be simultaneously used for impedance pneumography, allowing for cardiorespiratory monitoring with the same set of electrodes.

DISPLAY SYSTEMS AND RECORDERS
Visual display of collected data allows nursing personnel to observe one or more patients and still perform their required duties. The mainstay of this type of instrumentation has been the oscilloscope.

Cascade Oscilloscope
The cascade oscilloscope (Figure 2–7) converts the input signal (A), which is in analog form, to digital in the A–D converter (B) — analog being a signal voltage that is proportional to the variable being measured. It then stores and displays these data simultaneously. The mechanics of this manipulation are shown in the figure. After the digital storage register (C), which serves as a short-term memory for the system, receives information, it sends a signal to the digital analog converter (D), which in turn is displayed on the instrument scope (E). The character of the storage file al-

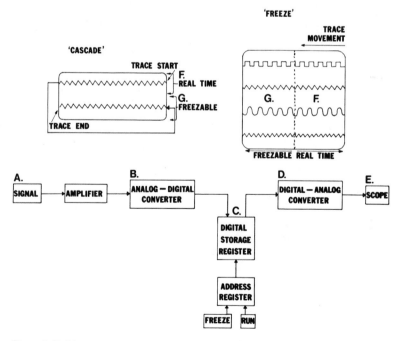

Figure 2–7. Displays: cascade, freeze, nonfade.

lows for either real time display or for long-term trend display. During real time operation (F), the entire register file is read, displayed, stored briefly, and discarded, whereas in the freeze mode (G), the storage register is not updated, and thus the same information continues to be read and displayed. The cascade oscilloscope displays two traces. The top trace cascades down to become the second trace. This second trace is freezable either under the control of an internal monitor or by operator command.

Cathode Ray Tube Oscilloscope

In the cathode ray tube oscilloscope (Figure 2–8) electrons from a hot cathode (A) are accelerated and focused into a beam (B) that passes between two vertical (C) and two horizontal (D) plates. The electric potential difference between the two horizontal plates causes the beam to deflect vertically, and the electric potential difference between the two vertical plates causes the beam to deflect horizontally. After passing through this electric field, the beam then strikes a fluorescent screen and produces a dot of light (E). Although primarily capable of operation in an X-Y format, the plates controlling the horizontal sweep of the beam are usually linked to a timing circuit to provide the more common time-amplitude format.

Long-persistence phosphor (F) that can be "erased" electrostatically allows for static display capabilities ranging from minutes to hours.

Typical cathode ray tube oscilloscopic display is in one color, usually orange or green. A new generation of oscilloscopes uses two fluorescent screens, one behind the other, each with a different phosphor color, and various electron intensities to provide up to three colors for display.

Galvanometric Recorders

For maximal efficiency and usefulness, once measured data must be clearly displayed and recorded, and be readily retrievable. Not all recording devices are capable of such performance, and frequently compromise is dictated by financial and space

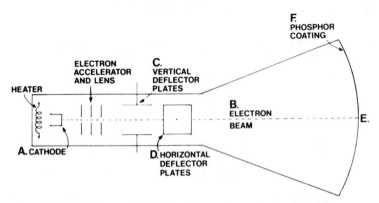

Figure 2–8. Cathode ray tube (CRT) oscilloscope.

limitations. Recording instruments vary from elementary to complex in character. The various common types of recorders are the galvanometric, potentiometric, light beam, and X-Y models.

The galvanometric recorder (Figure 2-9) is a simple, reliable, and accurate instrument commonly employed in such devices as the electroencephalograph and the electrocardiograph. Modern galvanometric recorders are the descendants of the D'Arsonval galvanometer. Their basic assembly consists of a rectangular coil of wire (A), usually wound on a bobbin of nonmagnetic material (B), mounted on a shaft supported by bearings and placed between the poles of a permanent magnet (C). The recording stylus (D) is attached either directly or through a mechanical linkage to the coil. When an electrical current is passed through the coil, a magnetic field opposing that of the permanent magnet is created, providing torque to move the stylus. The angular deflection of the stylus is linearly proportional to the magnitude of the input current. A stylus arm will transcribe an arc at its tip when it rotates on its pivot (E). A line written by this stylus would be curved if reproduced on stationary paper; this format is referred to as curvilinear. Although chart paper used with curvilinear recorders is usually marked with a curvilinear grid, wave forms are distorted and difficult to read.

A galvanometric recorder that transcribes a straight line on stationary chart paper is referred to as producing a rectilinear format. Many different methods of transposing the angular-linear outlet of the galvanometric stylus to perpendicular-linear have been developed. The simplest method of producing a rectilinear trace is to greatly extend the stylus arm, increasing the radius of the arc that the stylus transcribes. Although this trace is in essence curvilinear, the perpendicular linearity error can be made arbitrarily small. However, the longer the stylus arm is extended, the lower the frequency response of the system, thereby limiting the applications of this type of recorder. Another method consists of the use of a mechanical linkage that transforms pivotal motion to lateral motion. Finally, a very common method used

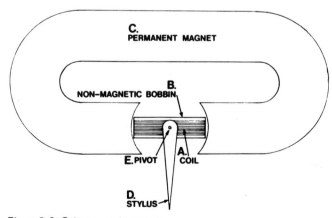

Figure 2-9. Galvanometric recorder.

is to draw chart paper over a knife edge with a stylus traveling along the tip of the knife edge, linearity being kept to within about 1 percent.

The actual trace recorded on chart paper can be produced by several different methods. Ink pen writers do not require special paper but tend to clog easily. In thermal writing, a resistance-heated stylus is used in conjunction with heat-sensitive paper to provide a relatively maintenance-free recording with good frequency response. Pressure writing uses pressure-sensitive paper with a round-tip stylus. Frequency response is limited by pen-paper friction.

Because of the momentum and finite torque of the stylus mechanism, frequency response of galvanometric recorders is generally limited to around 100 Hz, with some special systems capable of responses up to 400 Hz. This frequency response range is adequate for most physiologic signals encountered in the clinical setting.

Potentiometric Recorders

Potentiometric recorders (Figure 2–10) have been employed in a variety of biologic instruments such as flow-volume loop recorders and trend recorders. The signal input voltage (A) is compared with the slide-wire contact (B) voltage within the servo-amplifier (C). Any difference between the two voltages causes the servomotor (D) to be activated and to track until the difference is zero. The direction in which the servomotor tracks is determined by whether the slide contact voltage is less or greater than the signal input voltage. Because the pen (E) parallels the position of the

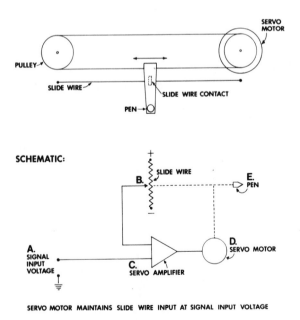

Figure 2–10. Potentiometric recorder.

slide wire contact, the signal input voltage determines the position of the pen on the graph paper.

Potentiometric recorders tend toward higher accuracy and linearity than galvanometric recorders. However, potentiometric recorders are inherently low-frequency devices and are usually limited to a frequency response of about 20 Hz.

An X-Y recorder is a potentiometric recorder with two perpendicular servosystems. Frequency response of an X-Y recorder is typically limited to about 10 Hz, depending upon the amplitude of the recording.

Writing is accomplished by either the ink method or the thermal method, with ink being the more common.

Light Beam Recorder

A light beam recorder (Figure 2–11) has a high frequency response, allowing measurement of rapid changes such as cardiac rate and rapid gas flow. A light beam recording system consists of a high-intensity projection-type cathode ray tube (CRT) (A) slaved to a display oscilloscope. The image produced by the slave CRT is projected onto light-sensitive paper (B) via a mirror (C), and this can be used in either the X-Y mode or the multiple trace mode. The paper travels through a developing solution bath (D) and dryer (E) prior to leaving the recorder. The frequency response of this system is limited by the intensity of the image and the sensitivity of the recording paper. The X-Y mode allows for a frequency response that is much higher than conventional recorders (about 1,000 Hz; in multiple-trace mode, frequency response is also 1,000 Hz).

A system using a light beam must be optically isolated from its local light-filled environment. Because of this isolation, and because the photosensitive paper must be developed and treated before use, there is a lag between the time a recording is

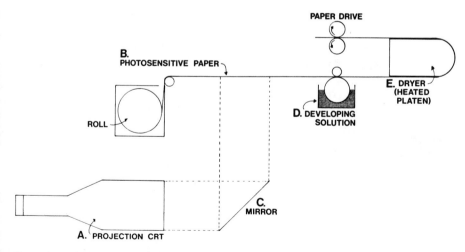

Figure 2–11. Light beam recorder.

made and the time it is available for viewing. This time lag, which is dependent upon paper speed, can range from a few seconds to several minutes.

Summary
In order to select a specific transducer (strain gauge or differential) or recording device (e.g., potentiometer vs. light beam), one must have an understanding of both the instrument and the task to be done.

MEASUREMENT OF BLOOD GASES AND pH
The capacity to determine arterial blood gases reliably and efficiently has greatly enhanced the ability to diagnose and treat patients with respiratory diseases. In addition to arterial blood gas and pH determinations, many laboratories are capable of measuring levels of oxygen saturation and carboxyhemoglobin. Nonetheless, intermittent blood gas determinations do not satisfy the need for continuous sampling of blood gases and acid-base balance. A variety of solutions for the problem of on-line continuous determinations have been proposed, among them the use of the mass spectrometer. The following section will describe the traditional methods used for intermittent sampling (PO_2, pH, PCO_2, oxyhemoglobin, carboxyhemoglobin), as well as proposed techniques for continuous measurement (muscle pH, blood and tissue oxygen and carbon dioxide).

Clark PO_2 Electrode
The Clark type PO_2 electrode (Figure 2–12) combines a thin platinum wire, or cathode (A), and a silver–silver chloride reference electrode, or anode (B), in a single unit. The electrode is placed in an electrolytic solution behind a plastic membrane (C), usually a polypropylene membrane, which is permeable only to oxygen. The electrolytic solution is a phosphate buffer to which some potassium chloride has been added to stabilize the potential of the anode. If a voltage of about –0.7 volt is applied between the platinum wire and the reference electrode, with the platinum wire being slightly negative (about –0.2 volt), oxygen reaching the surface of the platinum is reduced electrolytically.

$$2 H_2O + 2 e^- + O_2 = H_2O_2 + 2 OH^-$$

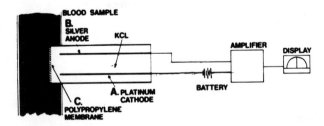

Figure 2–12. Clark PO_2 electrode.

This reduction process produces a current through the P_{O_2} electrode. Because the partial pressure of oxygen outside the membrane is the motive power in oxygen diffusion, the oxidation-reduction current obtained will be directly proportional to the concentration of oxygen within the sample, and the rate of reaction will be limited only by the rate of diffusion of oxygen to the surface of the cathode.

Because the characteristic of the oxygen electrode is linear, it can be calibrated simply by using an oxygen-free solution and another solution of a known oxygen concentration.

pH Electrode

The pH electrode (Figure 2–13) consists of a glass electrode (A) and a calomel reference electrode (B). The pH-sensitive element is a glass membrane (C) that allows the passage of only H^+ ions in the form of H_3O^+. This glass capillary is jacketed by an extremely acidic buffer solution (D) in which is enclosed a silver–silver chloride electrode (E). The connection between the potential measuring circuit and the solution being tested is completed through a potassium chloride salt bridge (F) and a calomel reference cell (G). Each of the two electrodes required to obtain the pH measurement, the glass electrode with a silver–silver chloride electrode inside a glass bulb and the calomel reference electrode, constitutes a *half-cell.* The saturated potassium chloride connects the two half-cells and completes the cell through which current can flow. The circuit is completed by a connection through a voltmeter (H). Across its membrane, the glass electrode develops an electric voltage that varies linearly with the pH of the solution being measured. Because the potential of the calomel electrode is constant, the electromotive force measured expresses the potential of the glass electrode. The potential developed is about 61.5 mv/pH unit at $32°C$.

Severinghaus P_{CO_2} Electrode

The Severinghaus P_{CO_2} electrode (Figure 2–14) uses the same principle as the pH electrode, because there is a linear relationship between the logarithm of the P_{CO_2}

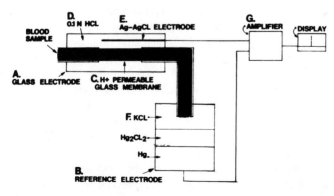

Figure 2–13. pH electrode.

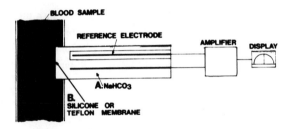

Figure 2-14. Severinghaus PCO_2 electrode.

and the pH of a solution. It is essentially a pH electrode surrounded by a membrane permeable to carbon dioxide. In this case, the electrode contains a bicarbonate buffer (A) and is separated from the sample by a Teflon or silicone membrane (B) selectively permeable to carbon dioxide. The space between the membrane and the glass electrode contains a matrix of nylon or glass wool. This serves as a wick to support the aqueous bicarbonate layer into which the carbon dioxide gas molecules can diffuse. Carbon dioxide diffusing through the membrane comes into equilibrium with the bicarbonate solution within the electrode. The carbon dioxide electrode actually measures the pH of this solution, which is altered according to the amount of H^+ ions formed:

$$CO_2 + H_2O \rightarrow H_2CO_3 \rightarrow H^+ + HCO_2$$

IL Model 182 Co-Oximeter

This instrument (Figure 2-15) simultaneously performs spectrophotometric analysis of the oxyhemoglobin, carboxyhemoglobin, and total hemoglobin concentrations at selected wavelengths. Because all three parameters measured have unique but overlapping absorption spectra, at any given wavelength the total absorbance is a summation of the absorbance of all three. Absorbance measurements are made at wavelengths at which the absorptivity of two or more species are equal. Changes in absorbance at specific wavelengths indicate changes in the relative concentrations of total hemoglobin (Hb), oxyhemoglobin (HbO_2), and carboxyhemoglobin (HbCO). Information obtained enters an electronic computational matrix that simultaneously solves three equations for the three unknowns and allows presentation on a digital display of the percentage of HbO_2, the percentage of HbCO, and the total Hb.

A 400-μl blood sample introduced into the sample port is drawn in via a peristaltic pump, diluted (9 parts blood to 1 part hemolyzing agent), then passed through a mechanical hemolyzing assembly, brought to a constant temperature, and pumped into the cuvette for measurement of absorbance. The sample then passes through the pump again and out as waste.

As shown in Figure 2-15, the path of light radiates from the lamp source through the cuvette to a lens that adjusts the path of the beam and directs it to the beam splitter.

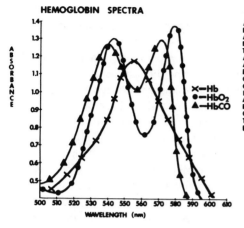

HEMOGLOBIN SPECTRA

X—Hb
●—HbO₂
▲—HbCO

DEOXYGENATED HEMOGLOBIN, OXYHEMOGLOBIN AND CARBOXYHEMOGLOBIN EACH HAVE UNIQUE BUT OVERLAPPING ABSORPTION SPECTRA. AT ANY GIVEN WAVELENGTH THE TOTAL ABSORBANCE IS A SUMMATION OF THE ABSORBANCE OF ALL THREE SPECIES. ABSORBANCE MEASUREMENTS ARE MADE AT WAVELENGTHS WHERE THE ABSORPTIVITY OF TWO OR MORE SPECIES ARE EQUAL. FROM THE ABSORBANCE AT 548 nm CHANGES IN ABSORBANCE ARE RELATED TO CHANGES IN THE TOTAL HEMOGLOBIN. A CHANGE IN ABSORBANCE AT 568 nm COMPARED TO THE ABSORBANCE AT 548 nm INDICATES A CHANGE IN THE RELATIVE CONCENTRATION OF CARB-OXYHEMOGLOBIN. A CHANGE AT 578 nm RELATIVE TO 548 nm INDICATES A CHANGE IN THE RELATIVE CONCENTRATION OF OXYHEMOGLOBIN.

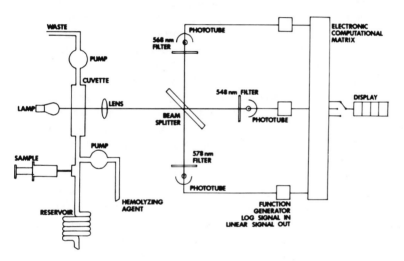

Figure 2–15. IL Co-Oximeter.

Continuous Blood and Tissue Gas Determinations

Continuous blood and tissue gas monitoring has been the goal of many investigators. Some have favored an indirect approach of extrapolating blood gas tensions from expired gases [10]. This is, of course, a less invasive technique than arterial puncture, but at this time it is a less than adequate method. The inability to obtain a true sample of alveolar gas from a diseased lung limits the use of this technique.

Satisfactory continuous arterial blood-gas analysis has been limited by (1) a contamination of the electrode surface (e.g., thrombogenesis); (2) change in the composition of the medium, which in turn changes the characteristics of the oxygen diffusion pathway; and (3) movement of the electrode causing a stirring artifact.

Ear oximeters show great promise as a noninvasive method. A fiberoptic ear probe directs narrow bandwidth light at the ear. The transmitted light is analyzed, and oxygen saturation values are obtained.

Attempts have been made [8, 11, 18] to withdraw blood from an artery, pass it through an electrode system, and return it to a vein. The need for systemic anti-coagulants and poor test reproducibility have been distinct disadvantages to this system. The introduction of a catheter or a probe directly into a blood vessel has also met with only limited success for the reasons cited above [5, 6, 17].

The most promising of all techniques for continuous monitoring of blood and tissue gases employs the use of the respiratory mass spectrometer. Both blood and tissue gas determinations using the mass spectrometer are theoretically possible. The procedure is as follows: With the membrane end of the catheter in the patient's blood vessel or tissue to be sampled, connect the opposite end to the vacuum outlet of the mass spectrometer. A minute amount of gas is constantly withdrawn through the diffusion membrane at a sampling rate varying from mass spectrometer to mass spectrometer within the range of 5×10^{-16} μl/sec. Only dissolved gases are drawn through the membrane, entering the catheter in quantities proportional to their partial pressures. These gases pass into the mass spectrometer, where they are quantitatively analyzed by molecular weight.

The basic difference between measurement of gases in tissue and in blood is one of gas flow. A catheter placed in the patient's artery is sampling the gas as it flows by the tip of the catheter. A catheter placed in the patient's tissue is sampling the bolus of static gas that surrounds the catheter. More important, however, is the problem of sensitivity of the mass spectrometer. In order to measure tissue gases, the sensitivity of the spectrometer must be considerably higher than that for measurement of arterial blood gases.

The elusive component in the search for on-line blood gas monitoring is the design of the sampling catheter. Technological advances in catheter design have not kept pace with advances in vacuum technology and electronics. The search for a reliable catheter has been joined by many and is indeed still continuing. Brantigan [1, 2] and co-workers have done considerable research into the design and structure of various types of catheters to be used in this fashion. Most catheters in use today are claimed to be thromboresistant without the need for a chemically bound heparin surface. This method will come of age when a catheter is perfected that can be implanted to sample accurately and safely for extended periods of time.

Muscle pH
The monitoring of muscle surface pH has been shown to be clinically valuable, capable of signaling an early warning of inadequate oxygen transport. The technique is simple because the insertion of the probe and the necessary equipment (pH probe and standard pH meter) are not elaborate.

Muscle tissue is typical of all aerobic tissue in that its metabolism proceeds anaerobically if its oxygen needs are not met. The end product of anaerobic metabolism is lactic acid, which dissociates to lactate and hydrogen ion. Therefore, a tissue's hydrogen ion concentration (pH) reflects the balance between oxygen supply and oxygen demand. Because a critical determinant of oxygen supply is perfusion, tissue pH is a direct indicator of local perfusion.

The muscle pH, normally 7.35 to 7.45, remains stable unless there is a local change in metabolism (oxygen supply) or a change in systemic pH. As a result, it can provide continuous monitoring of these parameters without requiring repeated blood samples. Continuous muscle pH monitoring could be used to follow any critically ill patient regardless of the underlying cause, because muscle pH reflects not only tissue perfusion but tissue oxygenation in general and overall acid-base status.

Instrumentation is similar to previously described pH systems. The electrodes are miniaturized for implantation.

Summary
The goal of any effective patient monitoring system remains—one that is capable of reliable and accurate continuous monitoring of both blood and tissue gases. For the present, we must settle for periodic sampling, which in most cases is sufficient to detect life-threatening change in the patient's status.

SPIROMETERS
Familiarization with the design and function of spirometers is essential for respiratory care personnel. The technology and instrumentation of spirometry has burgeoned in recent years, and there are currently available a number of spirometers of all sizes, shapes, and designs. The spirometers discussed include the following: water-seal, wedge, bellows, turbine, gear pump, hot wire, pneumotachograph, vane, and incentive.

Water-Seal Spirometer
The standard to which most forms of spirometers are compared for accuracy is the water-seal spirometer (Figure 2–16), which in essence consists of a movable bell placed open end down into a water-filled chamber with an inlet communicating to the interior of the bell. Two of the most common forms of water-seal spirometers are the counterweighted and the Stead-Wells spirometers.

In the counterweighted spirometer (Figure 2–16, left) the bell (A) is placed in a water-filled chamber (H), suspended by a chain (B) and pulleys (C), and counterbalanced by a weight (D). Breathing through the inlet-outlet (G) causes the bell to rise and fall a distance proportional to the volume of air breathed. A pen (E) attached to the weight produces tracings of the movement of the bells on the drum kymograph (F).

In the Stead-Wells spirometer (Figure 2–16, right) a light-weight plastic bell (A) is placed over guide rods (B) in a water-filled chamber. Patient exhalation through the inlet causes the bell to lift. The distance the bell moves is proportional to the volume exhaled. The linear gear (C) rises with the bell, turning the geared wheel (D)

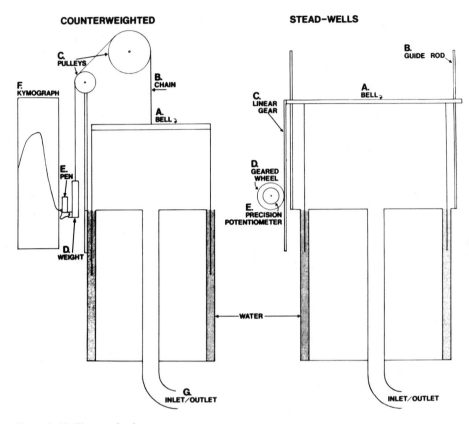

Figure 2–16. Water-seal spirometers.

on the precision potentiometer (E). In use, the amplitude of a voltage passing through the precision potentiometer changes with the position of the bell, producing an analog signal that is proportional to the volume of gas breathed into the spirometer. This signal in turn can be displayed on any graphic recorder.

Wedge Spirometer

The wedge spirometer, such as the Narco Vitalor (Figure 2–17), is a flat bellows spirometer with one side either fixed or weighted. When filling, the Narco Vitalor's bellows (A) expand radially around the pivot (B). The stylus (C), fixed to the leading edge of the bellows, marks its excursion on the kymograph (D) (shown perpendicular to the viewing field). Used in forced vital capacity (FVC) determinations, the Narco Vitalor registers a maximum of 5 liters. This instrument, however, has the advantage of being compact, portable, and durable. Other wedge spirometers are available with greater volume limits; unfortunately, they are more cumbersome. Reasonably high mechanical inertia and machine back pressure are the major dis-

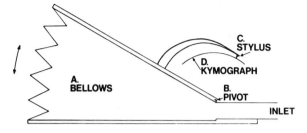

Figure 2-17. Wedge spirometer: Narco Vitalor.

advantages of wedge spirometers, but they are certainly capable of acceptable determinations of vital capacity and tidal volume. More sophisticated wedge devices
eliminate the problems of inertia and back pressure; however, they are somewhat
cumbersome and more suited for a pulmonary function laboratory.

Bellows Spirometer

The Jones Pulmonar is a horizontally mounted, square bellows type spirometer that
offers the advantages of being waterless, portable, relatively trouble free, and quite
accurate. A permanent record is provided by a direct writing pen, and a variable
speed control allows for the determination of a forced vital capacity and its timed
subdivisions along with maximal voluntary ventilation. Other portions of the flow
volume curve, such as maximum midexpiratory flow rate (MMFR) and maximum
expiratory flow (MEF), along with analysis of terminal flows, may be correctly calculated from the tracing.

The Bennett monitoring spirometer (Figure 2-18) is designed to monitor continuously the tidal volume of patients undergoing mechanical respiratory support.
This system utilizes the patient's expired air as its driving force to lift a bellows (A)
contained in a clear plastic case (B); during inspiration, air escapes from the bellows through a valve (C), preparing the spirometer for another cycle. In order to
activate the alarm (D), a flag switch (E) must be thrown. When the switch is in the
off position, the flag is up and clearly visible. Also, a flashing red light has been added in addition to the already available audible alarm system.

Alarm limits are set by the depth of the alarm rod (F), which is inserted into the
bellows guide rod (G). As the bellows fills, a magnet (H) on the tip of the alarm rod
passes a magnetic reed switch (J) and resets the alarm if the exhaled volume is greater than or equal to the alarm volume. If the alarm is not reset by the magnet, the
alarm will activate after the prescribed amount of time.

The accuracy of this spirometer is quite acceptable at approximately ±50 ml with
a measurement range between 100 and 2,200 ml. Ease of dismantling for cleaning
and sterilization is an additional desirable feature. Very few moving parts are involved in the operation of this type of spirometer. This instrumentation has proved
to be quite satisfactory if properly handled.

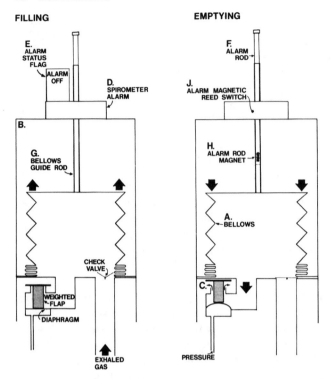

Figure 2-18. Bennett monitoring bellows spirometer.

This device can be used only by a patient who is receiving mechanical ventilation; as manufactured, it is inaccurate while intermittent mandatory ventilation (IMV) is in use. However, we have modified this spirometer to allow its use with IMV (see Chapter 12).

Wood et al. [20] have employed a Bird expiratory flow cartridge to feed the dumping mechanism of the Bennett spirometer during IMV breathing. This modification is of value only to determine the machine-generated tidal volumes, because it does not function during spontaneous breathing.

Optoelectronic Turbine Spirometer

The optoelectronic turbine spirometer (Figure 2-19) employs the rotational characteristics of a miniature turbine that is dependent upon gas flow. A light beam is focused on Polaroid film, translating the rotation of the turbine into a tracing representative of the vital capacity. Then a transparent plastic grid is placed over the tracing to calculate the numerical values. This device is lightweight, portable, and operates on either AC or battery power. It is quite easily adapted for use on patients with tracheostomies or for mass screening. The disposable sensors and films, however, are relatively expensive.

FLOW SENSOR

**INSP./EXP.
DISCRIMINATION**

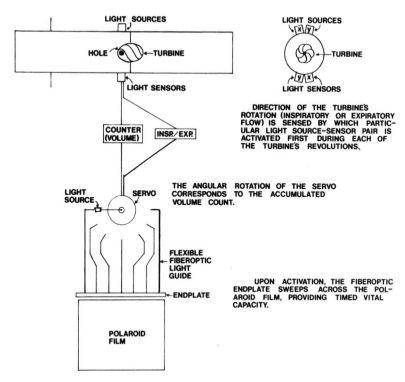

DIRECTION OF THE TURBINE'S
ROTATION (INSPIRATORY OR EXPIRATORY
FLOW) IS SENSED BY WHICH PARTIC-
ULAR LIGHT SOURCE–SENSOR PAIR IS
ACTIVATED FIRST DURING EACH OF
THE TURBINE'S REVOLUTIONS.

THE ANGULAR ROTATION OF THE SERVO
CORRESPONDS TO THE ACCUMULATED
VOLUME COUNT.

UPON ACTIVATION, THE FIBEROPTIC
ENDPLATE SWEEPS ACROSS THE POL-
AROID FILM, PROVIDING TIMED VITAL
CAPACITY.

Figure 2–19. Optoelectronic turbine spirometer: Marion Laboratories spirostat.

Gear Pump Spirometer

The gear pump principle is an accurate, reproducible method of measuring gas volume (Figure 2–20). During each revolution, the spirometer rotors will sweep out a fixed preset volume of gas. The Drager hand-held spirometer is just such an instrument. This spirometer, which is quite sturdy and relatively resistant to the effects of dust and humidity, can be autoclaved, tolerating temperatures up to 120°C. An optional timer is available for minute volume measurement.

Hot Wire Spirometer

Hot wire spirometers (Figure 2–21) utilize the principle of the thermistor, a device constructed of solid semiconductor material whose electrical resistance changes with a variation in temperature. The Monaghan M 700 spirometer employs just such a hot wire device. The heart of the apparatus is a thermistor heated to 170°F and kept isothermic by a linearizing circuit. And in this manner, a linear response to various flows is accomplished.

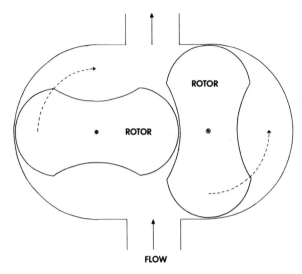

Figure 2–20. Drager gear pump spirometer.

DONTI/NCG SENSOR

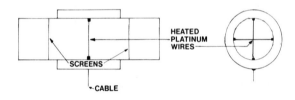

MONAGHAN SENSOR

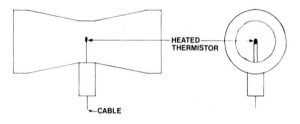

Figure 2–21. Hot wire spirometers.

The M 700 spirometer can be used with any respirator as long as care is taken to prevent substantial shift in temperature or gas density. This spirometer has been adapted to a continuous flow ventilation circuit (see Chapter 12). Because the M 700 does not detect direction flow, its use is limited. Nonetheless, this is an effective device, and it will sense small changes in volume and respiratory rates.

Fleisch Pneumotachograph

Because of the resistance imposed by the screen (A), gas flow through the Fleisch pneumotachograph (Figure 2-22, top) causes a pressure differential to be established between the upstream and downstream sides of the screen. A differential transducer (B) samples upstream and downstream pressures and, depending upon flow direction, produces a positive or negative flow signal that is linear over the rated range of the pneumotachograph. The flow signal is amplified and can be either displayed as flow or integrated to produce volume.

LSE Disposable Pneumotachograph

As with the Fleisch pneumotachograph, gas flow through the LSE Disposable Pneumotachograph (Figure 2-22, bottom) produces a pressure differential because of the resistance of the precision pore paper (A). However, unlike the Fleisch, this pressure difference is between the interior of the sensor and atmospheric pressure. A transducer (B) samples the internal pressure of the LSE pneumotachograph and,

FLEISCH PNEUMOTACHOGRAPH

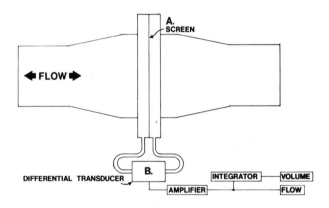

LSE DISPOSABLE PNEUMOTACHOGRAPH

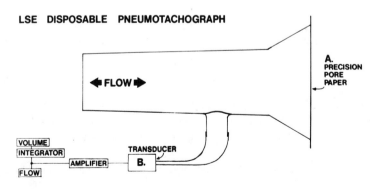

Figure 2-22. Pneumotachographs.

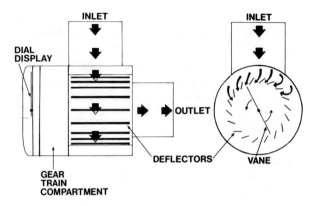

Figure 2-23. Wright vane spirometer.

depending upon flow direction, produces a positive or negative signal that is linear over the range of the sensor.

Vane Spirometer

A vane spirometer (Figure 2-23) employs a system of finely honed vanes that are moved by a flow of gas; because these are delicately balanced, the number of rotations is proportional to the amount of gas. Representative of this category of spirometers is the Wright respirometer. The delicacy of some of the instruments constitutes one of their major drawbacks. For example. Lunn and Hillard [12] reported an average of three repairs per year for each of their 25 respirometers. Because they are so delicate, minor jarring that is bound to be encountered in everyday use is enough to seriously disable the instrument.

Other vane type spirometers measure vane rotation optoelectrically, as does the Ohio Vortex respiration monitor. A light beam is interrupted by the blade of the vane as it rotates, producing an electrical pulse. The number of pulses is determined by the volume of gas analyzed.

Incentive Spirometers

Incentive spirometers are a group of new devices that are used to encourage a patient to breathe deeply. Preoperatively, the patient's maximum inspiratory volume is recorded. This record is used postoperatively as the goal the patient is encouraged to achieve.

Numerous devices are available, and they fall into two categories: high-cost, nondisposable units with disposable mouthpieces; and high-cost, completely disposable units. In some versions (Marion Laboratories, Bartlett-Edwards), an electronic volume indicator is used to visually display both the goal and the patient's achievements.

The patient is said to respond well to the visual incentive, and it is claimed that the inspiratory effort helps to prevent atelectasis and improve vital capacity. However, the therapeutic advantage of treatment by a therapist is lost with this method.

REFERENCES

1. Brantigan, J. W., Gott, V. L., and Martz, M. N.   A Teflon membrane for measurement of blood and intramyocardial gas tensions by mass spectroscopy. *J. Appl. Phys.* 32:2, 1972, pp. 276–282.
2. Brantigan, J. W., et al. A nonthrombogenic diffusion membrane for continous in vivo measurement of blood gases by mass spectrometry. *Appl. Physiol.* 28:3, 1970, pp. 375–377.
3. Dammann, J. F., Wright, D. J., and Updike, O. L. Physiologic monitoring and contributions to patient care. *Biomed. Sci. Instrum.* 5, 1969, pp. 17–27.
4. Fowler, K. T. The respiratory mass spectrometer. *Phys. Med. Biol.* 14:2, 1969, pp. 185–199.
5. Gertz, K. H., and Loeschcke, H. H. Electrode zur Bestimmung des CO_2-drucks. *Naturwiss enschaften,* 45, 1958, p. 160.
6. Heyrovsky, J. Electrolysis with the dropping mercury electrode. *Chemicke Listy* 16: 256, 1922.
7. Hilberman, M., Schill, J. P., and Peters, R. M. On-line digital analysis of respiratory mechanics and the automation of respirator control. *J. Thorac. Cardiovasc. Surg.* 58:6, 1969, pp. 821–828.
8. Hunt, T. K., Zederfelt, B., and Goldstick, T. K. O_2 and Healing. *Am. J. Surg.* 118, 1969, pp. 521–525.
9. Krekule, I., and Radil-Weiss, T. Simple computer technique for analysing the time relationships between cardiac activity and respiration. *Physiol. Bohemoslov.* 19, 1970, pp. 163–166.
10. Kruezer, F., and Nessler, C. G. Method of polargraphic in vivo continuous recording of blood O_2 tension. *Science* 128, 1958, pp. 1005–1006.
11. Ledsome, J. R., Linden, R. J., and Normal, J. The continuous measurement of pH and P_{CO_2}; a demonstration for teaching. *Proceeding of the Physiological Society,* April 14–15, 1967, 26 pp.
12. Lunn, J. N., and Hillard E. K. The effect of repairs on the performance of Wright spirometers. *Br. J. Anaesth.* 42, 1970, p. 1127.
13. Neely, W., et al. A computer analysis of pulmonary functions in surgical patients. *Ann. Thorac. Surg.* 11:6, 1971, pp. 565–569.
14. Osborn, J. J., et al. Continuous measurement of lung mechanics and gas exchange in the critically ill. *Med. Research Eng.* 1969.
15. Peters, R. M., and Stacy, R. W. Automatized clinical measurement of respiratory parameters. *Surgery* 56:1, 1974.
16. Powers, S. R., et al. Panel discussion: Monitoring. *J. Trauma* 10:11, 1970, pp. 1025–1040.
17. Stow, R. W., Baer, R. F., and Randall, B. F. Rapid measurement of CO_2 tension in blood. *Arch. Phys. Med.* 38, 1957, p. 646.
18. Sugioka, K.   A method for measuring continuous in-vivo blood P_{CO_2}, P_{O_2}, and pH in the intact animal. *Biomed. Sci. Instrum.* 4, 1968, pp. 185–189.

19. Van Bergen, F. H., Novak, A. L., and Cummings, J. F.   Analog computer for on-line determinations of ventilatory power, work and volume. *Med. Res. Eng.* 1970, pp. 7–12.
20. Wood, W. W., Greenwood, J., and Blodget, R.   Casebook spirometer modification for IMV. *Respir Ther.* 5:4, 1975.

Daniel J. Donovan
Richard P. Johnston
Kenneth F. MacDonnell

Gas Delivery Systems

3

Modern respiratory therapy has as one of its major tasks the provision of the equipment used for oxygen therapy. As a result, such items as gas regulators, cylinders, Venturi masks, and aerosols usually fall under the purview of the respiratory therapy department. Additionally, in some clinical situations proper respiratory care requires environmental manipulation to effect gas delivery that is relatively purified, for example, the removal of ragweed allergens from the air breathed by the patient suffering from ragweed asthma. For this reason, new air filtering devices, high-efficiency particulate air (HEPA) filters, will also be discussed in this chapter.

GAS FLOW AND PRESSURE REGULATORS

All gases exert pressure, which results from molecular activity. Pressure can be defined as the force applied to or distributed over a surface and measured as force per unit area, or pounds square inch (PSI). Regulators, which are employed to control gas pressures and which are also called *reducing valves*, can be divided into three categories: pressure preset, pressure adjustable, and multistage regulators. The pressure preset and the variable pressure regulators are the most commonly used (Figure 3-1). After connection to the source pressure, gas enters the reducing chamber (A) of the regulator; the pressure in this portion is determined by the amount of tension exerted by a spring (B) onto the diaphragm wall (C) of the chamber. When the preset pressure is attained, the diaphragm moves into the ambient chamber of the regulator; this in turn moves an armature (D), which occludes the feeding nozzle. Thus, gas flow ceases until pressure in the reducing chamber again falls below the desired

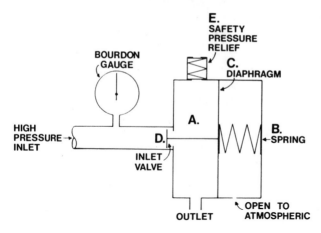

Figure 3-1. Preset pressure regulator.

level. The difference between a preset regulator and a variable regulator lies in the option to adjust pressure in the reducing chamber, adjustment being possible in the latter. A safety relief valve (E) with either a diaphragm or a ball spring arrangement prevents excessive pressure buildup in the reducing chamber.

Multistage regulators consist of a series of single-stage preset regulators. This system allows for a smoother and more specific regulation of pressure reduction and flow rate. Clinically, this type of regulator is of value in anesthesia apparatus. Flow rate is a measure of the movement of a fluid or gas volume per unit time. Velocity measures speed only; flow rate measures both speed and the amount of gas delivered, for instance, liters per minute. Flow meters allow for the accurate adjustment of rate over a narrow range usually from 0 to 15 liters/min. Such a system makes it possible to regulate specific concentrations of gas to the patient.

When a flow meter is used with a humidifier or any other piece of equipment, flow restrictions are created which can adversely affect proper gas delivery. All flow meters manufactured today are pressure compensated so that variations in back pressure will not have any effect on patient care.

GAS CYLINDERS
The containers or cylinders used to hold or ship compressed or liquid medical gases are given a letter designation according to size, measured in inches of diameter times height with a valve in place. The most frequently encountered are:

E	G	H & K
4¼ X 30	8½ X 55	9 X 55

The small cylinders employ a connector called a *yoke*, whereas the larger cylinders have a threaded outlet from their valves to which a nut attaches to a pressure regulator.

A color code for tanks to assure proper identification of the type of gas in each cylinder has been supported by the medical gas industry, the American Society of Anesthesiologists, and the American Hospital Association. The following color codes are in use today:

Kind of Gas	Color
air	blue or silver
oxygen	green or white
helium and oxygen	brown and green
carbon dioxide	gray
nitrous oxide	light blue
cyclopropane	orange
helium	brown
ethylene	red

Unfortunately, strict adherence to the color code has not been universal, and therefore, the therapist should verify the contents of each tank by reading the label. Tanks containing therapeutic gas mixtures are usually coded according to the general proportions of the gases; for example, a 95% oxygen with 5% carbon dioxide gas mixture would have a color code with 5% gray on top and 95% green on the bottom.

The duration of gas flow available at various flow rates from a gas cylinder may be determined using the following factors and equation:

	E	G	H & K
O_2 or compressed air	0.28	2.41	3.14
O_2-CO_2 mixture	0.35	2.94	3.84

$$\frac{\text{gauge pressure (PSI)} \times \text{factor}}{\text{liter flow}} = \text{duration (mins)}$$

OXYGEN DELIVERY SYSTEMS

Bendix model RSS is a mobile unit capable of manufacturing 90% oxygen at a 2 liters/min or 48% oxygen at 10 liters/min from room air. The RSS's ability to concentrate oxygen from ambient levels is made possible by the development of molecular sieves with highly accurate and reproducible aperture size. The fundamental building block of the molecular sieve crystal structure is a tetrahedron of four oxygen anions surrounding a smaller silicon or aluminum cation. Sodium ions or other cations serve to make up the positive charge deficit in the aluminum tetrahedra. Each of the four oxygen anions is shared with another silicon or aluminum tetrahedron, extending the crystal lattice in three dimensions. The resulting crystal is unusual in that it is honeycombed with relatively large cavities. Each cavity is connected with six adjacent ones through apertures. Exchanging the sodium ion with another cation, such as calcium, changes the aperture size, for example, from 3.5 to 4.2 angstrom units.

The RSS system incorporates two molecular sieves that exclude any molecule above mass 28 (N_2). Room air is drawn through the sieve, leaving an oxygen (mass 32)-enriched gas behind. The oxygen-enriched gas is stored in a holding tank, and the sieve is purged, leaving the system ready for the next enrichment cycle. The purge-enrichment cycle is alternated between the two molecular sieves.

The RSS uses 5 amp of current at 115 VAC. It weighs 195 pounds and stands 38 inches high by 20 inches wide by 30 inches deep. The RSS is also capable of providing compressed air at 30 cm H_2O.

VENTURI TYPE MASKS

The Venturi mask delivery system (Figure 3-2) was designed and is employed for those situations that demand exact concentrations of oxygen. The Inspiron Accurox is typical of many Venturi masks. Oxygen flow through a precision orifice in the jet (A) entrains room air through the dilution port (B), providing the patient with a constant FI_{O_2}. Oxygen concentration in the Venturi mask is dependent upon oxygen flow rate and orifice size. The aerosol collar (C), when used in conjunction with a compressed air aerosol generator, will humidify entrained air. Masks capable of delivery of 24, 28, 35, and 40% oxygen concentrations are the ones most commonly employed. The ratios of air to oxygen are 20:1, 10:1, 5:1, and 3:1, respectively.

Friedman [1], in an elegant report, disputes the accuracy of the currently employed Venturi mask system. Oxygen was measured by the Schollander method under two circumstances, first sampling gas from the mask orifice, and then collecting gas over several minutes in a bag and analyzing its oxygen concentration. Under these experimental conditions, oxygen concentrations were consistently higher than those claimed by the manufacturers. In a study done at our laboratory, using a res-

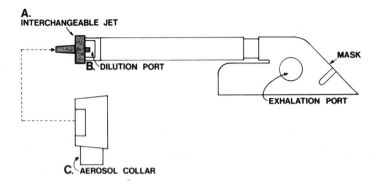

Figure 3-2. Inspiron Accurox Venturi mask.

piratory mass spectrometer attached to a nasal catheter, oxygen concentrations were measured in the posterior nasopharynx, with similar results.

The controversy over whether or not to humidify Venturi type masks has not been resolved. Friedman states that humidification of entrained air, using humidifier cuffs provided by the manufacturer and connected to a nebulizer, is preferable to direct oxygen humidification. Venturi masks humidified in that fashion, however, showed a decrease in delivered gas volume with a 2% increase in oxygen concentration. Mix-O-Masks' concentration did not change appreciably using this method of humidification.

OXYGEN CATHETERS, CANNULAS, AND MASKS
An oropharyngeal catheter is a green, pliable, plastic tube about 12 inches long. The tip is rounded with numerous holes through which oxygen can pass. The nasal catheter is not often used in respiratory therapy today. Nursing care is difficult. Gastric distention may be produced if the catheter is improperly inserted. At flow rates of 4 to 8 liters/min, concentrations of 25 to 40% oxygen may be achieved.

A nasal cannula is a tube lightly strapped to the patient's head in such a position that two ½-inch prongs protrude into the patient's nostrils. Humidification must be employed when using such a system in order to counteract oxygen's drying effect. At high flow rates, a patient may be subjected to sinus discomfort. Concentrations of 23 to 40% oxygen may be obtained over a range of 1 to 10 liters/min. The nasal cannula is frequently used to replace the simple oxygen mask, especially in elderly patients, who often complain of claustrophobia and will not tolerate a mask.

Oxygen masks are manufactured in long and short versions in an attempt to conform to different facial features. There are exhalation ports provided to prevent carbon dioxide buildup. Most masks have an adjustable metal strip across the bridge of the nose to reduce oxygen leakage. At flow rates of 6 to 10 liters per minute, concentrations of 35 to 55% oxygen are obtainable.

A partial rebreathing mask utilizes a reservoir bag to collect some of the patient's own expired gas. Because the exhaled gas contains about 14% oxygen, which is then mixed with 100% oxygen from the gas source, the patient receives a higher oxygen concentration than is provided by a simple mask.

Care must be taken to fit the mask properly and to not allow the bag to deflate completely during inhalation. If these precautions are not heeded, the therapy will inadvertently consist of a lower FI_{O_2} than desired. At flows of 8 to 15 liters/min, 40 to 70% oxygen can be delivered to the patient. A nonrebreathing mask employs a bag with a system of one-way valves. During exhalation, the bag fills with the source gas to provide a reservoir. A flutter valve at the patient orifice ensures that no exhaled gas enters the reservoir bag. Exhaled gas is directed out through one-way valves covering the exhalation ports on each side of the mask. Thus, when inhalation occurs, the patient breathes pure source gas from the reservoir bag. We have samples for oxygen concentrations at the external nares for several types of oxygen mask. Samples from normal volunteers were analyzed continuously with a mass

Table 3-1. Oxygen Concentrations at the External Nares with Various Types of Oxygen Mask

Mask	Concentration of O_2		Mean	Arithmetical Mean
100%	max.		97.5	79
	min.		60.5	
Regular O_2, 10 liters/min	max.		96.5	83.25
	min.		70	
Regular O_2, 6 liters/min	max.		87.5	69.75
	min.		52	
40% Venturi	max.		43.7	43.25
	min.		42.8	
35% Venturi	max.		37.5	37.25
	min.		37	
28% Venturi	max.		30.7	30.6
	min.		30.5	
24% Venturi	max.		27	27
	min.		27	
Rebreathing, 10 liters/min	max.		100	77.5
	min.		55	
Rebreathing, 6 liters/min	max.		97	67.5
	min.		38	

spectrometer, and care was taken to ensure a good mask fit. The results are shown in Table 3-1. It should be noted that the low concentration devices deliver a somewhat higher than desired concentration.

AEROSOL DELIVERY SYSTEMS

Aerosol masks are used in an attempt to deliver high humidity to the lung. Toward this end, they utilize large-bore tubing connected to aerosol generators whose FI_{O_2} is fixed at 0.4, 0.7, or 1.0. Prescribed flow rates must exceed the patient's minute volume.

In a study by Wexler et al. [2], direct measurements of intratracheal oxygen were made in patients whose tracheostomy tubes had been previously removed, but whose stomas were still open. A catheter was passed through a small plastic plug and both were inserted into the stoma, effectively sealing the opening.

Standard disposable aerosol masks were used. Low oxygen flow rates and air turbulence inside and outside the mask were found to be responsible for fluctuations in FI_{O_2}. Vents on either side of the mask were shielded from outside air currents in such a way as to maintain previous exhalation characteristics. Fluctuations were nearly eliminated, and concentrations of 100% oxygen were obtained at high flow rates.

Recent studies utilizing tagged water aerosols and lung scanners have shown that after inhalation through the nostrils, very little aerosol is deposited beyond the pharynx. Another portion of the experiment showed that even while the subject breathed through his mouth, the predominant deposition of water remained in his mouth.

Artificial humidification of the lungs is far more satisfactory in patients who have had tracheostomies performed, or whose course of therapy necessitates the insertion of an endotracheal tube. The Briggs adapter, more commonly called a *T-piece*, is used to replace the aerosol mask in most of these cases. The stem of the T is made to fit the so-called universal 15 mm endotracheal connectors. Oxygen concentrations obtainable are limited by the aerosol generator to which it is attached. Here again, flow rates should match or exceed the patient's minute volume.

An afterburner or reservoir tube may be added to the exhalation side of the T in order to maintain a properly humidified prescribed FI_{O_2}. If the T piece cannot be attached to the tracheostomy tube, a loose-fitting tracheostomy mask can be substituted that fits loosely over the tracheostomy site and that is held in place by a strap placed behind the patient's neck. Aerosol is generated in the same way as for the aerosol mask and Briggs adapter. The same precautions must also be considered.

Open-top face tents enclose the patient's face. They are used when large volumes of aerosol are required but specific gas concentrations are not. Even at high flow rates and 100% source oxygen, the maximum achievable FI_{O_2} is approximately 0.80.

HIGH-EFFICIENCY PARTICULATE AIR FILTERS

The prototype of the present-day high-efficiency particulate air (HEPA) or absolute filter was developed during World War I. Made of asbestos fibers with a matrix of esparto grass and Kraft fibers for strength, these filters were called Chemical Warfare Service (CWS) 6 filter media and were extremely efficient, being able to remove 99.95 percent of particles larger than $0.3\ \mu$. Approximately 30 years later, industry responded to the need of the Atomic Energy Commission for a filtering system with an increased rate of flow at the same efficiency level, and in 1960 the present laminar flow system came into use. Noncombustible glass fibers, now 99.97 percent efficient, have replaced the original matrix, and specific filters have been developed for specialized environments, for example, excess heat or humidity.

The flow of air entering a HEPA filter is broken up into many small streams as it passes through the narrow, convoluted passageways within the porous filter. Dust particles pass close to the filter elements. Deposition occurs throughout the filter, and under ideal circumstances a crust layer does not build up on the filter surface. The two major methods by which particles are removed are by diffusion (small particles) and impaction (larger ones).

Fibers within the filter are randomly oriented. Air, upon entering the filter, changes direction to conform with channels between two fibers. Particles, because of their inertia, resist directional change and become entangled in the fiber.

Minute particles respond as if they were a true gas. Particles diffuse from higher to lower regions of density, as do gases. As impaction clears the air of particles around the fibers, particulate density at these points is lowered and particles are attracted and trapped. HEPA filters increase in efficiency as more particles are trapped. Highest efficiency ratings are achieved just prior to replacement; however, flow rates are greatly reduced then.

An example of today's HEPA is the Flanders Filters, Inc., Model 9, which consists of a filter medium and precision-engineered separators. The upstream separator is set at an angle of 15 degrees off 90 degrees to the filter face. The downstream separator is set at 90 degrees to the face. The ridges of the separators cross over one another to cradle and support the filter medium. In this way, filter medium integrity is maintained and laminar flow is allowed.

Many efficiency test standards have been introduced in the last 40 years, the sophistication of which has paralleled advances in filter engineering. The National Bureau of Standards developed a procedure in 1938 for testing filter efficiency. Because it is not capable of examining HEPA filters, it is used primarily for prefilter testing. The dioctylphthalate (DOP) fog test passes uniform 0.3 μ DOP vapor droplets through a HEPA filter being tested and accurately measures by optical scanner the relative amount of light scattered by airborne particles before and after filtration. These tests yield comparative results only and may not reflect results seen in actual use. Proper matching of tests, types of filters, and conditions, however, assure the user of a high degree of uniformity among those filters in use.

Puritan-Bennett Corporation produces the Airclean S–99, which incorporates a series of filters said to be capable of cleaning and changing the air in a 3,200 square foot area 7 times per hour. Air is drawn into the back of the unit through a prefilter of nonwoven polyester fiber, rated 40 percent effective by NBS atmospheric dustspot test. It then passes through a carbon filter that suppresses odor and enters a blower powered by a 115-volt AC motor and is forced back into the room after passing through the HEPA filter. The rate of this movement of air can be varied from 0 to 450 cubic feet per minute. Puritan-Bennett Airclean S–99 filter will remove 99.97 percent of particles 0.3 μ or larger in size as assessed by the DOP test. The manufacturer also claims high efficiency protection, stating that most bacteria fall into the 0.3 μ or larger range. These units may be helpful for patients suffering with allergies caused by pollens and plant spores, most of which are 8 μ or larger. We have employed these filters in our respiratory intensive care unit.

REFERENCES
1. Friedman, S. A., et al. O_2 therapy: Evaluation of various air-entraining masks. *J.A.M.A.* 228, 1974, p. 474.
2. Wexler, H. R., Cooper, J. D., and Aberman, A. Mathematical model to predict inspired O_2 concentrations: Description and validation. *Can. Anaesth. Soc. J.* 22:4, 1975, p. 410.

New Diagnostic Techniques

2

Doraswamy Saroja Moorthi

Pulmonary Function Testing: New and Old

4

Total evaluation of the respiratory system requires adequate pulmonary function testing. The extent of this testing can vary from simple and cheap to complex and costly. All hospitals should have the facilities for at least simple lung function tests and blood gas analyses. Surely any metropolitan hospital should have the capacity to measure and evaluate all aspects of pulmonary function, for example, mechanics, distribution of gases, diffusion, perfusion, and ventilation. These tests are in no way meant to be substitutes for a careful clinical examination and evaluation; rather, they serve as valuable adjuncts in the management and diagnosis of respiratory illness. In order better to understand the most recently developed lung function tests, the subject of the second half of this chapter, a brief review of standard tests is first presented.

Standard pulmonary tests may be arbitrarily divided into a number of categories: mechanical properties, such as lung volumes and capacities, flow measurements, compliance, and resistance; diffusion characteristics, oxygen consumption, respiratory quotient; dead space and shunt fractions; ventilation and perfusion. The new lung function tests include closing volumes, flow-volume loops, maximal flow–static elastic recoil curve, $\dot{V}/\dot{Q}$ lung scanning with radioactive gases, and finally, the new refined tests for the integrity of the central and peripheral chemoreceptors.

STANDARD PULMONARY TESTS
Measurement of the various lung volumes and capacities is made with the use of a spirometer, which is a volume recorder. Some of these measurements are direct and

others are indirect. The various lung volumes and capacities are depicted in Figure 4-1.

Vital Capacity

One of the oldest yet most useful of the traditional lung function tests was first described in 1846 by John Hutchinson [29]. Noting that patients who were unable to move substantial amounts of air with maximal effort were not capable of maintaining their vital activities, the term *vital capacity* (VC) was coined and defined as the greatest volume of gas that can be expelled from the lungs by a voluntary effort after maximal inspiration. This volume is recorded on a low resistance spirometer and is corrected to BTPS (body temperature, pressure, and water saturation). Vital capacity measurements are accurate and reproducible; however, a normal subject may vary in his VC by as much as 20 percent from the predicted value. Tables are available that list predicted values for both sexes for varying age and stature. It is always important to state the nomogram upon which predicted values are based, because the older tables of predicted values greatly underestimated the expected level of performance.

A number of diseases may alter the vital capacity, which is decreased when the lung volume is encroached upon by either pulmonary or extrapulmonary factors such as resection of lung tissue, atelectasis, edema, infections, fibrosis, chest wall disease, pneumothorax, and pleural effusion. Thus, a decreased vital capacity does not in itself indicate the presence of, or type of, pulmonary disease.

Expiratory Reserve Volume

Expiratory reserve volume (ERV) is the maximal volume of gas that can be expelled from the resting end-expiratory position. In obesity, and in conditions that result in an increase in intraabdominal tension (e.g., pregnancy) the ERV may be decreased. The ERV may be calculated directly from the spirometric tracing.

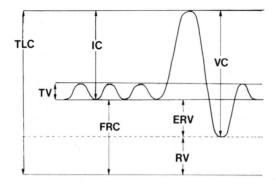

Figure 4-1. Lung volumes. TLC: total lung capacity; FRC: functional residual capacity; VC: vital capacity; IC: inspiratory capacity; RV: residual volume; TV: tidal volume; ERV: expiratory reserve volume.

Functional Residual Capacity

Functional residual capacity (FRC) is that volume of gas remaining in the lungs at the resting end-expiratory position. Functional residual capacity is increased in chronic obstructive pulmonary disease, especially emphysema, and may be decreased in restrictive diseases, especially if there are extensive bilateral infiltrations in the lung. The ERV and FRC have become significant clinical determinations, especially in the understanding and management of such disorders as adult respiratory distress syndrome (ARDS) (see Chapter 17). Unlike the ERV and VC, the FRC and residual volume (RV) are measured indirectly. There are a number of methods to measure FRC; to name a few: (1) helium (He) dilution using closed-circuit spirometry; (2) the open-circuit method of nitrogen (N_2) washout; and (3) body plethysmography. Once the FRC is determined, then one can calculate the RV by subtracting the ERV.

Closed-Circuit Helium Dilution Method

The patient breathes into a closed-circuit system containing known amounts of helium and air until equilibration is reached. Then the equation can be solved:

Before the test	*At the end of the test*
amount of He in lungs + amount of He in spirometer	=	amount of He in lungs + amount of He in spirometer

In the usual testing circumstance, the initial concentration of helium in the spirometer is 8 to 10 percent, and spirometer volume is around 6 liters. After equilibration between the patient and the spirometer, a final helium reading is observed. The FRC is then calculated as follows:

$$FRC = \text{spirometer volume} \times \frac{\text{initial He reading} - \text{final He reading}}{\text{final He reading}}$$

It is important to note the time taken for equilibration because it reflects the uniformity of gas distribution in the patient's lungs. For instance, in patients with chronic obstructive pulmonary disease and nonuniform gas distribution, equilibration time is delayed. If there are areas in the lung that do not participate in ventilation (bullae), then the FRC may be underestimated by this method.

Open-Circuit Nitrogen Method

Lung gas contains 81 percent nitrogen; hence, the volume of gas within the lungs when the patient begins breathing pure oxygen can be calculated if all the nitrogen in the lung is washed out, collected, and measured.

$$FRC = \frac{\text{ml } N_2 \text{ washed out of lungs}}{81}$$

Both the helium and the nitrogen methods are accurate and reproducible when properly performed. Further details on the above two techniques are readily available in the owner's manual obtained at the time of purchase of this equipment.

Body Plethysmography

To obtain an accurate determination of the volume of all the gases in the lung, both ventilated and nonventilated, body plethysmography is employed (Figure 4–2). The principle of measurement with the body box is based on Boyle's law: $P_1 V_1 = P_2 V_2$, at a constant temperature, where P = pressure and V = volume. The patient is seated in the airtight plethysmograph (body box) (A) and breathes normally and quietly from the air in the box. At the end of a quiet expiration, the mouthpiece is occluded by an electrically controlled shutter (B), and the patient is asked to pant, keeping his glottis open. During this maneuver, both mouth pressure and plethysmograph pressure are recorded on an oscilloscope using an X=Y plot (C). When the shutter is closed, the changes in volume of the patient's body (ΔV_1) is equal to the volume change in the plethysmograph (ΔV_2), and the increased or decreased pressure (ΔP_1) is reflected by an opposite change in plethysmograph pressure (ΔP_2) that is proportional to the change in its volume. So, if resting, thoracic volume = V_1, intrathoracic pressure = P_1, plethysmograph volume = V_2, and plethysmograph pressure = P_2, then,

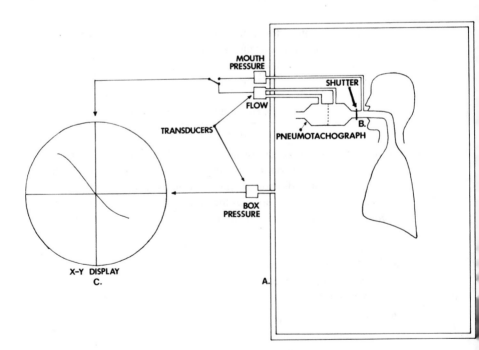

Figure 4–2. Plethysmograph.

$$P_1 V_1 = (P_1 + \Delta P_1) \times (V_1 + \Delta V_1).$$

At rest, $P_1 = P_2$, and during the cycle, $\Delta V_1 = \Delta V_2$. Therefore

$$V_1 = \frac{\Delta V}{\Delta P} \times P_1.$$

Because the slope of the oscilloscope equals

$$\frac{\text{change in mouth pressure}}{\text{unit change in plethysmograph volume}} = \frac{P}{V}.$$

Therefore,

$$V_1 = P_1 \times \frac{1}{\text{slope}} \times \frac{\text{plethysmograph calibration}}{\text{pressure calibration}}.$$

Thus, thoracic gas volume can be determined whether or not air spaces such as bullae are in ready communication with the airway.

The Total Lung Capacity and the RV-TLC Ratio

The total lung capacity (TLC) is that volume of gas contained in the lungs after a maximal inspiration. It is calculated by adding the residual volume to the vital capacity. TLC is decreased in restrictive lung disease and increased in obstructive diseases.

Because the residual volume bears a definite relationship to the TLC, varying somewhat with age, this ratio of RV to TLC is of some significance in the study of pulmonary disease. The normal values for this ratio in various age groups are 20 percent for 16–34 years, 23 percent for 35–49 years, and 31 percent for 50–69 years. An increased ratio is present in emphysema. However, an increased RV-TLC ratio is not specific for chronic obstructive pulmonary disease. Even in restrictive disease, this ratio may be increased if the degree of reduction in VC is more than that of RV.

Residual Volume

Residual volume (RV) is that volume of gas remaining in the lungs after a maximal forced expiration. This must of necessity be measured by indirect methods, usually by subtracting ERV from FRC.

Emphysema is the classic etiology responsible for an increase in RV and in the RV-TLC (total lung capacity) ratio. Both of these observations are a reflection of air trapping. Usually, RV and FRC increase together; however, there are circumstances in which the RV may be increased with a normal FRC, for example, if the ERV is decreased. The RV may be normal or decreased in diffuse pulmonary restrictive disease (such as sarcoid or pulmonary fibrosis). Caution must be exercised in the interpretation of the RV-TLC ratio, especially in restrictive lung disease. With restrictive lung disease the VC is reduced greater than the RV, leading to an increase in the RV-TLC ratio without any air trapping. There are a variety of methods employed to determine RV, and because of their interrelationship, the FRC, ERV, RV, and TLC are determined at the same time.

Tidal Volume

The tidal volume (TV) is that volume of gas exchanged during each breath at rest and during any stated activity. The tidal volume varies considerably even in normal subjects, and as such it is difficult to attach any significance to changes in the tidal volume except when it is considered along with the respiratory rate. When the tidal volume is extremely small, nearly approaching the dead space volume, the efficiency of ventilation is greatly impaired. Tidal volume determinations are of great importance in the patient being mechanically ventilated.

Minute Ventilation

The minute ventilation ($\dot{V}E$) is that volume of gas exhaled per minute calculated by multiplying the tidal volume by the number of breaths per minute; it is a helpful determination in working with the machine-assisted patient. By convention, a minute ventilation of less than 10 liters while on mechanical ventilation must be demonstrated before weaning is considered (see Chapter 12). Also, before mechanical ventilation is discontinued, the patient should be able to voluntarily double the resting minute ventilation.

Forced Expiratory Spirogram

The forced expiratory spirogram is the simplest and most commonly used measurement for flow determination in both office practice and hospital laboratories. Analysis of the forced expiratory tracing is facilitated by recording at a high kymograph speed. The patient is instructed to take as deep a breath as possible at the end of quiet exhalation and then exhale as rapidly and as forcefully as possible (Figure 4–3). Forced vital capacity (FVC) is the total volume of air exhaled as measured from a forced expiratory spirogram. The volume of air exhaled during 1, 2, and 3 seconds is called the *forced expiratory volume* in 1, 2, or 3 seconds (FEV_1, FEV_2, FEV_3). These are then expressed as a percent of the FVC. A normal young individual is able to exhale at least 75 percent in 1 second, 85 percent in 2 seconds, and 95 percent in 3 seconds (the FEV percentage decreases with age).

Another view of the same curve may be quite informative; for instance, the maximal midexpiratory flow (MMF) can be calculated. This is the measurement of the expiratory flow rate during the middle 50 percent of the vital capacity effort (see Figure 4–3).

$$MMF = \frac{VC}{2 \times time}$$

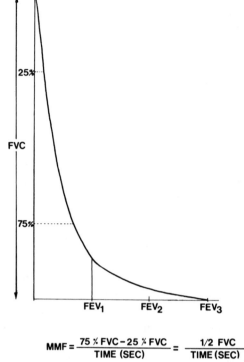

$$MMF = \frac{75 \text{ \% FVC} - 25 \text{ \% FVC}}{\text{TIME (SEC)}} = \frac{1/2 \text{ FVC}}{\text{TIME (SEC)}}$$

Figure 4-3. Timed vital capacity. MMF: maximal mid-expiratory flow rate; FVC: forced vital capacity; FEV_N: forced expired volume in N seconds.

The MMF is a very reproducible measurement because it is from the effort-independent portion of the expiratory curve (see p. 90). It is also a sensitive indicator of early obstructive pulmonary disease.

FEV_1, FEV_3, and MMF are decreased in obstructive pulmonary disease. In restrictive diseases the flow rates remain normal.

Peak Expiratory Flow Rate
Peak expiratory flow rate (PFR) is the point of highest flow during a maximal expiration. This test is dependent on full patient cooperation and effort. When this cooperation is obtained, the test is a simple, accurate, reproducible one. Using a Wright's peak flow meter, a relatively inexpensive, durable piece of equipment, the PFR is particularly useful in the office followup of patients suffering with bronchospasm.

Maximum Breathing Capacity or Maximum Voluntary Ventilation
The maximum breathing capacity (MBC) or maximum voluntary ventilation (MVV) is the maximal volume of air that a subject can breathe per minute. Usually, the

subject is asked to breathe maximally for 10 to 15 seconds, and from this the volume of ventilation for 1 minute is calculated. The disadvantages of this test are that it requires full cooperation and motivation on the part of the patient. It is also influenced by nonpulmonary factors such as muscle force and endurance. To obtain maximal values, a breathing frequency of 100/min is necessary. An indirect method of measuring MBC in those unable to perform the test is to multiply $FEV_{0.75}$ (FEV in 0.75 sec) by 40, or $FEV_{1.0}$ by 30.

Lung Compliance
Compliance of the lung is defined as that change in lung volume observed when the pressure gradient between pleura and alveoli is changed by 1 cm H_2O. Static compliance is measured when there is no flow, as in breath-holding, and dynamic compliance is measured during respiration. Pleural pressure is indirectly measured using esophageal pressure as an equivalent. Esophageal pressure is measured directly, using an esophageal balloon. A static pressure volume curve can be constructed using pressure measurements obtained at various lung volumes projected on an X-Y recorder (Figure 4–4). Compliance is represented as the slope of the middle portion of the curve.

Compliance is not a routine pulmonary function test because its clinical usefulness is limited, and it must be kept in mind that performance of the test requires the placement of an esophageal balloon, involving some discomfort for the subject. Compliance is decreased in restrictive diseases of the lung. In emphysema, static compliance is high (it must be corrected to lung volume).

In normal subjects, static compliance and dynamic compliance are equal at the same lung volumes if the breathing frequency does not exceed 60 to 90 per minute. Dynamic compliance is less than static compliance in patients with increased airway resistance to some lung units. In other words, compliance is frequency dependent. This is explained by the nonuniform distribution of ventilation to various

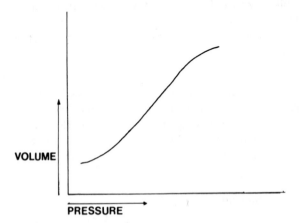

Figure 4–4. Static compliance curve of the lung.

lung units that have differing time constants, a *time constant* being the product of the compliance and resistance of that unit in the lung being observed. If the airway resistance to some units of the lung is increased, then these units require a longer time to fill and empty, and thus the time constant is prolonged (Figure 4-5). In Figure 4-5,B, there is a narrowed airway to one lung unit, i.e., this lung unit has increased resistance. If gas is breathed, the units in Figure 4-5,A will move symmetrically. The same is true for B only if the flow is slow. With increased flow, the unit with the narrowed airway ventilates less and less with increasing rates, resulting in a decrease in overall compliance at higher breathing rates. This concept of frequency dependence and time constants shows that the distribution of gases to various lung areas is determined by the interaction of resistance, compliance, and time constant. An area of lung with high compliance and low resistance will receive more ventilation than an area of low compliance and high resistance even when the time constant is equal in both areas. In Figure 4-5,C, the airways are normal, but

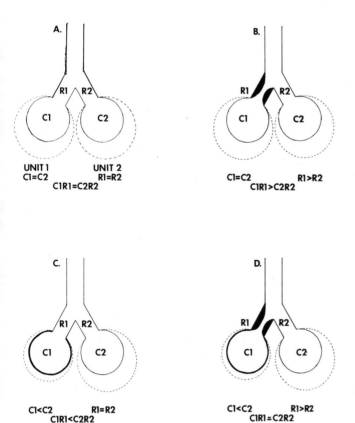

Figure 4-5. Concept of varying time constants (C X R) in varying lung units. C: compliance; R: resistance; CR: time constant.

one unit has decreased compliance because it is stiffer. This results in overall decreased lung compliance, but there is no frequency dependence. In Figure 4-5,D, there is a combination of events as seen in B and C — that is, compliance is decreased, and it is frequency dependent.

Frequency dependence of compliance is a very sensitive measurement in identifying dysfunction of small airways even when other routine tests remain normal [65]. The disadvantage of this measurement is the requirement of introducing an esophageal balloon, a factor that limits its usefulness as a routine measurement.

Absolute pleural pressures can also be used in the evaluation of parenchymal disease and pleural and chest wall disorders. When lung compliance measurement shows low values, sometimes it may be difficult to identify whether this is due to restrictive diseases of the lung or to diseases of the pleura and chest wall. It has been shown that the maximum static negative pressure developed in the pleura at total lung capacity (P_{max}) is higher than predicted in restrictive diseases of the lung, whereas in chest wall and pleural diseases it is very low [14]. In emphysema, P_{max} is low.

Airway Resistance

Airway resistance (R_{aw}) can be measured either by the body plethysmograph method or with the use of an esophageal balloon. The airway resistance is the pressure difference that must be applied between the pleura and the mouth to produce a flow at the mouth of 1 liter per second.

The resistance of airways smaller than 2 mm diameter is very small, contributing less than 10 percent of total R_{aw} in the normal situation. Thus, obstruction in the peripheral small airways will not be reflected in the airway resistance measurements until the obstruction is far advanced.

Another way of expressing airway resistance is to use the term *airway conductance* (G_{aw}), which is the inverse of airway resistance. The reason for the use of G_{aw} is that the relationship between R_{aw} and lung volume is hyperbolic. This means that the inverse of R_{aw} (G_{aw}) has a linear relationship to lung volume, permitting the lung volume to be taken into account. *Specific conductance* SG_{aw} is conductance per unit volume.

Air Velocity Index

The air velocity index (AVI) is a ratio of the percentage of the predicted maximal breathing capacity (MBC) and the percentage of predicted vital capacity:

$$AVI = \frac{\% \text{ predicted MBC}}{\% \text{ predicted VC}}$$

In normal subjects, this is 1. An index of less than 1 is seen in obstructive lung disease, and an index of greater than 1 in those with loss of functioning lung tissue.

Diffusing Capacity

Diffusing capacity is the capacity of the lung to transfer gas from air spaces to the red cells in the pulmonary capillaries. The factors affecting diffusion are [5] : (1) thickness of the alveolar membrane, (2) thickness of the lining cell, (3) permeability of the capillary wall, (4) thickness of the plasma between capillary wall and red cell, and (5) permeability of red cell membrane to oxygen or carbon monoxide. In addition, and of great importance, the diffusing capacity is most dependent on the number of alveoli available for gas exchange, the uniformity of ventilation to these alveoli, and their perfusion characteristics—in other words, their $\dot{V}/\dot{Q}$ balance.

The most commonly employed form of this test utilizes carbon monoxide. The behavior of carbon monoxide is similar to oxygen, and the measurement of carbon monoxide is technically easy. The pulmonary (lung) diffusing capacity for carbon monoxide is described by the formula

$$D_{L_{CO}} = \frac{\text{ml CO transferred from alveolar gas to blood per minute}}{\text{mean alveolar CO tension} - \text{mean capillary CO tension}}$$

The methods available for this determination are varied; they include (1) the single breath technique, (2) the steady state technique, (3) rebreathing, and (4) fractional carbon monoxide uptake. In the single breath method the subject takes a single deep breath of a mixture of carbon monoxide in air along with helium (used as a marker gas), then holds his breath for 10 seconds and exhales. The expired gas is analyzed for both carbon monoxide and helium. The calculation of $D_{L_{CO}}$ involves the following two equations. First, the calculation of alveolar concentration of carbon monoxide is given by the equation

$$F_{A_{CO}} = \frac{F_{I_{CO}} \times \% \text{ He in expired sample}}{\% \text{ He inspired}}$$

Once the alveolar concentration of carbon monoxide is known, then the diffusing capacity is calculated using Krogh's equation:

$$D_{L_{CO}} = \frac{\text{alveolar volume STPD} \times 60}{\text{breath-holding time (sec)} \times (P_B - 47)} \times \text{natural log} \frac{F_{A_{CO}}}{F_{E_{CO}}}.$$

Of these, alveolar volume is computed from the spirometric tracing of deep inspiration. $F_{A_{CO}}$ is the alveolar concentration of carbon monoxide, and $F_{E_{CO}}$ the final concentration of carbon monoxide after breath-holding. STPD means standard temperature, pressure, dry.

It is shown that in the same laboratory, variations among multiple measurements are minimal. Thus single-breath $D_{L_{CO}}$ can be used in situations where serial follow-up may be of use, as in following patients with sarcoidosis. The disadvantage of this method is that it can be done only in those patients who are able to hold their breath for 10 seconds. Also, in situations where alveolar volume is markedly reduced, error in measurement becomes enormous because of the inadequate sampling of the expired gas.

A steady state method may be used in situations where single breath DL_{CO} cannot be done. Fractional carbon monoxide uptake is simply a ratio of carbon monoxide absorbed to carbon monoxide inspired.

Measurement of Membrane Diffusing Capacity and Pulmonary Capillary Blood Volume

The total diffusing capacity of the lung (DL) and its relationship to its component membrane diffusing capacity (DM) and pulmonary capillary blood volume (vc) are expressed by the equation $1/DL = 1/DM + 1/\Theta vc$, where Θ is the volume of gas that will be taken up by red blood cells (RBC) in 1 ml of blood per minute for each torr pressure gradient between plasma and red cell. The value for Θ depends on the oxygen tension, and this affects the rate of uptake of carbon monoxide by the red blood cells. Nomograms that express the value of $1/\Theta$ for different oxygen tensions are available. If DL is calculated at two levels of oxygen tension, then the equation can be solved for both DM and vc.

Measurement of the oxygen diffusing capacity (DL_{O_2}) utilizes the formula

$$DL_{O_2} = \frac{\dot{V}_{O_2}}{PA_{O_2} - P\bar{c}_{O_2}},$$

where $\dot{V}_{O_2}$ is oxygen consumed, PA_{O_2} is the alveolar oxygen tension, and $P\bar{c}_{O_2}$ is the mean pulmonary capillary oxygen tension. $P\bar{c}_{O_2}$ is calculated with the Bohr integration procedure (see p. 83).

Measurement of Oxygen Consumption and Calculation of Respiratory Quotient

The amount of oxygen absorbed per minute defines oxygen consumption ($\dot{V}_{O_2}$), which can be calculated by measuring the oxygen concentration of expired air, the volume of expired air, and the minute ventilation. The test is performed by collecting all expired gas over a period of 2 minutes, then dividing the total volume by 2. This gas is then analyzed for oxygen and carbon dioxide. Oxygen consumption is the product of minute ventilation ($\dot{V}E$) and the oxygen concentration difference between inspired and expired air:

$$\dot{V}_{O_2} = \dot{V}E \times (FI_{O_2} - FE_{O_2}).$$

Similarly, the amount of carbon dioxide produced per minute ($\dot{V}_{CO_2}$) is the product of minute ventilation and the concentration of carbon dioxide in the expired gas:

$$\dot{V}_{CO_2} = \dot{V}_E \times F_{ECO_2}.$$

Thus, the respiratory quotient (RQ) or gas exchange ratio is determined as the ratio of carbon dioxide produced to oxygen absorbed:

$$RQ = \frac{\dot{V}_{CO_2}}{\dot{V}_{O_2}}.$$

The clinical usefulness of $\dot{V}_{O_2}$ measurement is mainly during exercise testing to determine the functional impairment of the cardiopulmonary system. In a normal individual, $\dot{V}_{O_2}$ is around 0.25 liter at rest. During strenuous exercise, this increases to 3 to 4 liters.

Dead Space Evaluation

Dead space is that portion of the tracheal bronchial tree that is not involved in gas exchange. The dead space is separated into anatomic and physiologic components. The anatomic dead space is that portion of lung without gas exchange units, such as the trachea or bronchi. On the other hand, physiologic dead space includes those sections in the lung that are ventilated but that do not participate in gas exchange. In order to measure physiologic dead space, the arterial carbon dioxide tension and the carbon dioxide tension of the expired gas must be determined.

A rough method of calculating anatomic dead space assumes that approximately 1 ml per pound of body weight is anatomic dead space. A more exact determination is to analyze the concentration of nitrogen in the expired gas after one single breath of 100% oxygen. The dead space formula states

$$V_D = \frac{(Pa_{CO_2} - PE_{CO_2})\dot{V}_E}{Pa_{CO_2}},$$

where V_D is the physiologic dead space, $\dot{V}_E$ is minute ventilation, and Pa_{CO_2} and PE_{CO_2} are the arterial and expired carbon dioxide tensions, respectively.

In a normal person, anatomic and physiologic dead space are the same and occupy about one-third of tidal volume, but in disease states such as chronic obstructive pulmonary disease and pulmonary embolism, physiologic dead space increases.

Estimation of Shunt Fraction

A right-to-left (R-L) shunt exists when blood bypasses the lungs and arrives in the systemic circulation. Whether intracardiac or extracardiac, the arterial blood cannot be completely saturated because it is mixed with venous blood. The shunt fraction ($\dot{Q}S$) is expressed by the equation

$$\frac{\dot{Q}s}{\dot{Q}T} = \frac{Ca_{O_2} - C\bar{c}_{O_2}}{C\bar{v}_{O_2} - C\bar{c}_{O_2}}$$

where $\dot{Q}s$ is the shunt flow, $\dot{Q}T$ is total blood flow, Ca_{O_2} and $C\bar{v}_{O_2}$ are oxygen content of arterial and mixed venous blood, respectively, and $C\bar{c}_{O_2}$ is the oxygen content of end capillary blood. This formula calculates the physiologic shunt, i.e., includes both anatomic arteriovenous communications along with any areas with very low ventilation-perfusion ratios.

The anatomic shunt alone can be calculated by giving the patient 100% oxygen to breathe so that all alveoli are washed out of nitrogen (in patients with severe obstructive pulmonary disease this might take 20 to 30 minutes). The alveolar P_{O_2} should be approximately 670 torr (barometric pressure 760 minus water vapor pressure 47 torr minus alveolar CO_2 pressure 40 torr). If one measures the arterial oxygen tension at this time. then solves for $\dot{Q}s$,

$$\frac{\dot{Q}s}{\dot{Q}T} = \frac{(PA_{O_2} - Pa_{O_2}) \times 0.0031}{(PA_{O_2} - Pa_{O_2}) \times 0.0031 + \text{arteriovenous oxygen content difference}}$$

A simple method for obtaining the approximate shunt fraction for a given arterial oxygen tension on 100% oxygen employs a nomogram (Figure 4-6). For example, a Pa_{O_2} of 225 torr indicates an approximate shunt fraction of 18 to 25 percent.

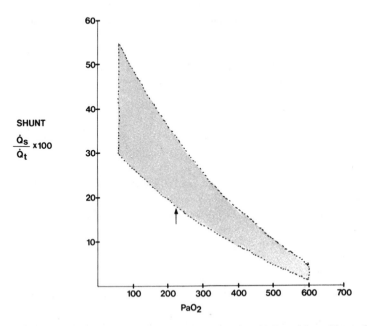

Figure 4-6. Nomogram for estimating shunt fraction. (Adapted from Moore, P. D., et al. *Post-Traumatic Pulmonary Insufficiency.* Philadelphia: Saunders, 1969.)

Hypoxemia from pulmonary shunting is associated with hyperventilation, resulting in arterial carbon dioxide tensions that are below normal, unless the shunt is enormous.

Alveolar-Arterial Oxygen Tension Gradient

The alveolar-arterial oxygen tension gradient ($AaPO_2$ gradient) is the difference between alveolar and arterial oxygen tension. The arterial oxygen tension can be measured directly, but the alveolar oxygen tension must be calculated using the alveolar air equation. In a simplified form,

$$PA_{O_2} = PI_{O_2} - \frac{Pa_{CO_2}}{R},$$

where PI_{O_2} is the inspired oxygen tension, Pa_{CO_2} is the arterial carbon dioxide tension, and R is the gas exchange ratio. For routine calculation, R is assumed to be 0.8. An alteration in the $AaPO_2$ gradient may be the first indication of faulty gas exchange. This is of special importance in diffuse interstitial disease, where the $AaPO_2$ gradient may be the only pulmonary function abnormality.

Compartmental Method Analysis of the Distribution of Ventilation, Perfusion, and Diffusing Capacity

In a homogeneous lung, when inspired gas is changed to 100% oxygen, the alveolar nitrogen concentration will change exponentially. This change in alveolar nitrogen concentration will give a straight line if plotted on semilog paper. In the normal lung with some degree of inequality in gas distribution, the nitrogen washout curve is not an absolute straight line. Based on this observation, a two-compartment model for the analysis of distribution of ventilation came into use. Hickam et al. utilized the term *slow space* to designate those alveoli that are poorly ventilated [26]. The term *fast space* is used to identify the well-ventilated alveoli. From the slope of the nitrogen washout curve, the volume and ventilation of both slow and fast spaces can be calculated [8] (Figure 4–7). With simultaneous measurement of arterial oxygen tension the perfusion to these spaces can also be calculated [21]. This permits the calculation of $\dot{V}A/\dot{Q}c$ to both the spaces.

The $\dot{V}A/\dot{Q}c$ ratio of both spaces determines the value of end capillary oxygen saturation. If the observed saturation is less than the calculated saturation, then this decrease must be due to diffusion impairment. To determine this component, the concept of Bohr integration is used [8]. The method of Bohr integration adds up to all the minute increases in saturation as red cells pass through the capillaries. A simple method of expressing this is

$$\text{Bohr integral} = \frac{\text{diffusing capacity} \times 100}{\text{blood flow} \times O_2 \text{ capacity}}$$

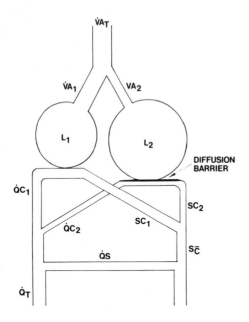

Figure 4-7. Compartmental analysis of slow space and fast space by the nitrogen washout method. $\dot{V}_{A_T}$: total alveolar ventilation; $\dot{V}_{A_1} \dot{V}_{A_2}$: ventilation to fast and slow spaces; $L_1 L_2$: volume of fast and slow spaces; $\dot{Q}_T$: total blood flow; $\dot{Q}_{c_1} \dot{Q}_{c_2}$: blood flow to fast and slow spaces; $\dot{Q}_S$: shunt fraction; $S_{c_1} S_{c_2}$: oxygen saturation of capillary blood from fast and slow spaces; $S_{\bar{c}}$: saturation of mean capillary blood.

Using this kind of analysis, King and Briscoe [35, 36] have shown that diffusing capacities to both the slow and fast spaces can be calculated.

In emphysema, the slow space has a very low diffusing capacity and moderate reduction in the $\dot{V}_A/\dot{Q}_c$ ratio; in chronic bronchitis, diffusing capacity is maintained but the $\dot{V}_A/\dot{Q}_c$ ratio is very low. The alveolar capillary block syndrome has either a low $\dot{V}_A/\dot{Q}_c$ ratio or a very low diffusion-perfusion ratio. Readers interested in obtaining more details on studying the $\dot{V}_A/\dot{Q}_c$ relationships and Bohr integration procedures are referred to King and Briscoe [8, 35, 36].

MOST RECENT LUNG FUNCTION TESTS

Closing Volume
At or near residual volume, the ventilation to the bases of the lung in the upright position is decreased. This is a result of the closure of the small airways in the dependent lung zones (i.e., the bases). Thus, closing volume (CV) [9–11] is that lung volume at which dependent small airways close, which in turn depends on the elastic recoil of the small airways.

There are two techniques used to measure airway closure: (1) the bolus technique, using a radioactive gas such as argon, xenon, or helium; and (2) the resident gas technique, in which the nitrogen concentration of expired air is measured following one breath of pure oxygen. In the bolus technique, the radioactive gas is inspired from residual volume and goes only to those lung units that are open. A slow, steady vital capacity maneuver, breathing room air, is then performed. The expired gas is continuously monitored for radioactivity. The concentration of radioactive gas is then plotted on an X-Y recorder against volume. The point at which there is a sudden rise in the concentration of radioactive gas represents the point of small airways closure.

The resident gas technique is a relatively simple method requiring only a spirometer, nitrogen analyzer, oxygen, and an X-Y recorder. The patient is asked to take a maximal inspiration from residual volume of 100% oxygen and then to slowly exhale to residual volume. The nitrogen concentration of the expired gas is plotted against volume on an X-Y recorder.

During the initial stages while the patient is breathing in, the dead space gas, which is room air, goes to open lung units. This is followed by the arrival of pure oxygen, which is now distributed to all lung units, for now they are all open (Figure 4-8A). The volume change during ventilation is greater at the lower lung zones so that the pressure at the base is less negative than that at the apex (B). Hence, the lower zones, which were closed at the beginning of inspiration, will contain a higher concentration of oxygen. Below the functional residual capacity (FRC), the pleural pressure at the base becomes gradually positive, causing closure of lung units in this region (Figure 4-8C). During slow exhalation, the initial dead space gas coming out of the mouth is 100% oxygen (phase I of the CV tracing) (Figures 4-9, 4-10). As the alveoli empty, the nitrogen concentration in the expired air increases (phase II). An

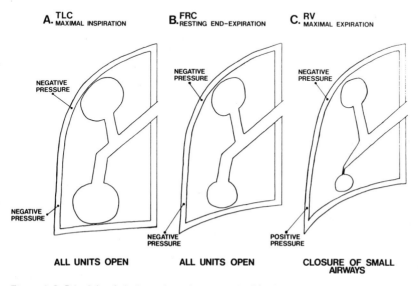

Figure 4-8. Principle of closing volume in a normal subject.

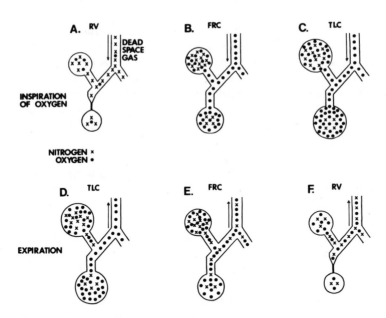

Figure 4-9. Resident gas technique of determining closing volume.

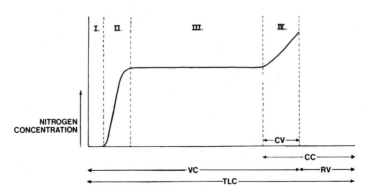

Figure 4-10. Closing volume tracing showing the various phases. Phase I: dead space gas; phase II: mixture of dead space and alveolar gas; phase III: alveolar gas from all lung units; phase IV: alveolar gas from open lung units. Closing capacity = closing volume + residual volume: CV% = CV/VC × 100; CC% = CC/TLC × 100.

alveolar plateau is reached (phase III), a result of the emptying of all alveoli. Toward the end of phase III, before residual volume is reached, the concentration of nitrogen increases (phase IV) because of the closure of small airways in dependent lung zones. The point at which the nitrogen concentration increases from phase III is the closing volume point. The distance from this point (using either technique) to the residual volume is the closing volume. If the residual volume is added to the closing volume, this is the closing capacity.

The closing volume tracing can also be used to calculate the dead space gas (from phases I and II). Phase III, or the alveolar plateau, gives an indication of the uniformity of distribution of ventilation in different lung spaces. If the distribution is nonuniform, as in chronic obstructive pulmonary disease, then the emptying rate of the units is also nonuniform. This causes a gradual rise in the slope of phase III, which is horizontal in normal persons. In this situation, one may not be able to recognize the change of slope from phase III to phase IV (Figure 4-11).

It has been estimated that the closing volume is around 10 percent of the vital capacity in the young, healthy nonsmoker. As one grows older, because of the gradual loss of elastic recoil, CV increases. Figure 4-12 shows the distribution of CV for various ages and both sexes. It has also been shown that in smokers the CV is, on an average, higher than in nonsmokers. In chronic obstructive pulmonary disease, alveolar units close at higher lung volumes (Figure 4-13); does this indicate loss of elastic recoil of small airways? Can one say that a smoker with abnormal closing volume will develop chronic obstructive pulmonary disease? These are questions for which answers are not yet clear.

The interrelationship between closing volume and functional residual capacity explains partially the abnormal gas exchange that one encounters with increasing age and in different positions. Craig and co-workers [17] showed that, on changing from the sitting to the supine position, functional residual capacity decreases, whereas closing volume remains the same. They divided their subjects into four groups based on the relationship between CV and FRC (Figure 4-14). In group 1, whose CV was below FRC in both seated and supine positions, the $AaPO_2$ gradient improved in the supine position because of the better $\dot{V}A/\dot{Q}c$ balance. In group 2, in whom CV remained below FRC in the sitting position but rose above it in the supine position, the $AaPO_2$ gradient became worse in the supine position. In groups 3 and 4, where

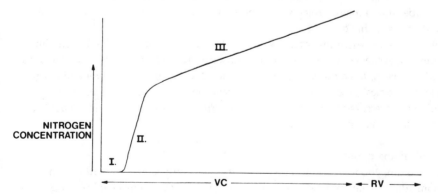

Figure 4-11. Closing volume in chronic obstructive pulmonary disease. Phase IV is not recognizable; closing volume cannot be determined.

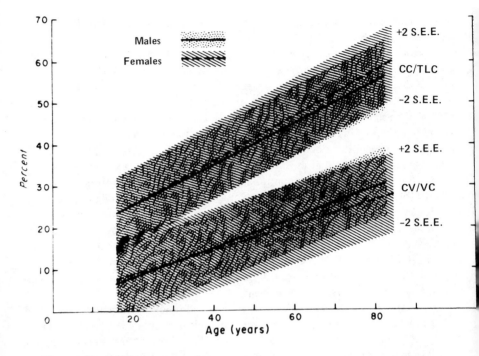

Figure 4–12. Closing volume for various age groups, both sexes. (Reproduced by permission from Buist, A. S. Regression lines plus or minus 2 standard errors of the estimate for the relation of closing capacity to total lung capacity and closing volume to vital capacity on age. Current concepts of the single breath nitrogen test. *New England Journal of Medicine* 293, 1975, p. 439. Fig. 2.)

CV was at or above FRC, the AaPo$_2$ gradients were always abnormal. These authors conclude that in many subjects, a change in position from supine to sitting could improve gas exchange.

Another area where the interrelationship between FRC closing volume and impaired gas exchange is important is in adult respiratory distress syndrome. Here, as FRC decreases, the closing volume goes above the tidal breathing level and gas exchange becomes grossly abnormal. Use of mechanical ventilation and positive end expiratory pressure increases FRC, thus reversing the relationship and producing better gas exchange.

Flow-Volume Loops
Flow-volume loops are determined by plotting instantaneous flow rates against lung volume during maximum effort. The curve measures overall mechanical properties of the lung. Reduced flow rates can result from either loss of elasticity and/or airways obstruction. The flow-volume loop is a fairly simple measurement techni-

A. TLC   **B.** FRC   **C.** RV

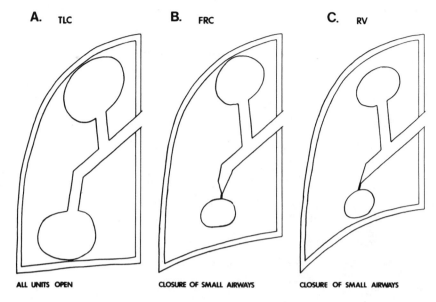

ALL UNITS OPEN   CLOSURE OF SMALL AIRWAYS   CLOSURE OF SMALL AIRWAYS

Figure 4–13. Closure of lung units even at rest expiration (B) in patients with chronic obstructive pulmonary disease (cf. Figure 3–8).

cally. Flow is recorded against volume using an X-Y recorder. In 1958 Hyatt and co-workers [32] described the isovolume pressure flow curve and showed that for a given lung volume the expiratory flow did not increase beyond a certain point ($\dot{V}_{max}$) even with increasing pressure. The reason for this flow limitation is due to the unique interrelationship among intramural pressure, pressure outside the airways, and the elastic property of the airways. Thus, flow rates are decreased not only as a consequence of airways obstruction but also as a result of the loss of elasticity, even when the airways are normal.

In order to better understand the flow characteristics of the expiratory limb of the flow-volume curve, a brief discussion of the equal pressure point (EPP) is necessary (Figure 4–15). The driving pressure for flow along the airways during expiration is the *alveolar pressure*. This pressure is the sum of the pleural pressure and the elastic recoil pressure of the lungs. During expiration, there is a pressure drop along the airways because of the flow of air. At one point, the pressure inside the airway must equal the pressure outside the airway (pleural pressure), the *equal pressure point*. The drop in pressure from the alveolus to this point is the *elastic recoil pressure*. Conceptually, the equal pressure point divides the airway into two segments, the upstream segment from the alveolus to it, and the downstream segment from it to the mouth [46, 47, 49]. The driving pressure in the upstream segment is the elastic recoil pressure, and in the downstream segment, the pleural pressure.

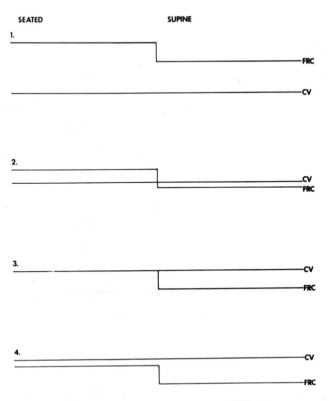

Figure 4-14. Relationship of closing volume and FRC in four groups of patients. (Adapted from Craig, D., et al. "Closing volume" and its relationship to gas exchange in seated and supine positions. *Journal of Applied Physiology* 31, 1971, p. 717.)

Also, in the upstream segment, the pressure inside the airways is positive relative to outside, and negative in the downstream segment except in the extrathoracic airways and sometimes part of the intrapulmonary airways [47]. During forced expiration or cough, compression of the airways in the downstream segment occurs.

During normal breathing, there is no EPP in the normal lung. With increasing force of expiration, as the pleural pressure changes from negative to atmospheric, the EPP appears at the airway opening [47]. With further increase in pleural pressure, the EPP moves upstream until $\dot{V}_{max}$ is reached and the EPP becomes fixed at the level of the lobar or segmental bronchi. This occurs in normal individuals when 25 percent of VC is exhaled. Beyond this, flow is independent of effort.

Pride and co-workers [54], in their analysis of mechanical events of the lung, compared the lung to a Starling resistor. When the pressure at the outlet of a collapsible tube is less than that of the surrounding pressure, the flow is dependent on the difference between the driving and surrounding pressures rather than between the driving and outlet pressures. In the lung, once $\dot{V}_{max}$ is reached, the flow is depen-

A.

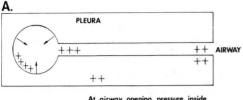

At airway opening pressure inside
airway equals pressure in the pleura

B.

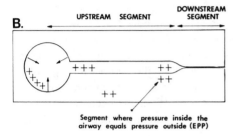

Segment where pressure inside the
airway equals pressure outside (EPP)

C. IN COPD

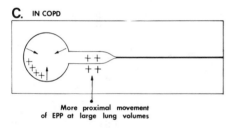

More proximal movement
of EPP at large lung volumes

Figure 4–15. Equal pressure point.

dent on the difference between the alveolar and the pleural pressures, i.e., on the
elastic recoil pressure of the lung, and is independent of the total pressure drop
from alveolus to atmosphere.

In normal individuals, these mechanical events are important only during coughing. The dynamic compression of the intrathoracic airways is an essential part of
an effective cough. The upstream movement of EPP helps to clear the secretions
from the collapsing downstream segment.

The information one obtains from a flow-volume loop is similar to that derived
from a forced expiratory spirogram. The curve is reproducible if effort is maximally
forceful over the same volume range. Reduction in flow at any given volume is
easily visualized. The peak point of expiratory flow is the *peak expiratory flow.*
This occurs usually at around 90 percent of vital capacity, and the normal value is
about 8 liters/sec. Flow at 50 percent vital capacity approximates the maximal
midexpiratory flow rate (MMF). Expiratory flow may be compared to inspiratory

flow at any given lung volume. Expiratory flow at lower lung volumes reflects the function of small airways. Available data in the literature so far seem to indicate that the ratio of expiratory to inspiratory flow is close to 1 at 50 percent vital capacity and near 0.5 at 25 percent vital capacity in healthy, nonsmoking individuals [3, 12, 61]. A decrease in these ratios might indicate dysfunction of small airways. Another ratio of some interest is $\dot{V}_{50}/\dot{V}_{25}$ [61]. During expiration, if the ratio is 2, then the curve is linear. If the ratio is more than 3, especially in a young individual, the curve is concave, indicating small airways dysfunction.

Figure 4–16 shows various types of flow-volume loops. Normal flow patterns (A) for various portions of the curve are presently under investigation, and there appears to be a wide variation in flow rates, even among normal individuals. However, the flow is fairly constant and maximal during major parts of inspiration. During expiration after breathing maximum (peak flow) the flow decreases uniformly. In chronic obstructive pulmonary disease (COPD), the flow limitation is seen throughout expiration (B). If tidal volume is superimposed, it is apparent that the patient is breathing at the MEFV level. Restrictive lung disease (C) causes decreases in the vital capacity, although not in flow; thus, the shape of the flow loop may look com-

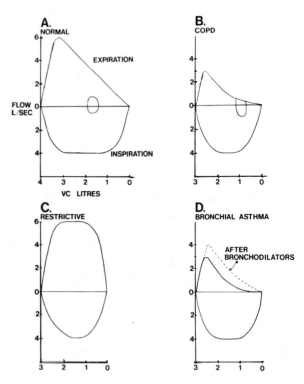

Figure 4–16. Flow-volume loops.

pressed from side to side. The pattern in bronchial asthma (D) is similar to that of COPD (B). Here, the expiratory flow may show improvement with the administration of bronchodilator drugs; similarly, the flow may decrease with allergenic challenge.

Extrathoracic obstructions display two patterns of abnormal flow. In fixed extrathoracic obstruction (E), as in cancer of the larynx and in tracheal stenosis, there is flow limitation during both inspiration and expiration. If there is variable extrathoracic obstructive lesion (F), then the flow limitation, which may still be present during both inspiration and expiration, is more marked during inspiration, with a slight decrease in expiratory flow at large lung volumes. Large airways intrathoracic obstructions (G) may be differentiated from COPD by the truncated appearance of the expiratory flow, which is reduced during expiration, mostly at large lung volumes. With intrathoracic lesions and COPD, the inspiratory portion of the loop remains normal. The use of a helium-oxygen mixture (H) improves flow during expiration at large lung volumes. The point at which flow becomes identical to that of room air is called *volume of isoflow* (V_{iso} $\dot{V}$).

The flow-volume curve is a simple, quick, reproducible test. There is no discomfort to the patient. It is particularly useful in detecting small airways dysfunction and central airway dysfunction.

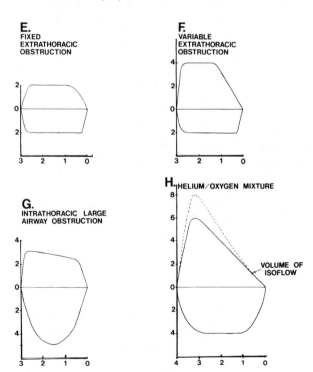

E.
FIXED
EXTRATHORACIC
OBSTRUCTION

F.
VARIABLE
EXTRATHORACIC
OBSTRUCTION

G.
INTRATHORACIC LARGE
AIRWAY OBSTRUCTION

H. HELIUM/OXYGEN MIXTURE

VOLUME OF
ISOFLOW

Effect of Alteration of Gas Density and Viscosity on the Shape of the Flow-Volume Curve

Schilder and colleagues [59], in an attempt to evaluate the role of various respiratory gases in determining the shape of the expiratory flow-volume curve, used gas mixtures of varying density and viscosity and then obtained flow-volume curves in normal subjects. They showed that when a light gas (helium) was exhaled, the $\dot{V}_{max}$ was higher during most of expiration. They also showed that $\dot{V}_{max}$ in normal persons is dependent on gas density at lung volumes greater than 25 percent of vital capacity. At these volumes the equal pressure point is in the larger airways and resistance of the upstream segment is caused mostly by convective acceleration and turbulence, both of which are density dependent. Thus, gas mixtures with low density, such as helium-oxygen mixtures, may be used to study the flow-volume relationship and determine the location of the equal pressure point. Several workers [2, 21] have used helium-oxygen mixtures in an attempt to identify the site of obstruction in chronic obstructive lung disease, bronchial asthma, and central airways disease.

The data seem to indicate that in chronic bronchitis, and in some instances of asthma, $\dot{V}_{max}$ does not increase with the helium-oxygen mixtures, suggesting that the equal pressure point is located peripherally and that the obstruction is in the peripheral airways in these patients. When small airways are obstructed, flow resistance is changed not so much by gas density as by viscosity. Helium is more viscid than room air, so that flow with a helium-oxygen mixture is less than that with air.

Other workers have shown, using helium-oxygen mixtures, that asthmatic patients may have either large airways obstruction or small airways obstruction. Those with obstruction in the large airways show an increase in $\dot{V}_{max}$ with a helium-oxygen mixture, whereas those who have predominantly small airways occlusion do not.

At very low lung volumes the expiratory flow is identical with room air and with a helium-oxygen mixture (see Figure 4-16). The point on the curve at which the flows become identical is designated as the volume of isoflow ($V_{iso}\dot{V}$) and is measured as a percentage of vital capacity [28]. The identity of the flow is attributed to the development of laminar flow at low lung volumes, the point at which flow becomes density independent. This point of $V_{iso}\dot{V}$ indicates the equal pressure point. In normal persons the peripheral movement of the equal pressure point occurs at volumes below 25 percent of vital capacity. With obstructive lung disease, the equal pressure point moves peripherally at higher lung volumes, as does their point of $V_{iso}\dot{V}$. Thus $V_{iso}\dot{V}$ is another sensitive measurement of small airways dysfunction.

Maximal Flow–Static Elastic Recoil Curve

The maximal flow–static elastic recoil curve (MFSERC) is determined by plotting maximal flow against static elastic recoil pressure [41]. This is useful in deciding whether $\dot{V}_{max}$ is decreased consequent to the loss of elasticity or from increased airway resistance, a determination that is relevant in treatment if the increased airway resistance is reversible.

Regional Lung Function Tests

Regional defects in the lung are not identified by routine physiologic measurements. Proper evaluation of local function requires the use of regional radiospirometry.

Prior to the introduction of radioactive gases by Knipping et al. [37], the only technique for obtaining unilateral pulmonary data was bronchospirometry, an invasive technique requiring significant technical skill and an obliging patient. The relative advantages and disadvantages of radiospirometery versus bronchospirometry have been reviewed by Miörner [50], whose analysis of cumulative data has established radiospirometry as a diagnostic method by which valid and reproducible measurements of pulmonary function can be made. The noninvasive nature of radioactive xenon analysis makes this method more acceptable to the individual being examined. Dynamic as well as static ventilation-perfusion information can be obtained in a matter of minutes.

Perfusion scanning alone with the use of macroaggregated albumin (MAA) tagged with radioactive material can be used when the evaluation of pulmonary circulation is important.

Perfusion Scanning

Perfusion scanning with macroaggregated albumin has become the standard in the diagnostic approach to pulmonary embolism. Radioactive iodine 131 has been replaced by technetium 99 in perfusion studies. In young patients without any cardiopulmonary disease, a normal chest x-ray, and a history compatible with pulmonary embolism, an abnormal scan is all that is needed to begin treatment. Multiple views (posterior, anterior, and right and left lateral) yield information concerning the regional distribution of blood flow to all of the lung.

It must be remembered that there are no pathognomonic lung scan abnormalities establishing the diagnosis of pulmonary embolus. Any disease causing an abnormality of the pulmonary microcirculation may result in an abnormal perfusion scan. In questionable cases, a simultaneous ventilation scan is of help. If ventilation is maintained to areas where perfusion is absent, this is diagnostic of pulmonary vascular occlusion.

Xenon 133 is the material that is used for ventilation-perfusion scanning. Xenon 133 emits a low-energy gamma ray, and it has a half-life of 5.27 days. When injected intravenously, 90 percent of the gas passes through the alveolar capillary membrane during the first passage (Figure 4-17, A). The patient is instructed to hold his breath for 10 seconds following injection, thus causing the radioactive gas to remain in the alveolar air. Activity is counted during this breathholding, and the perfusion pattern $\dot{Q}$ is determined. Then the patient rebreathes into a closed circuit spirometer for a few minutes to equilibrate the xenon in all lung zones. The count done following this maneuver is proportional to the aerating volume of the various areas in the lung (V). In Figure 4-17, B the patient washes the xenon out of his lung by breathing room air, and then inhales a single breath of ^{133}Xe in oxygen and holds his breath. The count obtained gives regional ventilation $\dot{V}$. Perfusion-volume, ventilation-volume, and ventilation-perfusion ratios [62] can also be expressed. Figure 4-18

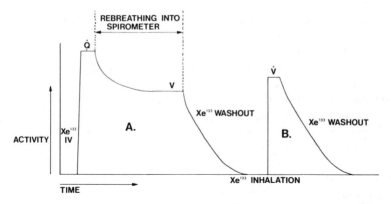

Figure 4–17. Radiospirometry using xenon 133. $\dot{Q}$: blood flow; V: volume; $\dot{V}$: ventilation.

shows the regional variation in ventilation and perfusion from the top to the base of the lung in the upright position. Regional ventilation increases from the apex to the base. Perfusion of blood also shows an increase from the apex to the base, the relative increase in perfusion being more than that of ventilation. At the extreme base of the lung there is some decrease in perfusion.

Measurement of regional lung volume requires adequate rebreathing so that the regional distribution is fairly complete. In extreme degrees of obstruction, regional volume measurements may not be accurate. Simultaneous measurement of regional ventilation, perfusion, and volume, and their interrelationships, can be used to diagnose localized disease. Parenchymal lung disease results in impairment of both ventilation and perfusion along with variations in regional volume. The preoperative use of radiospirometry in carcinoma of the lung to help select candidates capable of

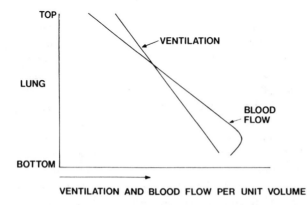

Figure 4–18. Regional gradient of ventilation and perfusion in the upright lung.

tolerating resectional surgery is still not widespread. This technique holds great promise in predicting the postoperative functional state of the lungs.

Evaluation of Respiratory Center and Peripheral Chemoreceptors

The lung has no inherent rhythmicity. A highly complex, sophisticated system based on the central nervous system receiving modulating influences from end organ and blood serve to adjust the respiratory pattern. A coarse respiratory rhythm is sustained as long as the medullary center is intact. The center contains both inspiratory and expiratory portions. This coarse respiratory pattern is modified under the influence of the apneustic and pneumotaxic center, which is located in the pons. The activity of these areas are influenced by the state of inflation of the end organ (lung). Further modification of the respiratory rhythm can result from cortical, reticular activating system (RAS), and hypothalamus activity. The central chemoreceptors are located superficially approximately 1 mm deep on the ventral lateral area of the medulla oblongata. These cells sample the cerebral interstitial fluid and are sensitive to alteration in pH. The peripheral chemoreceptors are located in the carotid and aortic bodies. They are responsible for the hypoxic ventilatory drive. It must be remembered that their response is also influenced by pH. From the preceding, it is clear that manipulation of pH and/or oxygen could be an effective means of determining the integrity of both central and peripheral chemoreceptors (Figure 4-19). Thus, the peripheral chemoreceptors may be assessed by monitoring the ventilatory response to hypoxemia or hyperoxemia. Normally, ventilation decreases when breathing high FI_{O_2} and increases with low FI_{O_2} (12 to 16% oxygen). This ventilatory response is immediate, and only the first breaths are considered in the evaluation. Following the immediate response, changes in PCO_2 may occur and affect the determination.

The central chemoreceptors may be tested by their response to the inhalation of carbon dioxide–enriched gases. When hyperoxic carbon dioxide gas mixtures are used, the influence of the peripheral chemoreceptors is eliminated, and any alteration in ventilation can then be attributed to the central chemoreceptors. When 7% carbon dioxide is used in oxygen, there occurs a rapid equilibration (in less than 1 minute) between the PCO_2 of the blood and of the cerebral interstitial fluid that allows the ventilatory response to be measured in a matter of 5 minutes. The carbon dioxide response curve in normal individuals is quite variable, with a range of response varying from 0.5 to 8 liters/torr change in CO_2 per minute.

In the presence of lung disease, chemoreceptor sensitivity cannot be assessed because abnormalities of respiratory mechanics impair the ventilatory response. An estimate that can be used as a guide states that if the FEV_1 is more than 1 liter, then carbon dioxide retention does not occur because of mechanical impairment of ventilation. So, if a patient has carbon dioxide retention and has FEV_1 greater than 1 liter, respiratory center depression should be considered as a possible reason for the carbon dioxide retention. A simple test that may help in defining the cause of carbon dioxide retention is to ask the patient to hyperventilate and then measure the arterial PCO_2. With severe lung disease, voluntary hyperventilation will not lower PCO_2; however, with primary hypoventilation the PCO_2 drops several torr. It must be remembered that this is nothing more than a gross estimate of chemoreceptor sensitivity, and each case should be judged on its own merits.

In recent years much interest has been focused on respiratory center activity. Among the newer tests are the evaluation of diaphragm electromyography and mouth occlusion pressure (MOP) during the initial 100 msec (0.1 sec) of inspiration (P_{100} or $P_{0.1}$) [20, 42, 66]. Diaphragm electromyography is measured by using a bipolar electrode placed in the esophagus straddling the diaphragm. This activity is a good method of measuring chemosensitivity when there is severe lung disease. The magnitude of diaphragm electromyography varies in normal subjects. However, there is a linear relationship between electrical activity and force of contraction of muscles.

MOP or P_{100} is a method of measuring respiratory drive. It reflects the force generated by the inspiratory muscles during the first 100 msec after the onset of inspiration against a closed airway. This MOP alteration with various stimuli such as hypoxia and hypercapnia has been shown to have a good correlation with diaphragmatic electrical activity and thus is a good index of respiratory efferent activity. The use of MOP as a measure of respiratory center activity requires that pressures be measured at the same lung volume and the same chest configuration [18].

Exercise Testing

Exercise can be used as a measure of cardiopulmonary reserve. Ventilation increases with increasing exercise in order to maintain an adequate oxygen supply to the alveolus to keep up with increased oxygen consumption. Pulmonary gas exchange in a normal person is very efficient during exercise, and Pa_{CO_2} remains reasonably constant during moderate exercise. But as lactic acid accumulates—a result of anaerobic metabolism—ventilation increases further and Pa_{CO_2} decreases. During this stage, more carbon dioxide is produced because of the buffering activity of bicarbonate against lactic acid. This increased carbon dioxide production results in an increase in gas exchange ratio that might exceed the metabolic respiratory quotient. The dead space–tidal volume ratio decreases during exercise, a result of improved $\dot{V}/\dot{Q}$.

To maintain adequate oxygen delivery, cardiac output increases by means of increases of both stroke volume and heart rate. The maximum obtainable heart rate in middle-aged men is around 180 per minute. Along with the increase in cardiac output, both the tissue extraction of oxygen and the arteriovenous oxygen content difference increase. These adaptations permit high oxygen delivery to the exercising muscles. Oxygen consumption may increase up to 3 to 4 liters/min during exercise from a resting level of 250 ml/min. The limiting factor for maximal oxygen delivery in the healthy subject resides in the cardiovascular system, not in the lungs.

Exercise testing may be performed using a variety of methods: (1) the standard step test; (2) walking up one or more flights of stairs; or (3) a more exact approach which quantifies different grades of exercise using either a cycle ergometer or a treadmill. With the cycle ergometer or treadmill, the work rate can be gradually increased until the limit of tolerance is reached. During the test, various measurements such as minute ventilation, oxygen consumption, carbon dioxide production, arterial blood gases, pulse rate, and expiratory flow rate can be measured.

With patients who are symptomatic, or with older individuals, submaximal levels of exercise should be employed. The increase in heart rate and cardiac output is linearly related to oxygen requirement, and nomograms are available to show the relationship between pulse rate and oxygen uptake [1]. Nomograms to predict oxygen consumption during treadmill exercise are also available [66, 67].

Exercise testing can help differentiate cardiac disability from respiratory impairment. With heart disease, the cardiac output is reduced, and the increase in heart rate is excessive. Hence, the ratio of oxygen consumption to heart rate is reduced [63]. In addition, metabolic acidosis because of lactic acid accumulation sets in earlier than normal because of the decrease in oxygen delivery to the tissues. This results in increasing $\dot{V}CO_2$ and increasing gas exchange ratio even with mild to moderate exercise. In a normal person, the lowest work rate at which this occurs is 60 watts.

In occlusive vascular diseases of the pulmonary circulation, the characteristic features with exercise are an increase in minute ventilation and the VD/VT ratio, exertional hypoxemia, increasing AaP oxygen and carbon dioxide gradients, along with a decrease in diffusing capacity. In disorders affecting lung parenchyma, especially obstructive diseases, expiratory flow patterns show the characteristic features of obstruction. Also, for a given heart rate, oxygen consumption is unusually high because of the increased work of the respiratory muscles.

Exercise testing may be valuable in unmasking malingering. A malingerer cannot prevent the normal respiratory and cardiovascular compensations.

Provocative Tests
In those patients with reversible airways disease, provocative tests may be useful to identify both the problem and the etiologic agent responsible for the airways obstruction. This includes inhalation challenge using various allergens or chemical dusts in very small concentrations followed by flow measurements. Another kind of provocation is to induce bronchospasm following exercise. The test results are regarded as positive if the flow decreases by 15 percent.

Inhalation Challenge
The patient inhales a small concentration of the challenging material and the VC, FEV_1, peak expiratory flow rate (PFR), and flow-volume curve measurements are made serially over the next 10 minutes and then followed for the next 24 hours with flow measurements periodically. A positive reaction may be either immediate or nonimmediate. The immediate reaction is maximal within 10 to 30 minutes and subsides by 1 to 1½ hours; the delayed reaction occurs by 3 to 4 hours after the challenge, is maximal around 6 to 7 hours, and lasts for about 24 hours. Some allergens may induce both immediate and nonimmediate reactions.

Exercise Provocation
Postexercise bronchoconstriction is a well-documented phenomenon in some patients with hyperreactive airways. The bronchoconstricting effects of exercise are maximal approximately 15 minutes after the end of the exercise. Hence, VC, FEV_1, PFR, and flow-volume curves should be measured 15 minutes after the exercise. It is of interest that the severity of bronchoconstriction is related to the type of exercise, being more common after running or with treadmill exercise. Patients are exercised on a treadmill for about 8 minutes, enough to raise the heart rate to about 90 percent of the predicted maximum. A reduction of 15 percent in the flow measurements is considered a positive test result. All exercise testing should be done with cardiac monitoring.

Measurement of Blood Gases
The measurement of arterial blood gases is a convenient yet accurate method of assessing the efficiency of the gas exchange function of the lung. Blood gas measurement of venous blood is not of much value because it is dependent on the metabolic needs of various tissues and also on the blood flow to the tissues. Also, samples of blood from various veins show varying results. However, in limited circumstances, a venous sample may be used to determine venous pH, which is 0.03 point lower than arterial pH. For this, the site should be warmed for 15 minutes before sample collection. Also, no tourniquet should be used.

The instrumentation employed in determining Pa_{O_2}, Pa_{CO_2}, and pH is discussed in Chapter 2.

An understanding of the clinical usefulness of blood gases requires a review of the general concepts of how any gas acts when mixed with other gases, when placed in solution, or both. The partial pressure of any gas contained in a mixture of gases is independent of those of the other gases in the mixture. Each gas acts as if it were alone. Expressed in another way, the total pressure exerted by a gas mixture is the sum of partial pressures of the gases that constitute the mixture. For example, in order to calculate the PI_{O_2} (partial pressure of inspired oxygen) at sea level, the barometric pressure must first be measured. The concentration of oxygen in room air is 21 percent, and the PI_{O_2} is expressed in the equation (water vapor pressure is 47 torr at $37°C$)

$$PI_{O_2} = (P_B - 47)\ 0.21.$$

PI_{O_2} is the partial pressure of inspired oxygen, and P_B is the barometric pressure. When the P_B is 760, then the PI_{O_2} is 150 torr.

The partial pressure of alveolar oxygen (PA_{O_2}) is less than the PI_{O_2} because of the addition of carbon dioxide from the blood. In normal subjects the PCO_2 added is around 40 torr, decreasing the alveolar PO_2 to 110 torr. In actuality, however, the PA_{O_2} is not 110 torr but is slightly lower, because the amount of carbon dioxide produced is a little less than the amount of oxygen consumed, i.e., the respiratory quotient (RQ) is 0.8 in normal subjects. A useful formula for estimating PA_{O_2} is

$$PA_{O_2} = PI_{O_2} - \frac{Pa_{CO_2}}{RQ}.$$

The PA_{O_2} of room air is approximately 100 torr. In fact, there are slight regional variations in ventilation-perfusion balance, along with some right-to-left shunting, thus explaining the observation in normal subjects of an alveolar-arterial oxygen tension gradient (AaP_{O_2}). In young individuals, normal Pa_{O_2} is in the 90 range, with an AaP_{O_2} gradient of less than 10 torr, whereas in older persons the Pa_{O_2} decreases and the AaP_{O_2} gradient increases.

Oxygen is carried in two forms, dissolved oxygen and oxygen in combination with hemoglobin. The reader is referred to Chapter 10 for a detailed discussion.

Carbon Dioxide Transport
Carbon dioxide is an end product of cellular metabolism. The majority of carbon dioxide is transported in the plasma in the dissolved form. The remainder is converted into carbonic acid (H_2CO_3) or carried as carbamino compounds. Carbonic acid is formed by the reaction

$$CO_2 + H_2O \rightarrow H_2CO_3$$

H_2CO_3 dissociates into

$$H_2CO_3 \rightleftharpoons H^+ + HCO_3^-$$

This reaction is more rapid in the red blood corpuscles because of the availability of the catalytic enzyme carbonic anhydrase. The free H^+ is buffered by hemoglobin and the HCO_3^- diffuses back into the plasma. In order to maintain electrical neutrality, chloride (Cl^-) enters the red blood corpuscles (the chloride shift). Thus, in the blood, carbon dioxide exists in three forms—dissolved CO_2, H_2CO_3, and carbmino compounds.

The Pa_{CO_2} is directly related to the amount of carbon dioxide produced and is inversely related to the amount of alveolar ventilation. The carbon dioxide dissociation curve is almost linear in the physiologic range. Because of this, the carbon dioxide content and Pa_{CO_2} of the blood reflect the state of ventilation (Fig. 4–19). Hyperventilation decreases the Pa_{CO_2} and hypoventilation increases it. With regional hypoventilation, there is hypercapnia of the blood returning from those areas; but a compensatory hyperventilation of the normal lung units may result in significant hypocapnia in the blood returning from those areas. The overall effect may well be the maintenance of a normal Pa_{CO_2}. Hyperventilation cannot correct the associated hypoxia because of the shape of the oxyhemoglobin dissociation curve,

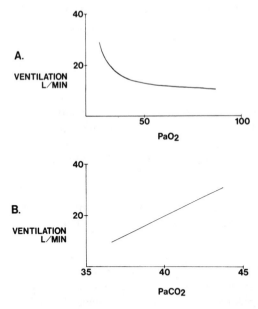

Figure 4-19. Relationship between blood gases and ventilation.

so in the proper clinical setting the combination of hypoxia and normocarbia indicates significant abnormality.

The pH Changes and Acid-Base Regulation

pH is defined as the negative logarithm to the base 10 of the hydrogen ion concentration. It describes the acidity or alkalinity of a substance. An acid is any substance that can donate a hydrogen ion (electron) to a solution. A base is a hydrogen ion (electron) acceptor.

   During the metabolic processes in different tissues, the waste products that are
produced are acid in nature. Theré are two kinds of acids produced: (1) nonvolatile
acids, mainly sulfate and phosphate (50–100 mEq/day); and (2) volatile acids, carbonic acid (20,000–25,000 mM/day). It is necessary that these acids be neutralized
or excreted to maintain normal cell function. Wide swings in cellular pH have an
adverse, indeed potentially lethal cellular effect. A system of body buffers serves to
neutralize some of the acid production, but the major and most efficient system of
rapid acid excretion (carbon dioxide) is by means of the lungs. The Henderson-
Hasselbalch equation relates pH to the bicarbonate-carbonic acid system:

$$pH = pK + \log \frac{HCO_3}{H_2CO_3}.$$

In the above equation, instead of H_2CO_3, PCO_2 can be used:

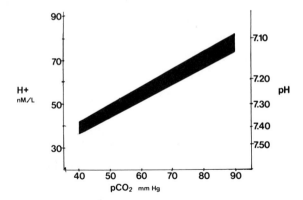

Figure 4-20. Significance bands showing the interrelationship among PCO_2, pH, and H^+ ion concentration for acute hypercapnia. (Reproduced by permission from Brackett, N. C., Jr., Cohen, J. J., and Schwartz, W. B. Carbon dioxide titration curve of normal man. *New England Journal of Medicine* 272, 1965, p. 6. Fig. 5.)

$$pH = pK + log \frac{HCO_3}{PCO_2 \times 0.03} \text{ ,}$$

where 0.03 is the solubility coefficient for carbon dioxide. Thus, pH is directly proportional to bicarbonate and inversely proportional to PCO_2. PCO_2 is regulated by the lungs and can change in minutes, whereas bicarbonate is regulated mainly by the kidney.

A primary disturbance in carbon dioxide excretion defines a respiratory acidosis or alkalosis (Figs. 4–20 and 4–21). A primary disturbance in bicarbonate excretion

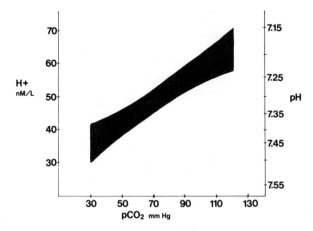

Figure 4-21. Significance bands showing the interrelationship among PCO_2, pH, and H^+ ion concentration for chronic hypercapnia. (Reprinted by permission from Schwartz, W. B., Brackett, N. C., Jr., and Cohen, J. J. The response of extracellular hydrogen ion concentration to graded degrees of chronic hypercapnia: The physiologic limits of the defense of pH. *Journal of Clinical Investigation* 44, 1965, p. 291. Fig. 5.)

defines a metabolic acidosis or alkalosis (Tables 4–1 through 4–4). Tables 4–5 through 4–9 illustrate typical pulmonary function profiles observed in various categories of lung disease — chronic obstructive pulmonary disease, restrictive disease, small airways disease, and hypoventilation and obesity.

Table 4-1. Respiratory Acidosis

Cause	Diagnosis
Insufficient central respiratory drive	
Drug overdose	Reversible with reversal of primary causes
Head injury; infections	
Primary hypoventilation	Poor response to CO_2 inhalation
Obesity with hypoventilation	Poor CO_2 response; obesity
Diseases of the lung	
Severe aireways obstruction from other causes	Increase in lung volumes and decrease in flow rates
Severe airway obstruction from other causes	Decrease in flow rates
Diseases of the chest wall	
Poliomyelitis, infective polyneuritis, myasthenia gravis	History and physical examination clue to diagnosis
Severe kyphoscoliosis	Physical examination clue to diagnosis

Table 4-2. Respiratory Alkalosis

Cause	Diagnosis
Hysterical hyperventilation	Normal function, normal $AaPO_2$ gradient
Hypoxia	
High altitude	History
Infiltrative diseases of the lung	History, physical examination, chest x-ray
Pulmonary edema	History, physical examination, chest x-ray
Adult respiratory distress syndrome	History, physical examination, chest x-ray
Right-to-left shunts	Pa_{O_2} on 100% oxygen and shunt calculation
Head injuries	History, physical examination
Cirrhosis of the liver	History, physical examination
Iatrogenic: mechanical ventilation	History

Table 4-3. Causes of Metabolic Acidosis

Increased Anionic Gap	Normal Anionic Gap
Diabetic ketoacidosis	Interstitial nephritis
Lactic acidosis	Diarrhea
Uremia	Renal tubular acidosis
Intoxications	Proximal — inability to absorb bicarbonate in the proximal lobule
Salicylate	Distal — decreased acid secretion
Ethylene glycol	
Methyl alcohol	Ureterosigmoidostomy

Table 4–4. Causes of Metabolic Alkalosis

Chloride-Responsive Causes	Chloride-Resistant Causes
Gastric suction	Primary hyperaldosteronism
Vomiting	Licorice ingestion
Diuretics	Severe potassium depletion
Villous adenoma of colon	
Base ingestion—antacid or IV bicarbonate	

Table 4–5. Characteristics of Chronic Obstructive Pulmonary Disease

	Chronic Bronchitis	Emphysema	Asthma
TLC	N↑	↑↑	N↑
FRC	↑	↑↑	↑
RV	↑	↑	↑
RV/TLC	↑	↑	↑
ERV	↓	↓	↓
VC	N↓	N↓	N↓
FEV_1	↓	↓	↓
MMF	↓	↓	↓
MBC (MVV)	↓	↓	↓
Bronchodilator response	N	N	↑
DL_{CO}	N	↓	N
C_{st}	N	↑	N
C_{dyn}	↓	↓	↓
R_{aw}	↑	N	↑
P_{max}	N	↓	N
CO_2 response	↓	↓	?↓
$AaPO_2$ gradient	↑	↑	↑
VD/VT	↑	↑	↑
$\dot{V}_{50}$	↓	↓	↓
$\dot{V}_{25}$	↓	↓	↓
CV	↑	↑	↑

Table 4-6. Characteristics of Restrictive Disease

	Parenchymal (Infiltrative)	Chest Wall and Pleura
TLC	↓	↓
FRC	↓	↓
RV	N↓	N↓
RV/TLC	N↑	N↑
ERV	↓	↓
VC	↓	↓
FEV_1	N	N
MMF	N	N
MBC (MVV)	N↓	N↓
DL_{CO}	↓	↓
DL_{CO}/lung volume	↓	N
C_{st}	↓	↓
C_{dyn}	↓ = C_{st}	↓ = C_{st}
R_{aw}	N	N
P_{max}	↑	↓
CO_2 response	N	N
$AaPO_2$ gradient	↑	N
$\dot{Q}s/\dot{Q}T$	↑	N↑
$\dot{V}_{50}$	N	N
$\dot{V}_{25}$	N	N
CV	↑	—

Table 4-7. Characteristics of Small Airways Disease

TLC	N
FRC	N
RV	N↑
RV/TLC	N↑
ERV	N
VC	N
FEV_1	N
MMF	N↓
MBC (MVV)	N
DL_{CO}	N
C_{st}	N
C_{dyn}	↓
R_{aw}	N
P_{max}	N
CO_2 response	N
$AaPO_2$ gradient	↑
$\dot{V}_{50}$	↓
$\dot{V}_{25}$	↓
CV	N↑
$V_{iso}\dot{V}$	↑

Table 4-8. Characteristics of Hypoventilation and Obesity

	Primary Hypoventilators, Nonobese	Obese Hypoventilators	Obese Nonhypoventilators
TLC	N	N↓	N↓
FRC	N	N↓	N↓
RV	N	N↓	N↓
RV/TLC	N	N↑	N↑
ERV	N	↓	↓
VC	N	↓	↓
FEV_1	N	N	N
MMF	N	N	N
MBC (MVV)	N	N↓	N↓
DL_{CO}	N	N	N
C_{st}	N	N↓	N↓
C_{dyn}	N	N↓	N↓
R_{aw}	N	N	N
P_{max}	N	N↓	N↓
CO_2 response	↓	↓	N
$AaPO_2$ gradient	N	↑	↑
CV	—	↑	↑

Table 4-9. Characteristics of Miscellaneous Pulmonary Disorders

	Bronchiectasis	CHF	Pulmonary Emboli
TLC	N↑	↓	N
FRC	N↑	↓	N
RV	↑	N↓	N
RV/TLC	↑	N↑	N
ERV	↓	↓	N
VC	N↓	↓	N↓
FEV_1	↓	N↓	N↓
MMF	↓	N↓	N↓
MBC (MVV)	↓	↓	N
DL_{CO}	N↓	N↓	↓
C_{st}	N↓	↓	N
C_{dyn}	↓	↓	N
R_{aw}	N↑	N↑	N
P_{max}	N	N↑	N
CO_2 response	N↓	N	N
$AaPO_2$ gradient	↑	↑	↑
V_D/V_T	↑	↑	↑
CV	↑	↑	N

REFERENCES

1. Astrand, P. O., and Ryhming, I. A nomogram for calculation of aerobic capacity (physical fitness) from pulse rate during submaximal work. *J. Appl. Physiol.* 7, 1954, p. 218.
2. Barnett, T. B. Effect of helium and oxygen mixtures on pulmonary mechanics during airway constriction. *J. Appl. Physiol.* 22, 1967, p. 707.
3. Bass, H. The flow volume loop—normal standards and abnormalities in chronic obstructive pulmonary disease. *Chest* 63, 1973, p. 171.
4. Bates, D. V., Macklem, P. T., and Christie, R. V. *Respiratory Function in Disease.* Philadelphia: Saunders, 1971.
5. Bedell, G. N., et al. Plethysmographic determination of the gas volume trapped in the lungs. *J. Clin. Invest.* 35, 1956, p. 664.
6. Bentivoglio, L. G., et al. Regional pulmonary function studies with xenon in patients with bronchial asthma. *J. Clin. Invest.* 42, 1963, p. 1193.
7. Brackett, N. C., Jr., Cohen, J. J., and Schwartz, B. Carbon dioxide titration curve of normal man. Effect of increasing degrees of acute hypercapnia on acid-base equilibrium. *N. Engl. J. Med.* 272, 1965, p. 6.
8. Briscoe, W. A., and King, T. K. C. Analysis of disturbance in oxygen transfer in hypoxic lung disease. *Am. J. Med.* 57, 1974, p. 349.
9. Buist, A. S. Early detection of airways obstruction by the closing volume technique. *Chest* 64, 1973, p. 495.
10. Buist, A. S. Current concepts—the single breath nitrogen test. *N. Engl. J. Med.* 293, 1975, p. 438.
11. Buist, A. S., and Ross, B. Predicted values for closing volume using a modified single breath nitrogen test. *Am Rev. Respir. Dis.* 107, 1973, p. 744.
12. Carilli, A., Denson, L. J., Rock, F., and Malabanan, S. The flow volume loop in normal subjects and diffuse lung disease. *Chest* 66, 1974, p. 472.
13. Cherniack, N. S., and Fishman, A. P. Abnormal breathing patterns. *DM,* July, 1975.
14. Colp, C., Reichel, J., and Park, S. S. Severe pleural restriction—the maximum static pulmonary recoil pressure as an aid in diagnosis. *Chest* 67, 1975, p. 658.
15. Comroe, J. H., Jr., et al. *The Lung. Clinical Physiology and Pulmonary Function Tests.* Chicago: Year Book, 1962.
16. Cotes, J. E. *Lung Function—Assessment and Application in Medicine.* Philadelphia: Davis, 1968.
17. Craig, D. B., et al. "Closing volume" and its relationship to gas exchange in seated and supine positions. *J. Appl. Physiol.* 31, 1971, p. 717.
18. Derenne, J. P., et al. Occlusion pressures ($P_{0.1}$) in normal supine man. *Am. Rev. Respir. Dis.* 111, 1975, p. 907.
19. Despas, P. J., Leroux, M., and Macklem, P. T. Site of airway obstruction in asthma as determined by measuring maximal expiratory flow breathing air and a helium oxygen mixture. *J. Clin. Invest.* 51, 1972, p. 3235.
20. Ellis, J. H., Jr., Perera, S. P., and Levin, D. C. A computer program for calculation and interpretation of pulmonary function studies. *Chest* 68, 1975, p. 209.
21. Emmanuel, G., Briscoe, W. A., and Cournand, A. A method for the determination of the volume of air in the lungs: Measurements in chronic pulmonary emphysema. *J. Clin. Invest.* 40, 1961, p. 329.

22. Filley, G. F. *Acid-Base and Blood Gas Regulation*. Philadelphia: Lea & Febiger, 1971.

23. Fowler, W. S.   Breaking point of breathholding. *J. Appl. Physiol.* 6, 1954, p. 539.

24. Fry, D. L., and Hyatt, R. E.   Pulmonary mechanics: A unified analysis of the relationship between pressure, volume and gasflow in the lungs of normal and diseased human subjects. *Am. J. Med.* 29, 1960, p. 672.

25. Godfrey, S., and Campbell, E. J. M. Control of breathholding. *Respir. Physiol.* 5, 1968, p. 385.

26. Hickam, J. B., Blair, E., and Frayser, R.   An open circuit helium method for measuring functional residual capacity and defective intrapulmonary gas exchange. *J. Clin. Invest.* 33, 1954, p. 1277.

27. Holmgren, A., and Linderholm, H. Oxygen and carbon dioxide tensions of the arterial blood during heavy and exhaustive exercise. *Acta Physiol. Scand.* 44, 1958, p. 203.

28. Hucheon, M., et al. Volume of isoflow—a new test in detection of mild abnormalities of lung mechanics. *Am. Rev. Respir. Dis.* 110, 1974, p. 458.

29. Huchinson, J., Esq. On the capacity of the lungs and on the respiratory functions with a view of establishing a precise and easy method of detecting disease by the spirometer. *Med. Chir. Trans.* (London) 29, 1846, p. 137.

30. Hyatt, R. E. The interrelationships of pressure flow and volume during various respiratory maneuvers in normal and emphysematous subjects. *Am. Rev. Respir. Dis.* 83, 1961, p. 676.

31. Hyatt, R. E., and Black, L. F. The flow volume curve. A current perspective. *Am. Rev. Respir. Dis.* 107, 1973, p. 191.

32. Hyatt, R. E., Schilder, D. P., and Fry, D. L. Relationship between maximum expiratory flow and degree of lung inflation. *J. Appl. Physiol.* 13, 1958, p. 331.

33. Jones, N. L. Current concepts: Exercise in pulmonary evaluation. Clinical applications. *N. Engl. J. Med.* 293, 1975, p. 541.

34. Jones, N. L. Current concepts: Exercise in pulmonary evaluation. *N. Engl. J. Med.* 293, 1975, p. 647.

35. King, T. K. C., and Briscoe, W. A.   Bohr integral isopaths in the study of blood gas exchange in the lung. *J. Appl. Physiol.* 22, 1967, p. 659.

36. King, T. K. C., and Briscoe, W. A. Abnormalities of blood gas exchange in COPD. *Postgrad. Med.* 54, 1973, p. 101.

37. Knipping, H. W., et al. Eine neue Methode zur Prufung der Herz- und Lungenfunktion. Die regionale Funktionsanalyse in der Lungen- und Herzklinik mit Hilfe des radioaktiven Edelgases [133]Xenon. *Dtsch. Med. Wochenschr.* 80, 1955, p. 1146.

38. Leblanc, P., Ruff, F., and Milic-Emili, J.   Effect of age and body position on airway closure in man. *J. Appl. Physiol.* 28, 1970, p. 448.

39. Lefcoe, N. M., Carter, R. P., and Ahmed, D. Post exercise bronchoconstriction in normal subjects and asthmatics. *Am. Rev. Respir. Dis.* 104, 1971, p. 562.

40. Lopata, M., Evanich, M. J., and Lourenco, R. V. Relationship between mouth occlusion pressure and diaphragm electromyogram in normal man. *Am. Rev. Respir. Dis.* 111, 1975, p. 908.

41. Macklem, P. T.   Current concepts. Tests of lung mechanics. *N. Engl. J. Med.* 293, 1975, p. 339.

42. Macklem, P. T., Fraser, R. G., and Brown, W. G. Bronchial pressure measurements in emphysema and bronchitis. *J. Clin. Invest.* 44, 1965, p. 897.

43. Macklem, P. T., and Mead, J. Factors determining maximum expiratory flow in dogs. *J. Appl. Physiol.* 25, 1968, p. 159.

44. Macklem, P. T., and Wilson, N. J. Measurement of intrabronchial pressure in man. *J. Appl. Physiol.* 20, 1965, p. 653.

45. McFadden, E. R., Jr., and Linden, D. A. A reduction in maximum midexpiratory flow rate. A spirographic manifestation of small airways disease. *Am. J. Med.* 52, 1972, p. 725.

46. McNeill, R. S., et al. Exercise induced asthma. *Quart. J. Med.* New Series XXXV 137, 1966, p. 5567.

47. Mead, J., et al. Significance of the relationship between lung recoil and maximum expiratory flow. *J. Appl. Physiol.* 22, 1967, p. 95.

48. Miller, R. D., and Hyatt, R. E.   Evaluation of obstructing lesions of the trachea and larynx by flow volume loops. *Am. Rev. Respir. Dis.* 108, 1973, p. 475.

49. Mills, E. Spectrophotometric and fluorometric studies on the mechanism of chemoreception in the carotid body. *Fed. Proc.* 31, 1972, p. 1394.

50. Miörner, G. Xe^{133} radiospirometry. A clinical method for studying regional lung function. *Scand. J. Respir. Dis.* (Suppl) 64, 1968, p. 5.

51. Mitchell, J. A., Sproule, B. J., and Chapman, C. B. Factors influencing respiration during heavy exercise. *J. Clin. Invest.* 37, 1958, p. 1693.

52. Pepys, J. Current concepts: Inhalation challenge in asthma. *N. Engl. J. Med.* 293, 1975, p. 758.

53. Peters, R. M. Coordination of ventilation and perfusion. *Ann. Thorac. Surg.* 6, 1968, p. 570.

54. Pride, N. B., et al. Determinants of maximal expiratory flow from the lungs. *J. Appl. Physiol.* 23, 1967, p. 646.

55. Rebuck, A. S., and Campbell, E. J. M.   A clinical method for assessing the ventilatory response to hypoxia. *Am. Rev. Respir. Dis.* 109, 1974, p. 345.

56. Saroja, D., MacDonnell, F., and Berman, B. Effect of exercise on lung function tests in hay fever. *Ann. Allergy* 34, 1975, p. 286.

57. Schilder, D. P., Roberts, A., and Fry D. L. Effect of gas density and viscosity on the maximal expiratory flow volume relationship. *J. Clin. Invest.* 42, 1963, p. 1705.

58. Schwartz, W. B., Brackett, N. C., Jr., and Cohen, J. J. The response of extracellular hydrogen ion concentration to graded degrees of chronic hypercapnia: The physiological limits of the defence of pH. *J. Clin. Invest.* 44, 1965, p. 291.

59. Serino, T. V., et al. Differential vital capacity determinations with radioactive xenon. *J. Nucl. Med.* 15, 1974, p. 625.

60. Solliday, N. H., et al. The lazy respiratory center—or how to recognize a tired horse. Clinical conference in pulmonary disease. *Chest* 66, 1974, p. 71.

61. Takishima, T., et al. Direct writing recorder of the flow volume curve and its clinical application. *Chest* 61, 1972, p. 262.

62. Trevis, S., Strieder, D. J., and Adelstein, S. J. *Scintillation Camera Radiospirometry in Regional Pulmonary Function in Health and Disease.* Progress in Nuclear Medicine vol 3. Baltimore: University Park Press, 1973.

63. Wasserman, K., and Whipp, B. J. Exercise physiology in health and disease—state of the art. *Am. Rev. Respir. Dis.* 112, 1975, p. 219.

64. Whitelaw, W. A., Derenne, J., and Milic-Emili, J. Occlusion pressure as a measure of respiratory center output in conscious man. *Respir. Physiol.* 23, 1975, p. 181.

65. Woolcock, A. J., Vincent, N. J., and Macklem, P. T. Frequency dependence of compliance as a test for obstruction in small airways. *J. Clin. Invest.* 48, 1969, p. 1097.

66. Workman, J. M., and Armstrong, B. W. Oxygen cost of treadmill walking. *J. Appl. Physiol.* 18, 1963, p. 798.

67. Workman, J. M., and Armstrong, B. W. A nomogram for predicting treadmill walking oxygen consumption. *J. Appl. Physiol.* 19, 1964, p. 150.

Mauricio J. Dulfano
Don E. Davis

Sputum and the Respiratory Therapist

5

The respiratory apparatus is directly exposed to a variety of noxious environmental substances in the course of its normal daily function. Evolutionary adaptation has led to the development of several defense mechanisms that provide adequate protection from most naturally occurring potentially harmful environmental factors. The first and most important line of defense is provided by the mucosal barrier, more specifically, the mucociliary system, which extends from the nasal cavity down to the terminal bronchioles. The constant beating of the respiratory cilia maintains a steady mucous flow upward and out of the lungs in a mechanical cleansing action. The second line of defense consists of wandering alveolar macrophage cells, which provide in situ defense against foreign invaders that managed to penetrate the first line of defense.

That most respiratory therapists are cognizant of the need of clearing or thinning out secretions is evident in their methods of treating airways obstruction phenomena. However, few have learned to associate these therapeutic maneuvers with information that can be provided by appropriate examination of the respiratory secretions [18]. In recent years the respiratory therapist's curriculum has rapidly expanded to incorporate the study of respiratory physiology, blood gas analysis, and principles of intensive care and physiotherapy. Unfortunately, inattention to the subject of sputum analysis has left a great gap in the respiratory therapist's training. Years of experience have convinced us that judicious interpretation of the appearance and composition of respiratory secretions is fundamental to the understanding of respiratory pathology and to the selection of therapeutic intervention.

This chapter is an attempt to bridge this gap by introducing the respiratory therapist to the discipline of sputum analysis.

STRUCTURE OF RESPIRATORY MUCOSA

The respiratory mucosa consists of an epithelial layer, under which there is alveolar connective tissue that binds the epithelium to the next layer, the lamina muscularis mucosae, which contains bundles of smooth muscle fibers. The mucosa is well supplied with blood vessels and capillaries, which extend upward to the epithelial cells on the surface. Pseudostratified columnar epithelium lines the lumen of the larynx as well as that of the trachea and bronchi. It is composed of columnar ciliated and cuboidal basal cells interspersed with mucus-producing goblet cells [21] (Figure 5-1). The surface elements of this epithelium are dramatically visualized by scanning electron microscopy, as portrayed in Figure 5-2. Respiratory secretions are generated by various structures. The goblet cells produce the layer of surface mucus, and the ciliated cells provide the action that propels this layer. The basal cells undergo replication, providing replacements for either of these differentiated cells. Deeper, within the mucosa, we find the bronchial glands, which normally supply the bulk of the respiratory mucus. These glands are under the control of the autonomic nervous system and secrete their contents when activated by vagal stimulation. The respiratory tract mucus is a complex fluid, the physicochemical composition and structure of which are incompletely understood [2].

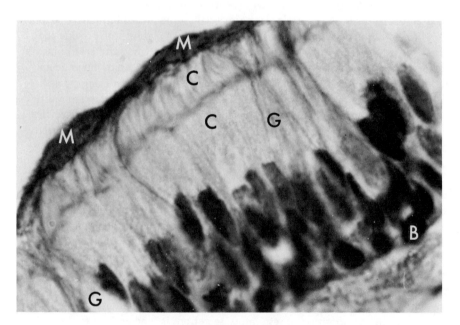

Figure 5-1. Mammalian mucosa. × 1,000, hematoxylin-alcian blue. M: mucous blanket; C: ciliated cell; G: goblet cell emptying into M; B: basal cell.

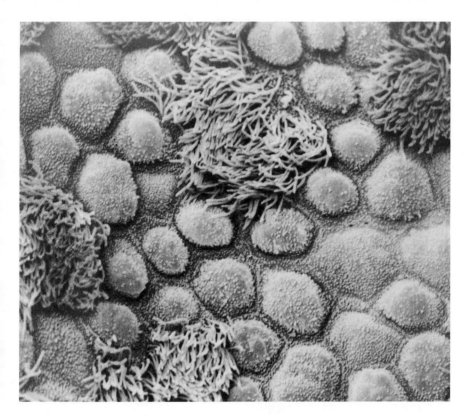

Figure 5–2. Tracheal surface. Scanning electron micrograph, X 2,600. Clusters of cilia interspersed with the nonciliated cells covered with microvilli.

THE MUCOUS BLANKET

After secretion, the mucus spreads itself along the respiratory lumen in a more or less continuous fashion from which the term *mucous blanket* is derived. It is generally believed, although never actually demonstrated, that this mucous blanket is composed of two layers, a stiff, adhesive gel of high tensile strength that rides on top of the cilia, and a more fluid layer (sol) that surrounds the cilia shafts [13] (see Figure 5–1). The mucous gel matrix consists of long glycoprotein chains from which extend short lateral carbohydrate chains crosslinked by disulfide and hydrogen bonds in an aqueous medium (Plate 1, facing page 120). The thickness of the mucous blanket in man has not been determined; however, it is not uniform, and it thins out progressively from the trachea down to the small bronchi, seeming to disappear at the alveolar level.

Propulsion of the mucus depends on the ciliated epithelial cells, which are distributed wherever the mucus is produced. The cilia beat rhythmically, but not in unison, at a rate of approximately 1,000/min. The beating action, called *meta-*

Table 5-1. Respiratory Mucociliary Flow

Accelerated by	Retarded by
Acetylcholine	Dehydration
ATP, AMP	Alcoholism
Catecholamines	Trauma
Potassium iodide	Cold $< 12°$ C
Temperature 28–33° C	Oxygen too high or too low
Negative ions	Bacterial bronchitis
	Viral infections
	Atropine
	Positive ions
	Sulfur dioxide
	Nitrous dioxide

chronal beating, is coordinated in such a manner as to produce a continuous propagation of waves along the tracheobronchial tree [11, 20]. Thus the mucus rides on top of the cilia and never ceases to advance. This mechanical escalator continually transports mucus from bronchioles to the pharynx, where it is automatically swallowed. Thus, under normal conditions, no mucus is ever expectorated. Damage to or loss of cilia, changes in ciliary beating pattern or frequency, changes in the physicochemical characteristics or quantity of the mucus, and injury to respiratory epithelial cells all reduce mucus transport [1]. Other major factors that affect mucus transport can be seen in Table 5-1.

RESPIRATORY TRACT CLEARANCE

Many factors are involved in our defense against invaders of the tracheobronchial tree. The major mechanisms of lung clearance are phagocytosis and mucous transport.

At the alveolar level the epithelial elements are concerned with in situ defense against environmental elements, the primary mechanism being one of phagocytic activity. Thereafter, the ingested particles and intact macrophages are either removed from the alveoli to the nearest bronchiole, where they either follow the regular ciliary escalator pathway or are transported to regional lymph nodes draining the lung. Here they may remain sequestered, or are dissolved and then removed by lymph or blood, or are bound as molecules to cells in the lung or elsewhere. At any rate, macrophages probably process the majority of the particles except some of those that are removed in a few hours. Macrophages, or *histiocytes* as they are also called, will be described below, with the other cellular elements of the sputum.

THE MUCUS

Samples of normal respiratory tract mucus in its pure form are difficult to obtain because of the very nature of the substance and the absence of expectoration in the normal individual. Consequently, we are dependent on the expectorated material, or sputum, for interpretation of the respiratory secretions. Clearly, they are not exactly alike, for the sputum also contains all the accumulated debris resulting from the clearance mechanisms defending the respiratory mucosa [8].

The sputum is a semisolid substance of gelatinous consistency. Its color, translucency, odor, and other characteristics change from patient to patient as well as from expectoration to expectoration. The quantity of sputum produced in a 24-hour period varies greatly and depends on many factors, such as general body hydration and the ratio between expectorated and swallowed mucus.

Evaluation and analysis of the sputum depends on proper collection procedures. Regardless of who performs this task (physicians, or respiratory therapists or other paraprofessional personnel), the following precautions should be taken:

1. The patient must be made aware of the importance of examination of his sputum, and of the need for cooperation in its collection.
2. The patient should be instructed to maintain good oral hygiene to minimize contamination from the mouth.
3. Emphasis should be placed on collecting only that sputum produced by a deep chest cough, disregarding mouth saliva or nasal secretions.
4. A graded, transparent container with lid should be provided.

Whereas expectorated sputum collected under the above conditions should suffice for most bacteriologic or cytologic analyses, other methods should also be considered under special circumstances.

The respiratory therapist is often requested to obtain respiratory tract mucus by passing a sterile catheter into the trachea and aspirating the mucus into a sterile sputum trap. This method does not avoid contamination, because the catheter must pass through the nose or mouth. However, in patients who are unable to cough or in those subjected to endotracheal intubation, this is a practical compromise. Under these conditions, the validity of the specimen as a sample of lower respiratory tract flora is increased if the upper passages are cleared of exudate and if a relatively large amount of fluid is aspirated.

Transtracheal aspiration is an invasive method that should be performed by physicians in patients who are unable to cough productively. A 14-gauge needle with a short bevel is quickly inserted through the cricothyroid membrane and mucus aspirated from the trachea. The advantage to this procedure is that the mucus is not contaminated by flora from the upper respiratory tract or by saliva from the mouth. The main disadvantages of transtracheal aspiration are failure to obtain an adequate specimen through the small bore needle, difficulty with the uncooperative patient, and patient discomfort [19].

For most purposes analysis of sputum should be carried out on freshly expectorated material. If this is not feasible, the collection period is extended to include several forced coughs over a period of 30 to 60 minutes. Within such periods of time there is no need to add preservatives; the bacteriologic content as well as the cell morphology will remain intact within the natural wet environment. If, on the other hand, examination of the sample will be delayed for several hours or more, collection of the specimen into a jar containing 70% alcohol will preserve the material for cytologic examination. However, under no circumstance should bacteriologic cultures be performed on "old sputum" because of the rapid emergence of contaminants. The only common exception is culture for acid-fast bacilli.

The critical steps in the examination of sputum begin with the gross observation of the specimen, preferably in a transparent, flat container. One should look for the solid particles, plugs, or blood flecks that represent the best aliquots. Basically this is a matter of individual experience. In many cases, specimens are sampled by trial and error, and in some laboratories a minimum of two to four selected sputum aliquots are simultaneously prepared on separate slides. If the sputum is to undergo cytologic examination, particularly Papanicolaou staining, it is imperative to avoid drying the thin film of sputum because that will quickly alter the morphology of the cells [17]. Thus, no time should be wasted between the preparation of the smear and the immersion of the slide into a fixative mixture of 95% ethyl alcohol and ether, where it is left for at least 1 hour. In this form the sputum can be preserved almost indefinitely, transported, or otherwise handled until ready for staining.

We have found the traditional clinical gross classification of sputum into mucoid or purulent to be meaningful in terms of some clinical laboratory correlation. In our daily work, expectoration that looks essentially colorless, clear and transparent to light, and usually containing air bubbles, is called *mucoid.* Those of a yellow or green tint, dense and opaque to light, are called *purulent.* Samples displaying characteristics of both groups are classified as *mucopurulent* [8] (Figure 5-3). Each of these groups shows remarkably consistent characteristics. The mucoid expectorations have a much lower cell population density and percentage of neutrophil leukocytes than do the purulent sputums. The percentage of solids by dry weight, the pH, and the viscosity are also lower in the mucoid samples. The elastic recoil is higher in mucoid than in purulent sputum. The distribution of these differences is shown in Table 5-2.

Whereas the above characteristics demonstrate the existence of a clear difference between mucoid and purulent sputum at the macroscopic level as well as at the microscopic level, there are no such clear-cut differences to characterize different respiratory pathologic conditions producing sputum similar in macroscopic appearance (Table 5-3).

We have learned that a careful appraisal of the expectoration at bedside can be very useful in the management of patients even before detailed quantitative analytical observations of sputum are made. This information is routinely provided by the respiratory therapist working in our respiratory care center.

Several methods for observation and identification of the cells in sputum are available. The time-honored examination of unstained specimens is still widely in use. Although with it the definition of the cells is not precise, this method offers the advantages of simplicity, of simultaneous visualization of noncellular structures, and of rapid identification of the general source of the sputum, namely, whether it originates in the lower respiratory tract or is highly contaminated by saliva, or both. The simplest unfixed wet preparation is best examined with the addition of aqueous-

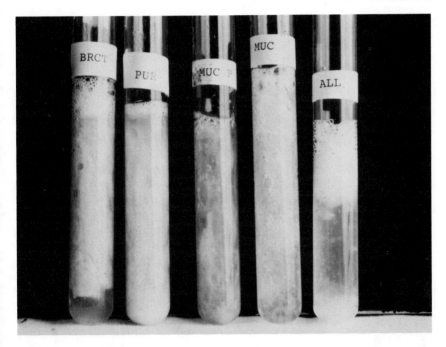

Figure 5-3. Sputum, gross appearance. BRCT: bronchiectasis; PUR: purulent; MUCP: muco-purulent; MUC: mucoid; ALL: allergic.

buffered crystal violet [5]. An amount of stain equal to the volume of the sputum aliquot is added to the slide, and the two are gently mixed before the coverslip is replaced on top of the specimen. The presence of large histiocytes (macrophages) and of ciliated epithelial cells confirms the lower tracheobronchial tree origin of the sputum specimen.

For more refined cytologic observations, the classic Papanicolaou stain is still the best available method and should be used for final diagnosis [17]. Some laboratories are interested not only in the differential counts but also in the quantities of each and of all cell types [5]. For that purpose, it is necessary to obtain 24-hour collections of sputum. However, this method may introduce very significant errors, and it is not recommended.

CELLS FOUND IN MUCUS
The cells found in respiratory tract mucus comprise those derived from the reticulo-endothelial system that appear in response to specific stimuli, and the cells sloughed off from the tracheobronchial tree. Together they reflect the degree and type of inflammation of the respiratory mucosa and help in the differential diagnosis of bronchial diseases [15].

Bronchial epithelial cells originate in various bronchial epithelial layers from the basal to the superficial columnar layers. Although the nuclei of the epithelial cells

Table 5-2. Comparative Characteristics of Mucoid and Purulent Sputum

Gross Appearance	Cells per Low-Power Field	Differential Cytology	Dry Weight (%)	pH	Viscosity	Elastic Recoil at 100 dynes/cm^2
Mucoid	Occupies 1/2 or less	PMN <60%	Between 2 and 5%	Avg, 7.59	Low (large range)	High (avg, 6.98)
Purulent	Occupies 2/3 or more	PMN >70%	Between 6 and 10%	Avg, 7.83	High (large range)	Low (avg, 4.41)

Table 5-3. Physical Properties of Sputum in Stable Bronchial Diseases

Property	"Normal"	Chronic Bronchitis	Bronchial Asthma
Color	Colorless	Usually yellow or greenish	Colorless
Odor	Nonodorous	Varies according to the kind of infection	Usually nonodorous
pH	7.45 to 8.15	6.3 to 7.9	5.4 to 7.6
Viscosity, at 1 sec^{-1} shear rate		<400 poises	<400
Elastic recoil, at 100 dynes/cm^2		4–8 S$_R$ units	4–8 S$_R$ units

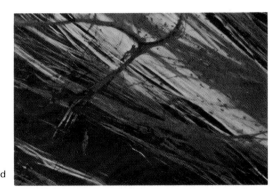

Plate 1 Mucous matrix composed of glycoprotein bundles. ✕ 1,000, toluidine blue observed under polarized microscopy.

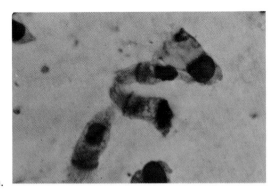

Plate 2 Ciliated bronchial epithelial cells in sputum. ✕ 1,000, Papanicolaou.

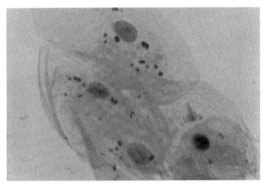

Plate 3 Sputum from upper respiratory tract showing large squamous epithelial cell and bacteria. ✕ 1,000. Papanicolaou.

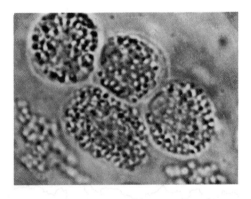

Plate 4 Unfixed, wet sputum smear showing eosinophils with prominent and refractile cytoplasmic granulations obscuring the nuclei. ✕ 1,000.

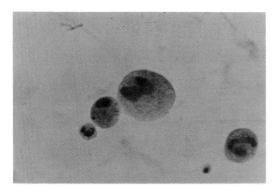

Plate 5   Sputum from lower respiratory tract showing large macrophages with eccentric nuclei and polymorphonuclear neutrophils (below and to right). X 400, Papanicolaou.

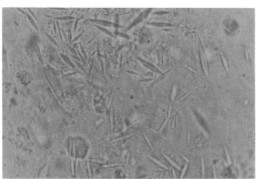

Plate 6   Charcot-Leyden crystals. Unfixed, wet sputum. X 400.

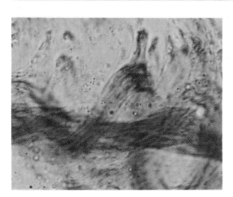

Plate 7   Curschmann's spirals in sputum. X 1,000, Papanicolaou.

remain the same, their cytoplasmic morphology differs. Typical ciliated bronchial epithelial cells are shown in Plate 2 (facing page 120). Bronchial epithelial cells of the nonciliated variety most commonly belong to the goblet type. It should be remembered that bronchial epithelial cells of all varieties are clearly different from the squamous epithelial cells characteristic of the upper respiratory tract epithelium (Plate 3, facing page 120). The presence of squamous epithelial cells in the smear should alert the observer to the fact that the sputum sample did not originate in the lower respiratory tract.

The most abundant cells in sputum are those derived from the reticuloendothelial system. Among them, the most representative from a functional standpoint are the polymorphonuclear leukocytes, or neutrophils; the eosinophils; and the histiocytes or macrophages. Knowing their respective counts is of considerable help in interpreting the nature and the evolutionary stage of various bronchial inflammations.

Eosinophils, which have been described as cells of beauty and mystery, are found in sputum in small numbers (Plate 4, facing page 120). From their appearance and conglomeration in tissues exposed to the environment, it is apparent that the eosinophilic leukocyte is involved in the host's defense. Although eosinophils can be observed in many inflammatory diseases of the respiratory tract, a marked increase is most commonly associated with bronchial asthma [9].

Mast cells are difficult to identify in sputum, and their significance seems to parallel that of the eosinophils. This is supported by their similar distribution in tissue exposed to the environment and subjected to immunologic exchanges.

Polymorphonuclear leukocytes are the most abundant of these cells and represent the most common indicator of the extent or acuteness of bronchial inflammation. As discussed above, these types of cells clearly differentiate purulent from mucoid sputum. They usually appear as multilobulated, contain fine granules, and may phagocytize small particles. Their morphology is compared to that of the histiocyte in Plate 5 (facing page 121). Their obvious function is to ingest and destroy bacteria in parallel or in conjunction with the histiocyte.

Histiocytes or macrophages, the large cells found in sputum, are principally responsible for in situ defense against microorganisms or particulate material breathed in (see Plate 5). In general terms, a large number of histiocytes in sputum is usually associated with adequate cellular defenses, and therefore these cells are more numerous after acute infections have been overcome. The absence or a low level of these scavengers is usually indicative of the beginning of an acute exacerbation of disease or of failure to respond adequately to invasion of the respiratory tract.

Noncellular elements sometimes found in sputum are Charcot-Leyden crystals and Curschmann's spirals, which are usually associated with bronchial asthma. Charcot-Leyden crystals seem to originate from the disintegration of eosinophils, basophils, or mast cells. Readily detected in wet, unfixed preparations (Plate 6, facing page 121), they may also appear in the sputum of chronic bronchitic and asthmatic patients, as well as in that of those afflicted with other inflammatory respiratory

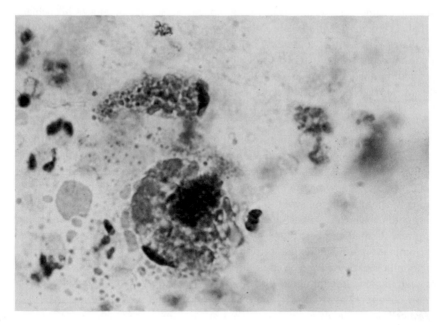

Figure 5–4. Sputum lipid-soluble material ingested by the macrophages and also free. X 400, Sudan IV.

conditions, but they are always found in association with increased eosinophilia [9].

Curschmann' spirals (Plate 7, facing page 121) are usually associated with the presence of eosinophils and Charcot-Leyden crystals. Appearing as twisted spirals of mucinous material around a central thread, they are composed of proteins, cells, crystals, and other debris. The spirals seem to originate in the smaller bronchioles because of inspissated secretions [9].

One of the most common respiratory problems in the chronically ill elderly patient is food aspiration. This diagnosis is commonly missed or made very late. Simple examination of the sputum for the presence of foodstuffs will clarify this point. However, precautions should be taken to avoid contamination by mouth contents prior to collecting the sputum sample.

Lipid-laden macrophages in the sputum are an indication that fat substances have been aspirated deep into the tracheobronchial tree and have caused an acute or chronic pneumonia. The identification of lipid-laden macrophages in the sputum is based on the staining with lipid-soluble dyes (Sudan III or IV) and lipid extraction with fat solvents. The nuclei of macrophage cells stain blue with Nile blue, and the cytoplasmic lipids are stained red (Figure 5–4). Neutral fats stain bright orange to red with Sudan dyes but show no birefringency. Fatty acids can be demonstrated by polarized microscopy because fatty acids are birefringent. Thus cholesterol crystals can be recognized by their characteristic Maltese cross appearance [10].

The aspiration of foreign bodies and particulate matter can create a variety of pathologic alterations, such as atelectasis and lung abscesses.

Because beans are frequently part of the average diet, the diagnosis of aspiration can also be made by demonstrating particles of this vegetable in the sputum. Beans can be readily identified by gross and microscopic examination. Although their structure under the microscope is distinctive, the simplest way to identify them is by exposing the sputum to iodine. If starch is present, the amylose component stains blue and the amylopectin, reddish (Figure 5-5).

PHARMACOTHERAPY OF PHYSICAL PROPERTIES OF SPUTUM

Terms such as *expectorant, mucolytic,* or *bronchomucotropic* are confusing to respiratory therapists and most other medical personnel. Unfortunately, this confusion is compounded by inappropriate usage and inaccurate claims on the labels of some medical products. The following definitions were offered by Boyd, and it may be useful to restate them here [3].

Expectorant

Expectorant is a term derived from the Latin that means "out of the chest." The word appears to date back to the sixteenth century. Michael Servetus, for example, reported in 1546 on the use of syrup of horehound for what may be translated to mean "purging through the sputum." The word has been used to refer to a drug that increases the amount of sputum or that increases the output of bronchial or tracheobronchial secretions. In 1954 Boyd defined an expectorant in pharmacologic terms as a drug that augments the volume output of demulcent respiratory tract fluid in therapeutic doses [3]. The term *expectorant,* therefore, has many connotations.

Respiratory Tract Fluid Augmenting Agents

The definition of this term is basically the same as that given by Boyd for *expectorant* in 1954 [3]. It refers to a measurable pharmacologic action and is more specific than the old term expectorant. *Bronchomucotropic* has the same meaning because respiratory tract fluid contains an abundance of mucins. Bronchomucotropic agents may be classified as: (1) systemic agents, which augment the output of respiratory tract fluid when given orally or by parenteral injection, or (2) inhaled agents, which augment the output of respiratory tract fluid following inhalation [4].

Antibronchomucotropic Agents

These are agents that inhibit the production of respiratory tract fluid. It should be emphasized that these are terms subject to pharmacologic demonstration in laboratory animals. Clinical pharmacologic trials in man have been confined mainly to measuring the effect of drugs on cough or volume of sputum. A bronchomucotropic agent can obtund coughing only if coughing is due to a decreased production of respiratory tract fluid.

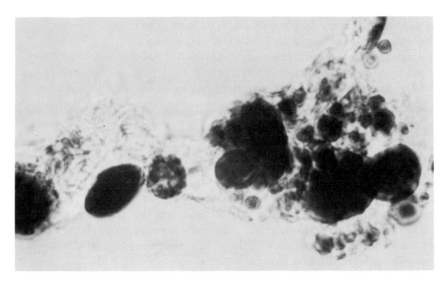

Figure 5–5. Sputum containing bean residues. X 1,000, iodine.

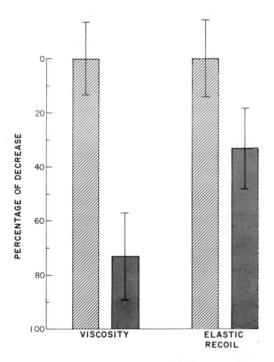

Figure 5–6. Changes in viscoelastic properties of sputum exposed in vitro to acetylcysteine. Effect of Mucomyst on sputum flow properties (average for 18 patients).

Mucolytic Agents

Mucolytic agents should act specifically on the mucin's glycoprotein and cause their depolymerization. Theoretically this effect can be obtained in several ways, i.e., by attacking disulfide bonds (acetylcysteine), by acting as or stimulating protease activity (deoxyribonuclease, trypsin, iodine), or by other, not yet defined mechanisms. In the case of agents such as guaifenesin, Alevaire, and certain detergents, there is no adequate substantiation of a true mucolytic action (Table 5-4).

The claimed beneficial effects of mucolytic agents are based on clinical trials. In the cases where validation of effects by rheologic tests (measurement of viscoelastic properties of sputum) were undertaken, the results are extremely difficult to appraise because of the very different methodologic procedures. Although many drugs seem to have some mucolytic effect in vitro, it is very difficult to prove a true effect in patients under controlled conditions. Therefore, one should temper fleeting clinical enthusiasm until we have a standard methodology for appraisal. The conditions of the clinical evaluation should be standardized in terms of hydration, temperature, humidity, and medication to which the patient is subjected. Changes in the volume of expectoration should be assessed separately from specific rheologic effects. Pulmonary function tests and other fashionable procedures are no substitutes for proper rheologic measurements in assessing the effects of a drug on the physicochemical character of mucus. An example of a clear-cut pharmacologic effect in vitro could be seen in our studies with N-acetyl-L-cysteine (Figure 5-6). Under controlled conditions, this drug proved to have an effect when exposed directly to the sputum.

Water as a Mucolytic Agent

The therapeutic effects of superhydration by means of increased water intake by mouth or by local bronchial humidification are highly controversial. Since time immemorial the therapeutic merits of humidification have not been challenged. However, proof for such a contention is still lacking, particularly in regard to the aerosol route, as demonstrated by the widespread discussion in the literature [12, 14, 16, 22]. The controversy is generated for several reasons: (1) methodologic differences in the rheologic measurements, (2) the substitution of clinical or physiologic parameters for rheologic measurements, and (3) the lack of uniformity in ensuring similar degrees of underlying hydration and ambient humidity. In a controlled evaluation of the aerosol route it would also be necessary to indicate the type of water generator, its output and particle size, the amount actually delivered to the lower respiratory tract, exposure time, environmental temperature, and relative humidity. Such a study in patients represents a formidable task and has not yet been undertaken.

In vitro studies of the rheologic effects of water on sputum are of some help in understanding these effects. If water is mixed with sputum, a predictable decrease in viscosity is obtained [12]. However, other evidence shows that sputum exposed for 24 hours to 100% relative humidity at 37°C does not seem to incorporate water when judged by weight changes [6].

Table 5-4. Agents Affecting Physical Properties of Mucus

Agent	Constituents	Site of Action	Mechanism
Water		Mucus	Dilution
Normal saline solution	0.9% NaCl	Mucus	Dilution
Sodium bicarbonate	2.5–5%	Surface of mucus	Alkalosis
Mucomyst	N-acetyl-L-cysteine	Disulfide bonds	Decreases viscosity
Dornavac	Deoxyribonuclease	Protein moiety	Proteinase
Tryptar	Trypsin	Protein moiety	Proteinase
Iodine	Saturated solution of potassium iodide	Respiratory mucosal glands	Stimulation of secretion
Robitussin	Guaifenesin	Respiratory mucosal glands	Stimulation of secretion

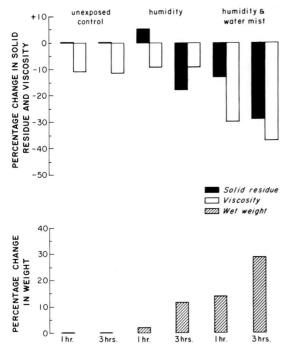

Figure 5-7. The difference between exposure of sputum to 100% humidity versus that of exposure to 100% humidity plus water mist. The difference in effect is clearly seen in terms of dilution and viscosity changes.

Recent work in our laboratory has shed some light on this subject. Freshly expectorated samples of sputum were exposed for definite periods of time to an environment of 100% relative humidity at 70°F. In addition, other aliquots in the same environment were also exposed to directly nebulized water mist. Under these conditions the amount of water incorporated and the rheologic changes could be assessed both for humidity alone and for humidity plus water mist (Figure 5-7). The results indicate that sputum incorporates water more slowly and in lesser quantity from plain humidity than from water mist. It also showed that exposure to humidity alone does not decrease the viscosity of sputum, whereas significant mucolytic effects are seen when water mist is added to humidity [7]. Of course, from the respiratory therapist's point of view, the real question remaining is whether enough water can be made to be deposited in the lower respiratory tract to obtain a similar effect in actual practice.

REFERENCES

1. Asmundsson, T., and Kilburn, K. H. Mechanisms of Respiratory Tract Clearance. In Dulfano, M. J. (ed.). *Sputum, Fundamentals and Clinical Pathology.* Springfield, Ill.: Thomas, 1973.
2. Boat, T. F., and Matthews, L. W. Chemical Composition of Human Tracheo-

bronchial Secretions. In Dulfano, M. J. (ed.). *Sputum, Fundamentals and Clinical Pathology.* Springfield, Ill.: Thomas, 1973.

3. Boyd, E. M. Expectorants and respiratory tract fluid. *Pharmacol. Rev.* 6, 1954, p. 521.

4. Boyd, E. M. Pharmacological Agents and Respiratory Tract Fluid. In Dulfano, M. J. (ed.). *Sputum, Fundamentals and Clinical Pathology.* Springfield, Ill.: Thomas, 1973.

5. Chodosh, S. Examination of sputum cells. *N. Engl. J. Med.* 282, 1970, p. 854.

6. Cragg, J., and Smith, S. G. Some properties of respiratory tract mucus. *Arch. Intern. Med.* 107, 1961, p. 81.

7. Dulfano, M. J., Adler, K., and Wooten, O. Physical properties of sputum. IV. Effects of 100 percent humidity and water mist. *Am. Rev. Respir. Dis.* 107, 1973, p. 130.

8. Dulfano, M. J., and Philippoff, W. Physical Properties. In Dulfano, M. J. (ed.). *Sputum, Fundamentals and Clinical Pathology.* Springfield, Ill.: Thomas, 1973.

9. Dulfano, M. J., and Rodriguez, A., Respiratory Secretion in Bronchial Asthma. In Weiss, E. G., and Segal, M. S. (eds.). *Bronchial Asthma: Mechanisms and Therapeutics.* Boston: Little, Brown, 1976.

10. Jiminez, F. A. Special Examinations of Sputum. In Dulfano, M. J. (ed.). *Sputum, Fundamentals and Clinical Pathology.* Springfield, Ill.: Thomas, 1973.

11. Kilburn, K. H., and Asmundsson, T. Anatomy of the Mucociliary Apparatus. In Dulfano, M. J. (ed.). *Sputum, Fundamentals and Clinical Pathology.* Springfield, Ill.: Thomas, 1973.

12. Lifshitz, M. I., and Denning, C. R. Quantitative interaction of water and cystic fibrosis. *Am. Rev. Respir. Dis.* 102, 1970, p. 456.

13. Lucas, A. M., and Douglas, L. C. Principles underlying ciliary activity in the respiratory tract. II. A comparison of nasal clearance in man, monkey and other mammals. *Arch. Otolaryngol.* 20, 1934, p. 518.

14. Matthews, L. W., and Dsershuk, C. F. Mist tent therapy in the obstructive pulmonary lesion of cystic fibrosis. *Pediatrics* 39, 1967, p. 176.

15. Midici, T. C., and Chodosh, S. Nonmalignant exfoliative sputum cytology. In Dulfano, M. J. (ed.). *Sputum, Fundamentals and Clinical Pathology.* Springfield, Ill.: Thomas, 1973.

16. Palmer, K. N. V. Reduction of sputum viscosity by a water aerosol in chronic bronchitis. *Lancet,* 1, 1960, p. 91.

17. Papanicolaou, G. N. *Atlas of Exfoliative Cytology.* Cambridge, Mass.: Harvard University Press, 1954.

18. Rodman, T., and Sterling, F. H. *Pulmonary Emphysema and Related Lung Diseases.* St. Louis: Mosby, 1969.

19. Seligman, S. J. Bacteriology. In Dulfano, M. J. (ed.). *Sputum, Fundamentals and Clinical Pathology.* Springfield, Ill.: Thomas, 1973.

20. Sleigh, M. A. Some aspects of the comparative physiology of cilia. *Am. Rev. Respir. Dis. (Suppl.)* 93, 1966, p. 16.

21. Tuttle, W. W., and Schottelius, B. A. *Textbook of Physiology.* St. Louis: Mosby, 1969.

22. Wolfsdorf, J., Swift, D. L., and Avery, M. E. Mist therapy reconsidered, an evaluation of labelled water aerosols produced by jet and ultrasonic nebulizers. *Pediatrics,* 43, 1969, p. 799.

Kenneth F. MacDonnell
Doraswamy Saroja Moorthi

Bronchoscopy

6

The technique of bronchoscopy has been employed as a diagnostic tool for many years, and the introduction of the flexible fiberoptic instrument has greatly enhanced the value of this procedure. At present, two kinds of bronchoscopes are in general use: rigid and flexible (Table 6-1). The relative merit of each will be discussed.

RIGID BRONCHOSCOPY

The rigid bronchoscope is a hollow metallic tube that has been used for many years to examine the tracheobronchial tree. Rigid bronchoscopy may be performed with either general or topical anesthesia. Visualization of the lower-lobe segmental bronchi is quite adequate, but upper lobe segments are not well visualized. Rigid bronchoscopy is mainly indicated for diagnostic purposes in children and for the removal of foreign bodies. In situations of massive hemoptysis the rigid bronchoscope allows for more adequate suctioning, thus better visualization and identification of a bleeding site. Apart from these special circumstances, flexible fiberoptic bronchoscopy is the method of choice whenever endoscopic examination of the bronchial tree is undertaken.

FLEXIBLE FIBEROPTIC BRONCHOSCOPY

Fiberoptic bronchoscopy examination offers the unique capability of direct and prolonged viewing of the tracheobronchial tree along with observation of the tracheobronchial tree in a dynamic state. Sackner and associates [4, 5] have utilized

Table 6-1. Clinical Applications of Bronchoscopy

Fiberoptic Bronchoscope	Rigid Bronchoscope

Laryngeal obstructions
  Edema
  Ulceration
  Tumors
	Foreign body removal
	Massive hemoptysis
	Evaluation of lung lesion in children

Tracheal examination
  During and after intubation
  Tracheomalacia
  Tracheostenosis	

Persistent lung lesions
  Tumors
  Coin lesions ⎫ For biopsy, brushings,
  Diffuse lesions ⎭ washings	

Hemoptysis	
Bacteriology of lower respiratory tract, especially unusual organisms	
Tracheobronchial toilet and segmental lavage	
Selective bronchography	
Aid to endotracheal intubation	
Pleural lesions (thoracoscopy)	

Research purposes
  Tracheal mucous velocity
  Tracheobronchial dynamics	

this capability to study tracheal mucous velocity in dogs and the effects of various stimuli, such as oxygen, on mucous flow. Also, the optics of this instrument are of a quality that allow motion pictures and fine still photographs to be taken. This may be of particular interest in patients with tracheomalacia, tracheal stenosis, or emphysema. These observations may then be recorded, analyzed, and stored. Advantages of the fiberoptic bronchoscope over the rigid variety are (1) ease with which the instrument can be introduced—no intubation, (2) better patient tolerance, and (3) better visualization of all segments and subsegments of the bronchial tree— views are magnified and very sharp.

All fiberoptic materials have a core and a cladding. When glass is melted by heat and rapidly pulled apart, the melted portion forms long silklike threads with well-defined optic properties. *Cladding* is the process of coating bundles of fibers externally with a glass of lower refractive index. Then the fibers are tightly fixed at both ends. When light passes through these bundles it shifts direction when it crosses the interface between two media of different densities. Thus optic fibers repeatedly redirect light (Figure 6-1). The bronchoscope has two fiberoptic bundles, a light-carrying bundle and an image-carrying bundle. The light-carrying bundle consists of many fibers arranged at random. The image-carrying bundle has fibers aligned so that a sharp image is produced. A lens is present at both ends of

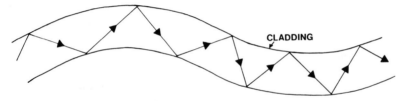

Figure 6-1. Movement of light through an optic fiber.

the image-carrying bundle. There are several models of fiberscope available, such as Olympus, Machida, or ACMI (Figure 6-2).

TECHNIQUE OF FIBEROPTIC BRONCHOSCOPY

The patient is given nothing by mouth for 3 to 4 hours prior to the procedure. Usually premedication, including atropine and a narcotic, is given approximately 30 minutes before bronchoscopy. Many physicians give intravenous diazepam (Valium) immediately before the procedure to reduce patient anxiety. Although fiberoptic bronchoscopy can be done at the bedside, the procedure is better yet performed in a special room provided with a comfortable adjustable chair, adequate suctioning equipment, and proper lighting. If a fluoroscope is available, better localizing of brushing can be accomplished.

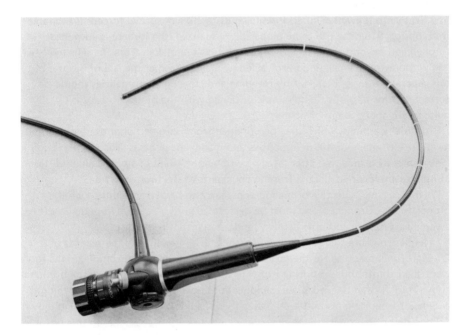

Figure 6-2. Olympus model bronchoscope.

The patient usually sits comfortably in a chair, and the operator stands in front of the patient. In subjects who are not able to sit, this procedure is performed with the patient supine. Topical anesthesia is first applied to the nasopharynx, which is sprayed with 1 percent lidocaine (Xylocaine), using a hand bulb nebulizer. The bronchoscope may be introduced nasally or orally, most operators preferring the nasal route. For oral introduction, prior intubation with an endotracheal tube is required. This may be done with the use of a standard or flexible endotracheal tube, which may be inserted with the bronchoscope and left in position throughout the entire procedure, allowing for multiple insertions of the bronchoscope. Also, in a patient with marginal lung function, assisted ventilation will be easier if required when there is an endotracheal tube in place. For anesthetizing the vocal cords many operators use a 4% soluton of Xylocaine. Once the bronchoscope is introduced into the trachea, either through the endotracheal tube or alone, Xylocaine is used as needed by direct injection through the bronchoscope's aspiration channel. Usually we use about 150 to 200 mg of Xylocaine throughout the entire procedure. All parts of the bronchial tree should be visualized systematically on both sides.

In severely ill patients who are being mechanically ventilated through an endotracheal tube or tracheostomy, fiberoptic bronchoscopic examination can be done with the use of special T adaptors so as to maintain an airtight seal during the procedure.

Through the bronchoscope bronchial brushing, biopsies, and washings can be performed. Slide preparations for cytologic examination require immediate immersion in a fixative to prevent cellular drying and distortion. A special forceps is available for biopsies. After the site to be biopsied is visualized, the forceps is advanced through and beyond the bronchoscope. A bite is then taken from the selected site and withdrawn. A small amount of bleeding may be seen at the site of biopsy, but this generally is insignificant. Any bleeding and clotting abnormalities should be corrected prior to biopsy. The sample obtained with the biopsy forceps is usually quite small, about 2 mm of tissue.

Bronchial washings, which may be obtained from a segmental or a subsegmental level, are extremely useful in infectious and malignant diseases. The sample is collected into a Luken's trap after lavaging with about 10 ml of sterile saline solution. Multiple samples are collected from various parts of the bronchial tree.

When indicated, selective bronchography can also be performed through the bronchoscope. Bronchoscopy must be performed with great care in patients with severe heart disease, extreme debility, and intercurrent acute disease.

In a questionnaire survey Credle and associates [1] examined the records of 24,521 bronchoscopies for the incidence of complications. The complications found were divided into those resulting from anesthesia, and those related to the bronchoscopy. They further divided these complications into minor (not life-threatening) and major (requiring resuscitation) categories (Tables 6-2 and 6-3; also Figure 6-3).

The fiberoptic bronchoscope may also be used as a thoracoscope. In this procedure the bronchoscope is inserted through a chest tube for a visual evaluation of the pleural space.

Table 6-2. Complications Related to Premedication or Anesthetic Agent

Type of Complication	Minor (number)	Major (number)	Mortality (number)
Adverse reaction to premedication			
Respiratory depression	1	4	
Transient hypotension	5		
Syncope	2		
Hyperexcitable state	1		
Adverse reaction to local anesthetic			
Respiratory arrest		3	
Seizures		3	
Methemoglobinemia		1	
Cardiovascular collapse			1
Laryngospasm	1		
Other	2		

Note: Numbers are total numbers of incidences from a grand total of 24,521.
Source: Reproduced with permission from Credle, W. F., Jr., Smiddy, J. F., and Elliott, R. C. Complications of fiberoptic bronchoscopy. *American Review of Respiratory Disease* 109, 1974, p. 68. Table 2.

Table 6-3. Complications Related to the Bronchoscopic Procedure

Type of Complication	Minor (number)	Major (number)	Mortality (number)
Laryngospasm	31		
Bronchospasm	4	2	
Respiratory compromise	4	4	1
Syncope		1	
Cardiac arrest			1
Bradycardia		1	
Premature contractions	8		
Ventricular tachycardia		1	
Postprocedure fever	8		
Pneumonia		2	
Epistaxis	12		

Note: Numbers refer to numbers of incidences from a grand total of 24,521.
Source: Reproduced with permission from Credle, W. F., Jr., Smiddy, J. F., and Elliott, R. C. Complications of fiberoptic bronchoscopy. *American Review of Respiratory Disease* 109, 1974, p. 69. Table 3.

The patient with hypoxia should receive supplemental nasal oxygen during and after the procedure, the FI_{O_2} being titrated according to the patient's blood gases. Careful cardiac monitoring is also required.

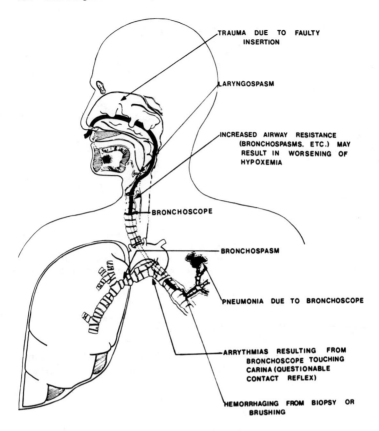

TRAUMA DUE TO FAULTY
INSERTION

LARYNGOSPASM

INCREASED AIRWAY RESISTANCE
(BRONCHOSPASMS. ETC.) MAY
RESULT IN WORSENING OF
HYPOXEMIA

BRONCHOSCOPE

BRONCHOSPASM

PNEUMONIA DUE TO BRONCHOSCOPE

ARRYTHMIAS RESULTING FROM
BRONCHOSCOPE TOUCHING
CARINA (QUESTIONABLE
CONTACT REFLEX)

HEMORRHAGING FROM BIOPSY OR
BRUSHING

Figure 6–3. Complications after fiberoptic bronchoscopy.

REFERENCES

1. Credle, W. F., Jr., Smiddy, J. F., and Elliot, R. C. Complications of fiberoptic bronchoscopy. *Am. Rev. Respir. Dis.* 109, 1974, p. 67.
2. Ikeda, S. *Atlas of Flexible Bronchofiberscopy.* Baltimore: University Park Press, 1974.
3. Levin, D. C., Wicks, A. B., and Ellis, J. H., Jr. Transbronchial lung biopsy via the fiberoptic bronchoscope. *Am. Rev. Respir. Dis.* 110, 1974, p. 4.
4. Sackner, M. A. Bronchofiberscopy — state of the art. *Am. Rev. Respir. Dis.* 111, 1975, p. 62.
5. Sackner, M. A., Warner, A., and Landa, J. Applications of bronchofiberscopy. *Chest* 62, 1972, p. 70S.
6. Senno, A., et al. Thoracoscopy with the fiberoptic bronchoscope. A simple method in diagnosing pleuropulmonary disease. *J. Thorac. Cardiovasc. Surg.* 67, 1974, p. 606.

Clinical Topics

3

Bernard D. Kosowsky

Hemodynamic Aspects of Respiratory Care

7

CARDIOLOGIC ASPECTS OF RESPIRATORY CARE

The lungs and heart form a closely integrated system for providing oxygenated blood to the general circulation. The lungs, situated functionally between the right and left sides of the heart, receive blood from the right ventricle through the pulmonary arteries and deliver blood to the left atrium through the pulmonary veins. Abnormalities of cardiac or pulmonary function can markedly alter the dynamics of this pulmonary circulation.

With the advent of cardiac catheterization techniques, it became possible to measure pressures in and sample blood from various portions of the cardiopulmonary vascular system. Pressure determinations can be obtained by using strain gauge transducers or by fluid-filled manometers. Intravascular pressures are usually recorded with reference to atmospheric pressure at the level of the right or left atrium. Net right heart pressures can be recorded with reference to intrathoracic pressure by means of an intraesophageal balloon. This latter technique is cumbersome and is usually not required for most clinical situations, although patients with chronic obstructive lung disease and with marked alterations in intrathoracic pressure may demonstrate falsely elevated mean pressures [18].

Intravascular pressures demonstrate phasic alterations related to cardiac systole and respiration. In low pressure chambers and vessels, it is often difficult to identify distinctly the components of the pressure pulse. In such situations, the mean pressure is utilized. These recordings are obtained through electronic processing of the pulse recording, or by utilizing a highly damped catheter system.

In the normal adult subject, the right atrial pressure ranges between 0 and 5 torr (0 to 7 cm H_2O). This reflects venous filling pressure from the superior and inferior venae cavae and is identical to the central venous pressure (see below). This pressure will vary with the capacitance of, and the blood volume within, the systemic venous system, as well as with the back pressure from the right ventricle and tricuspid valve. Central venous pressure (CVP) is usually monitored through a fluid-filled catheter or polyethylene tube connected to a calibrated manometer. The tip of the catheter is positioned at the junction of the superior vena cava and the right atrium, and the zero point of the manometer is placed at the level of the mid-right atrium, approximately 5 cm vertically below the angle of Louis, but varying somewhat with chest wall configuration.

The right ventricle generates a systolic pressure of 15 to 25 torr; the pressure normally falls to zero during diastole. In the absence of right ventricular outflow obstruction, the pulmonary artery systolic pressure is identical to that of the right ventricle, whereas the pulmonary artery diastolic pressure is approximately 10 torr.

Pulmonary artery pressure will be raised by increases in pulmonary blood flow or volume, pulmonary vascular resistance, or pulmonary venous pressure. Pulmonary blood flow is increased most often as a result of congenital left-to-right cardiac shunts. Pulmonary blood volume may be temporarily increased following rapid infusion of blood or colloid. Pressure will also rise when a normal amount of blood is forced to flow through a decreased vascular space. Although pulmonary artery pressure may not rise significantly following surgical removal of an entire lung, it will rise as a result of extensive diminution in effective vascular volume as seen in chronic obstructive lung disease. Enhanced pulmonary vascular resistance can result from intravascular obstruction such as in pulmonary emboli, with vasoconstriction secondary to hypoxemia or serotonin, or structural restriction of the vascular lumina.

The effect of the pulmonary venous dynamics on cardiopulmonary function is not well understood. The pulmonary veins are rich in receptors and may play an important role in the response to hypoxemia. Elevated pulmonary venous pressure often results from abnormalities of left heart function. Left atrial pressure may be elevated because of mitral valve disease or may reflect an elevated left ventricular diastolic pressure seen in left ventricular congestive failure. There is no simple means for monitoring left atrial pressure directly. In order to place a catheter in the left atrial cavity, one must traverse the intraatrial septum through a patent foramen ovale or by transseptal needle puncture. Alternatively, one may enter the left atrium by means of the mitral valve using the retrograde left-heart catheterization technique. These methods generally require the facilities and talents of a catheterization laboratory and are not suited for bedside use.

The left atrial pressure can be very closely approximated by recording the pulmonary capillary wedge pressure (PCWP). When originally described, this technique entailed the use of an end-hole woven Dacron catheter passed into a peripheral branch of the pulmonary artery and advanced farther while the patient took a deep inspiration [7]. With a catheter thus wedged within the vessel, the lumen no longer reflects the pressure in the surrounding pulmonary artery but rather the pressure in the vascular tree ahead of it, which is in continuity with the left atrium. The validity of this technique has been confirmed in many studies, including those of patients with chronic pulmonary disease [31]. Reliable results can be anticipated when a characteristic left atrial pressure pulse is obtained in the wedge position and when blood sampled from the wedged catheter has an oxygen saturation consistent with pulmonary venous blood. However, in patients with pulmonary hypertension, or severe segmental pulmonary disease, it may be extremely difficult to obtain reliable recordings.

Determination of PCWP has been greatly facilitated by the use of flow-directed balloon-tipped catheters (Swan-Ganz) [27]. Once positioned in the superior vena cava, the partially inflated balloon will usually follow the blood flow through the right heart, guiding the catheter into the pulmonary artery. The catheter tip is then positioned in the right or left pulmonary artery or in the proximal portion of one of the lobar branches. In this location, pulmonary artery pressures can be recorded from the catheter lumen, which extends beyond the deflated balloon tip. When the balloon is fully inflated in this position, the artery is temporarily occluded and the catheter records pressures distally, representing the PCWP. It is important to avoid prolonged wedging of the catheter, because pulmonary infarction has been reported following extended obstruction to flow.

Normal PCWP ranges up to 12 torr. Patients with chronic congestive heart failure may have PCW pressures as high as 25 torr. Pulmonary edema is often associated with pressures above 25 torr, but this relationship is also affected by the plasma oncotic pressure and the permeability of the pulmonary vasculature [4]. Slight differences in right heart and PCW pressures may signify major physiologic alterations. Yet caution must be exercised in interpreting these data because of the high propensity to error in making these measurements. A 5 torr difference in the recording of a PCWP theoretically may differentiate a patient with left ventricular congestive failure from a normal subject. However, this amount of error could readily result from malposition of the transducer in relationship to the true location of the left atrial cavity. Ideally, the site at which the transducer system is opened to air to obtain a zero reading should be at the same level as the left atrium when one is recording PCWP. Furthermore, pressure transducers designed for systemic arterial pressure recordings may not be accurate at the low end of the scale at which right heart and PCW pressures are recorded. Thus, such transducers should be recalibrated in the low pressure range. A saline solution–filled CVP manometer can be utilized to check the accuracy of low pressure recordings. 20 cm H_2O pressure corresponds to approximately 15 torr.

Measurements of PCWP can be extremely valuable in the management of patients with acute respiratory failure [30]. It is often impossible to distinguish those patients with severe cardiac failure from those with predominant pulmonary disease. The critically ill cardiac or respiratory patient may present with dyspnea, tachycardia, diffuse rales, cardiomegaly, venous engorgement, a diffuse alveolar filling pattern on chest roentgenogram, and hypoxemia. The adult respiratory distress syndrome is an extreme form of respiratory failure that closely mimics classic pulmonary edema. There has been considerable controversy over the status of left ventricular function in patients with chronic obstructive lung disease [5]. Although the gross performance of the left ventricle appears to be normal in most patients, sophisticated analyses of ventricular metabolism and functions reveal abnormalities in the presence of chronic respiratory disease. Despite these alterations in left ventricular function, the left ventricular end-diastolic pressure and therefore the pulmonary artery and pulmonary capillary wedge pressures are usually normal in such cases. Thus, patients with primary pulmonary disease with abnormally high pulmonary precapillary vascular resistance will have elevated pulmonary artery systolic and diastolic pressures with a normal PCWP. Normal individuals or those with primary cardiac failure will demonstrate no sizeable gradient between PA diastolic pressure and PCWP.

Further useful information may be garnered by obtaining mixed venous blood from a pulmonary artery line and comparing it to a systemic arterial sample. Calculation of the arteriovenous oxygen content difference (A-VO_2) provides a rough guide to the total cardiac output that helps distinguish between left ventricular failure and hypervolemia as the cause of an elevated PCWP [26]. A hypotensive patient with cardiac failure may have normal PCWP in the presence of hypovolemia. However, in this case, the A-VO_2 difference will be elevated.

Precise cardiac output determination using the Fick method can be obtained by measuring oxygen consumption in conjunction with the A-VO_2 difference. This technique is cumbersome and is difficult to perform accurately at the bedside. Recent advances in instrumentation allow one to obtain cardiac output determination at the bedside, utilizing the indicator dilution principle. One such method is the thermodilution technique, which uses a flow-directed double-lumen balloon-tipped catheter placed in the pulmonary artery. An aliquot of cold saline solution is injected into a lumen positioned in the right atrium, and the temperature change is recorded by a thermistor at the catheter tip in the pulmonary artery. A small computer instantaneously calculates the cardiac output. This procedure can be repeated frequently and does not require the withdrawal of blood. However, unless one pays meticulous attention to the details of the technique, erroneous results can be obtained.

PULMONARY EMBOLISM

Pulmonary embolism is a frequently occurring cause of death or disability in patients with underlying cardiac or pulmonary disease. Despite major advances in diagnostic techniques, pulmonary embolism often escapes identification until postmortem examination.

Most pulmonary emboli arise from venous thromboses in large veins in the legs. Although the source may be identifiable by the accompanying local venous distention, tenderness, edema, discoloration, pain, or warmth, in the majority of cases the diagnosis cannot be made clinically [20]. Half of those patients with extensive thrombosis display no clinical signs or symptoms, whereas 30 to 50 percent with a "positive" clinical diagnosis in fact have normal deep veins. More precise diagnosis can be achieved by employing ultrasonic techniques, electric impedance plethysmography, and especially venography. In approximately 10 to 15 percent of cases, thrombi arise in the right side of the heart. The presence of a cardiac catheter, a pacemaker electrode, or a septal myocardial infarction may predispose to such an occurrence.

Acute pulmonary embolism results in obstruction to flow within the pulmonary circulation; in only a minority of instances, this produces pulmonary infarction. Unfortunately, the signs and symptoms of these two entities are often confused by the physician, thus resulting in misdiagnosis.

The hemodynamic effect of pulmonary embolism will depend to a great extent on the patient's underlying cardiopulmonary status [13]. In previously normal patients, hypoxemia is the most common manifestation of acute pulmonary embolism. This can result from venous admixture and diminished diffusion, or from ventilation-perfusion imbalance. Hypoxemia is noted even with relatively small obstructions. Thus, the finding of a normal PO_2 makes the diagnosis of pulmonary embolism unlikely.

Pulmonary hypertension occurs with somewhat larger degrees of obstruction. This results from one or a combination of several mechanisms, including (1) mechanical obstruction to flow, (2) vascular spasm, (3) vasoconstriction secondary to serotonin release from clots, and (4) vasoconstriction secondary to hypoxemia. In previously normal patients, the mean pulmonary artery pressure rarely exceeds 40 torr even in the presence of massive emboli. The degree of hypoxemia and pulmonary hypertension correlate to the extent of vascular obstruction.

Right ventricular failure with subsequent elevation of right atrial and venous pressures occur only in the presence of significant pulmonary hypertension. The cardiac index is usually normal or elevated in previously normal patients with acute pulmonary embolism [14].

The extent of the hemodynamic response to acute pulmonary embolism are less predictable in patients with previous cardiopulmonary disease. Such patients show disproportionately more hypoxemia, pulmonary hypertension, and right ventricular failure when compared to previously normal patients with similar degrees of obstruction. The cardiac index is often depressed in these patients.

Acute pulmonary embolism usually does not directly affect left ventricular function. Although hypoxemia and low cardiac output may adversely affect perfusion and contractility, there is only scant evidence to support a direct effect of pulmonary hypertension or right ventricular failure on left ventricular function. Recent echocardiographic studies show reversal of normal interventricular septal motion in acute right ventricular overload [10].

The most common presenting symptom of acute pulmonary embolism is dyspnea, sometimes accompanied by severe substernal chest pain that mimics acute myocardial infarction. Other findings may include shock, cyanosis, diaphoresis, and syncope. The patient will often display tachypnea, tachycardia, rales, and findings consistent with pulmonary hypertension and right heart failure such as an accentuated P2 and right ventricular gallop sounds. Patients with previously stable chronic obstructive lung disease may merely show signs of clinical deterioration without specific findings to point to a diagnosis of acute pulmonary embolism. Thus, pulmonary embolism should be suspected whenever a patient with chronic respiratory insufficiency unexplainedly decompensates.

Some patients will progress to develop pulmonary infarction following acute pulmonary embolism. In such cases, one notes pleuritic chest pain, fever, and hemoptysis, with physical and x-ray findings of consolidation. Most laboratory tests are of little help in aiding the diagnosis of pulmonary emboli and pulmonary infarction. There are no characteristic biochemical abnormalities. The electrocardiogram shows no specific changes, and recent reports demonstrate that the previously heralded finding of right axis deviation and right ventricular strain are rarely seen. In fact, left axis deviation occurs as commonly as right axis deviation in acute pulmonary embolism [25]. Chest roentgenograms are helpful in diagnosing pulmonary infarction, but they may not aid in the diagnosis of pulmonary embolism.

The perfusion lung scan is the most sensitive test for pulmonary embolism [29]. An abnormal scan in an appropriate clinical setting, especially in patients without prior cardiopulmonary disease, is usually sufficient evidence to diagnose pulmonary embolism, whereas a negative lung scan effectively rules out significant vascular obstruction. Patients with underlying chronic obstructive lung disease may show patchy abnormalities in vascular perfusion as a result of parenchymal destruction without pulmonary embolism. In such cases, simultaneous ^{133}Xe ventilation scanning can be helpful to assess if the perfusion defects match the areas of ventilation abnormalities. In doubtful cases, pulmonary angiography is valuable in confirming the diagnosis.

The mainstay of therapy is heparin anticoagulation [6]. When anticoagulation is contraindicated or unsuccessful, venous interruption is advisable if the source of the thrombi can be identified [3].

CARDIAC ARRHYTHMIAS

Cardiac arrhythmias occur frequently in patients with pulmonary disease. Estimates of the incidence of rhythm disorders vary considerably and depend to a great extent on the patient population selected and the technique of arrhythmia determination. Whereas 7 percent of a large group with severe chronic lung disease displayed arrhythmias or tachycardia on routine hospital electrocardiograms [28], 84 [11] to 89 [8] percent of hospitalized patients with chronic obstructive pulmonary disease demonstrated arrhythmias when long-term ambulatory monitoring techniques were utilized.

The type of arrhythmia noted in such studies range from premature atrial contractions to ventricular fibrillation. Supraventricular and ventricular arrhythmias are equally common.

Arrhythmias result from diverse etiologies. Occasionally, the occurrence of arrhythmias can be ascribed to specific events such as tracheal suction, isoproterenol inhalation, or lung surgery. Both atrial and ventricular arrhythmias occur frequently during tracheal suction when the patient is breathing room air. Pretreatment with 100% oxygen breathing renders tracheal intubation less arrhythmogenic [21]. Isoproterenol inhalation by means of aerosolized sprays can produce ventricular irritability. Excessive exposure may result in myocardial injury and infarction [1]. Chronic high-level exposure has been implicated as a cause [24] of sudden death, presumably from ventricular fibrillation. Atrial arrhythmias frequently complicate the postoperative course of patients who undergo lung resection. Such arrhythmias are especially prevalent in patients who have left pneumonectomies [15].

Generally, the precise etiology of arrhythmias in patients with pulmonary disease is not clearly known. Often, patients have underlying cardiac disease; are receiving drugs such as digitalis, theophylline, and catecholamines; or have major blood-gas abnormalities.

The precise relationship of blood-gas and acid-base derangements to arrhythmias is not known. Ventricular irritability is often attributed to the presence of hypoxemia. Some investigators [23] report a direct relation between the incidence of ventricular ectopic beats and the degree of hypoxemia, whereas other studies fail to show a correlation among hypoxemia, hypercapnia, and ventricular arrhythmias. Acute hypoxemia often results in bradycardia and conduction disturbances, terminating with cardiac arrest because of an increased vagal tone, mediated by hypoxic stimulation of chemoreceptors [2]. Studies in dogs show an increase in the ventricular fibrillation threshold in the presence of hypoxemia and respiratory acidosis [19]. Hyperventilation may be a physiologic response to hypoxemia and other stimuli, or it may be iatrogenically induced by mechanical respiratory therapy. The associated alkalosis may cause tissue hypoxia by shifting the oxyhemoglobin dissociation curve to the left (Bohr effect). Alkalosis also enhances the rate of firing of pacemaker cells and increases myocardial sensitivity to circulating catecholamines. Hypokalemia associated with alkalosis can be responsible for diverse arrhythmias, especially in a digitalized patient. Arrhythmias developing as a consequence of profound alkalosis are, for the most part, supraventricular in origin [12].

Although supraventricular arrhythmias, per se, are "benign," insofar as they rarely are a primary cause of death, such disturbances can severely aggravate the condition and management of the critically ill pulmonary patient. At rapid rates, cardiac and tissue ischemia may be produced as a result of increased work of the heart and a diminution in cardiac output. Furthermore, these rhythms may be premonitory to more serious arrhythmias, including cardiac arrest.

There is a wide range of supraventricular arrhythmias seen in patients with respiratory disease. The most prevalent supraventricular rhythm disorder is sinus tachycardia. Arbitrarily defined as a sinus rate of greater than 100 per minute, this rhythm is found in the majority of patients with chronic pulmonary disease, especially when this is complicated by acute respiratory insufficiency or infection. Sinus tachycardia is identified by the preservation of a normal P wave morphology and P-R interval. The sinus rate is usually not constant, and the heart rate will vary with the patient's course and activity. There is no specific treatment for this arrhythmia other than the correction or control of underlying medical problems which stimulate the tachycardic response.

Premature supraventricular ectopic beats can be recognized in approximately 50 percent of patients with chronic respiratory disease. This rhythm disorder is of little clinical significance, although the patient may notice "skipped beats" or an irregular pulse. Of greater importance is the fact that these beats may be the harbinger of more serious arrhythmias such as paroxysmal atrial tachycardia or atrial flutter and fibrillation.

The electrocardiographic hallmark of an atrial premature beat (APB) is an abnormal P wave occurring early in the cardiac cycle followed by a QRS complex with the same morphology as the sinus beats. Occasionally, the QRS configuration will be aberrated when the APB is very premature. Extremely early APBs may not be able to conduct to the ventricle. Such blocked APBs result in pauses between sinus beats that simulate sinus arrest or heart block. This can be especially confusing when the ectopic P wave is concealed in the T wave of the previous beat. The P-R interval of APBs is always equal to or greater than that of normal beats. When a QRS complex follows a P wave with a shorter than normal P-R interval, one must consider premature junctional or ventricular beats to be occurring.

Atrial tachycardias are the most common sustained abnormal supraventricular rhythm in patients with pulmonary disease. Classic paroxysmal atrial tachycardia (PAT) can occur with or without heart block. Although digitalis excess and hypokalemia can contribute to the occurrence of this arrhythmia, in most reports neither of these factors can be implicated.

The atrial rate in PAT is usually between 160 and 240 per minute. The atrial rate is constant and the P waves, when identifiable, differ in morphology from the underlying sinus beats. The ventricular rate will depend on the degree of atrioventricular block present. In the presence of digitalis excess, AV block is usually present. However, just the presence of such block is not enough to implicate glycosides as an etiologic factor. In digitalis-induced PAT, the P waves are generally of small amplitude and the P-P intervals show slight beat-to-beat variability. The atrial rate in this situation tends to vary directly with the degree of toxicity.

Paroxysms of atrial tachycardia can often be terminated by such vagal maneuvers as carotid sinus massage, Valsalva's maneuver, or gagging. These interventions, when successful, will abruptly terminate the arrhythmia. Careful examination of the electrocardiogram, however, will usually reveal a slight slowing of the atrial rate immediately prior to the cessation of the rhythm. If tachycardia persists despite these maneuvers, and if the patient is symptomatic, cholinergic drugs such as neostigmine or edrophonium can be utilized. Pressor amines may be useful, especially in the presence of hypotension, but must be used cautiously in patients with underlying cardiac disease. Emergency conversion of PAT can be attained using synchronized electric countershock.

Digitalis therapy will augment the efficacy of vagal maneuvers in terminating PAT. It is also the drug of choice for preventing recurrence. One should not hesitate to use digitalis so long as one can be certain that the drug is not the cause of the arrhythmia. Because patients with respiratory dysfunction appear to be likely to develop digitalis toxic arrhythmias, this drug must be used with extreme caution in patients already receiving digitalis. A digoxin blood level of less than 1.5 ng per milliliter with a normal serum potassium level would militate against digitalis toxicity. Paroxysmal atrial tachycardia with block thought to be caused by digitalis is best treated with intravenous potassium with the possible additional use of diphenylhydantoin, procainamide, or quinidine.

Variant forms of atrial tachycardia are especially prevalent in patients with acute and chronic pulmonary disease or cor pulmonale. Multifocal atrial tachycardia (MAT) is defined as an atrial rate greater than 100 per minute with well-organized discrete P waves of varying morphology from at least three different foci [22]. The P-P intervals display irregular variations, and the baseline between P waves is isoelectric. Chaotic atrial mechanism is a more general term depicting the same rhythm abnormality with or without tachycardia [17]. Although digitalis rarely causes these arrhythmias, it is of little or no value in the treatment of such disorders. It is important to distinguish MAT from atrial fibrillation. The latter rhythm is best controlled by the administration of digitalis, whereas increments of digitalis often produce high grade AV block, atrial tachycardia with block, or nodal and ventricular irritability in patients with MAT. Control of this arrhythmia depends on the management of the underlying ventilatory and metabolic derangements. Reduction in the use of arrhythmogenic bronchodilator drugs may help alleviate this arrhythmia, for which standard antiarrhythmic drugs are not reliably useful. The ultimate prognosis of patients with this arrhythmia is poor.

Atrial flutter can complicate the management of patients with severe pulmonary disease. In this rhythm, the atria depolarize at a rate of 240 to 360 beats per minute. Fortunately, the AV node interposes a degree of block, so that usually no more than every other beat reaches the ventricles. However, at slower flutter rates, e.g., 200 to 220 per minute, there may be 1:1 conduction, especially in patients treated with quinidine. At faster flutter rates, even 2:1 block may result in ventricular rates between 160 and 180 per minute. Such rapid rates, in the presence of pulmonary or cardiac insufficiency, can be very deleterious. Ventricular rates may vary sporadically as the degree of block changes from 1:1 to 2:1 to 4:1. Intermediate rates with irregular rhythms may be noted in situations in which block occurs at two levels in the junctional region, such as Wenkebach period at one level and 2:1 block at the lower level in the AV node.

Atrial flutter is diagnosed by noting a rapid regular atrial rate without distinct P waves. The electrocardiographic baseline is not isoelectric, and the undulating flutter waves present a sawtooth appearance. In the presence of 2:1 block, one of the flutter waves may be obscured by the QRS or T wave, thus simulating PAT or sinus tachycardia. Carotid sinus stimulation can be utilized to transiently increase the level of block and thus unmask the characteristic flutter waves. This is especially valuable in the presence of aberrated conduction, in which the rhythm may be mistaken for ventricular tachycardia unless flutter waves are recognized. Atrial flutter can occur paroxysmally and may progress to atrial fibrillation either spontaneously or as a result of therapeutic intervention.

Digitalis is the primary drug in treating atrial flutter. It may be valuable in preventing paroxysms and it will enhance atrioventricular block so as to control the ventricular rate. In acutely ill patients, however, it is usually necessary to use large doses of digitalis in order to adequately slow the ventricular rate. This often produces signs and symptoms of digitalis toxicity, which can be extremely dangerous in patients with hypoxemia and metabolic disorders. Digitalis may convert atrial flutter to normal sinus rhythm, but more commonly, it will alter the rhythm to atrial fibrillation. Often the atrial fibrillation will then revert to sinus rhythm. However, even if fibrillation persists, the ventricular rate is more easily controlled with this rhythm than with flutter.

Quinidine is useful in preventing and terminating paroxysms of atrial flutter. It should be used only in patients who are adequately digitalized because quinidine may accelerate the ventricular rate by its vagolytic effect on AV conduction or by slowing the atrial rate and thus facilitating 1:1 conduction.

Beta adrenergic-blocking drugs may be used to slow the ventricular rate in patients who are unresponsive to subtoxic doses of digitalis. However, marked ventilatory abnormalities have been observed in patients with bronchial asthma during beta adrenergic blockade with propranolol. This has produced a reluctance to use this agent in patients with any significant respiratory dysfunction. Nonasthmatic patients with chronic obstructive lung disease with or without heart disease, in fact, show little change in respiratory function when treated with propranolol [16]. Thus, propranolol can be administered cautiously to patients without bronchospastic tendencies to treat debilitating arrhythmias. Several pure $beta_1$ antagonists have been used successfully to treat arrhythmias without affecting bronchial smooth muscle; however, no such drug has yet been approved for use in the United States.

In an emergency situation, atrial flutter with a rapid ventricular response can be terminated by synchronized electrical countershock. Low energies (25 to 100 joules) are usually successful and are preferable in patients receiving digitalis. Very low energies (1 to 5 joules) may convert atrial flutter to fibrillation.

Atrial fibrillation can be seen in patients with pulmonary heart disease, but its presence should raise the question of possible thyrotoxicosis or concomitant rheumatic or coronary disease. Atrial fibrillation is characterized electrocardiographically by an irregularly irregular ventricular rate with fibrillatory atrial activity. Coarse atrial fibrillation can simulate atrial flutter, but careful analysis fails to reveal a consistent relationship between atrial and ventricular depolarizations. This rhythm can also be confused with chaotic atrial mechanisms.

The ventricular response in atrial fibrillation is totally dependent on the degree of block in the AV nodal region. The ventricular rate in untreated patients with normal AV node function will generally be greater than 140 per minute. Ventricular conduction is usually normal. When two closely coupled beats occur after a relatively long pause, the second such beat may be conducted aberrantly, thus simulating a ventricular premature contraction. At times it is impossible to differentiate these two phenomena, although aberrated beats will tend to have a right bundle branch block configuration and a triphasic pattern in lead V_1 with a normal initial deflection and will occur only with long-short cycle sequences.

The treatment of atrial fibrillation is similar to that of flutter. Because digitalis is the drug of choice, it is important not to withhold therapy because of aberrated beats in the mistaken thought that toxicity is at hand. Toxicity must be suspected when the ventricular rate is slow and when the abnormal beats display fixed coupling to the previous depolarizations. Regularization of the ventricular response may represent nodal tachycardia, a dangerous manifestation of digitalis excess. Determination of digitalis concentration in the serum is often helpful, but electrophysiologic toxicity can occur at supposed normal blood levels in extremely ill patients with metabolic and ventilatory abnormalities.

Major ventricular arrhythmias carry a grave prognosis in patients with severe respiratory failure [9]. These disorders are usually anticipated by the appearance of ventricular premature beats (VPBs). The occurrence of early VPBs which interrupt the preceding T wave or couplets and triplets are especially ominous. The emergence of ventricular irritability should alert the physician to a possible deterioration in the patient's ventilatory or metabolic status or the excessive use of arrhythmogenic drugs. Correction of such abnormalities is usually necessary before the ventricular arrhythmia can be suppressed. Antiarrhythmic therapy is of limited usefulness especially in established ventricular tachycardia and fibrillation. Even electric countershock is often unsuccessful once this degree of arrhythmia is reached.

Ventricular tachycardia is usually identifiable by a fairly regular ventricular rhythm with widened QRS complexes that have no direct relationship to the atrial activity. Occasionally, retrograde conduction through the AV node will result in there being a P wave for each QRS complex, making it difficult to differentiate from supraventricular tachycardia with aberrancy. Careful examination of the initiation or termination of this rhythm or the response to vagal maneuvers may be helpful in elucidating the nature of the rhythm. If in doubt, it is usually wise to treat the patient as if the rhythm were ventricular tachycardia. Bidirectional tachycardia refers to a rapid regular ventricular rhythm with alternation in the polarity of the QRS complexes. This rhythm often reflects an advanced stage of digitalis toxicity and carries an ominous prognosis.

Lidocaine is the drug of choice to suppress irritability. It is administered as an intravenous bolus followed by continuous infusion. Procainamide can be utilized orally as well as intravenously in an attempt to forestall serious ventricular disorders. The treatment of ventricular tachycardia will depend on the clinical status of the patient. Rapid ventricular tachycardia with hemodynamic compromise is best treated by a high energy defibrillatory shock (200 to 400 joules). If there is adequate time, and if the QRS complexes are distinctly identifiable, synchronized countershock with lower energies (10 to 100 joules) can be utilized. In less urgent situations, intravenous lidocaine or procainamide therapy can be tried before countershock. These drugs are useful in patients who do not respond to counter-shock alone, or who have recurrent arrhythmias after successful defibrillation. Patients with severe respiratory insufficiency who develop ventricular fibrillation are often able to be resuscitated.

REFERENCES

1. Aelony, Y., Laks, M. M., and Beall, G. An electrocardiographic pattern of acute myocardial infarction associated with excessive use of aerosolized isoproterenol. *Chest* 68, 1975, p. 107.
2. Ayres, S. M., and Mueller, H.   Hypoxemia, hypercapnia, and cardiac arrhythmias: The importance of regional abnormalities of vascular distensibility. *Chest* 63, 1973, p. 981.
3. Crane, C. Venous interruption for pulmonary embolism: Present status. *Prog. Cardiovasc. Dis.* 17, 1975, p. 329.
4. daLuz, D. L., et al. Pulmonary edema related to changes in colloid osmotic and pulmonary artery wedge pressure in patients after acute myocardial infarction. *Circulation* 51, 1975, p. 350.
5. Ferrer, M. I. Cor pulmonale (pulmonary heart disease): Present day status. *Am. Heart J.* 89, 1975, p. 657.
6. Genton, E., and Hirsh, J. Observations in anticoagulant and thrombolitic therapy in pulmonary embolism. *Prog. Cardiovasc. Dis.* 17, 1975, p. 239.
7. Hellems, H. K., Haynes, F. W., and Dexter, L.   Pulmonary "capillary" pressure in man. *J. Appl. Physiol.* 2, 1949, p. 24.
8. Holford, F. D., and Mithoefer, J. C. Cardiac arrhythmias in hospitalized patients with chronic obstructive pulmonary disease. *Am. Rev. Respir. Dis.* 108, 1973, p. 879.
9. Hudson, I. D., et al. Arrhythmias associated with acute respiratory failure in patients with chronic airway obstruction. *Chest* 63, 1973, p. 661.
10. Kerber, R. E., Dippel, W. F., and Abboud, F. M. Abnormal motion of the inter-ventricular septum in right ventricular volume overload. *Circulation* 48, 1973, p. 86.
11. Kleiger, R. E., and Senior, R. M. Long term electrocardiographic monitoring of ambulatory patients with chronic airway obstruction. *Chest* 65, 1974, p. 5.
12. Lawson, N. W., Butler, G. H., and Ray, C. T. Alkalosis and cardiac arrhythmias. *Anesth. Analg.* (Cleve) 52, 1973, p. 951.
13. McIntyre, K. M., and Sasahara, A. A. Determinance of right ventricular function and hemodynamics after pulmonary embolism. *Chest* 65, 1974, p. 534.
14. McIntyre, K. M., and Sasahara, A. A. Hemodynamic and ventricular responses to pulmonary embolism. *Prog. Cardiovasc. Dis.* 17, 1974, p. 175.
15. Mowry, F. M., and Reynolds, E. W. Cardiac rhythm disturbances, compli-cating resectional surgery of the lung. *Ann. Intern. Med.* 61, 1964, p. 688.
16. Nordstrom, L. A., MacDonald, F., and Gobel, F. L. Effect of propranolol on respiratory function and exercise tolerance in patients with chronic obstruc-tive lung disease. *Chest* 67, 1975, p. 287.
17. Phillips, J., Spano, J., and Burch, G. Chaotic atrial mechanism. *Am. Heart J.* 78, 1969, p. 171.

18. Rice, D. L., et al. Wedge pressure measurement in obstructive pulmonary disease. *Chest* 66, 1974, p. 6.
19. Rogers, R. M., et al. Vulnerability of canine ventricle to fibrillation during hypoxia and respiratory acidosis. *Chest* 63, 1973, p. 986.
20. Sasahara, A. A. Current problems in pulmonary embolism. *Prog. Cardiovasc. Dis.* 17, 1974, p. 161.
21. Shim, C., Fine, N., Fernandez, R., and Williams, M. H. Cardiac arrhythmias resulting from tracheal suctioning. *Ann. Intern. Med.* 71, 1969, p. 1149.
22. Shine, K. I., Kastor, J. A., and Yurchak, P. M. Multifocal atrial tachycardia. *N. Engl. J. Med.* 279, 1968, p. 344.
23. Sideris, D. A., et al. Type of cardiac dysrhythmias in respiratory failure. *Am. Heart J.* 89, 1975, p. 32.
24. Speizer, F. D., Doll, R., and Heaf, P. Investigation into the use of drugs in preceding death from asthma. *Br. Med. J.* 1, 1968, p. 339.
25. Stein, P. D., et al. The electrocardiogram in acute pulmonary embolism. *Prog. Cardiovasc. Dis.* 17, 1975, p. 247.
26. Stevens, P. M. Assessment of acute respiratory failure: Cardiac vs. pulmonary causes. *Chest* 67, 1975, p. l.
27. Swan, H. J. C., and Ganz, W. Catheterization of the heart in man with the use of a flow directed balloon tipped catheter. *N. Engl. J. Med.* 283, 1970, p. 447.
28. Thomas, A. J., and Valabhji, P. Arrhythmia and tachycardia in pulmonary heart disease. *Br. Heart J.* 31, 1969, p. 491.
29. Tow, D. E., and Simon, A. L. Comparison of lung scanning and pulmonary angiography: The detection and followup of pulmonary embolism: The urokinase-pulmonary embolism trial experience. *Prog. Cardiovasc. Dis.* 17, 1975, p. 239.
30. Unger, K. M., Shibel, E. M., and Moser, K. M. Detection of left ventricular failure in patients with adult respiratory distress syndrome. *Chest* 67, 1975, p. 8.
31. Walston, A., and Kendall, M. E. Comparison of pulmonary wedge and left atrial pressure in man. *Am. Heart J.* 86, 1973, p. 159.

Bernard A. Berman
John M. O'Loughlin

Immunologic Processes in Respiratory Disease

8

Many commonly encountered respiratory diseases are better understood by a therapist if his or her expertise is buttressed by a familiarity with the basic principles of allergy and immunology.

Human immunologic development begins in utero. The infant's first year of life is spent acquiring this defense system and developing it into an efficient entity. There are two basic types of acquired immunologic process: cell-mediated and humoral, the first involving small lymphocytes of thymic origin, and the second involving circulating antibodies (immunoglobulins). A primary stem cell is responsible for the development of both the humoral system and cell-mediated functions. Deficiencies in either type, or in both types, are detected in both neoplastic and nonneoplastic diseases, and in congenital disorders.

Participating in cellular immunity are the thymus-controlled lymphocytes, or T cells. Believed to be independent of thymus control are the B cells, or those primarily responsible for antibody release. It is also commonly believed by medical scientists that T and B cells have their origin in a common stem cell in the embryo and that they differentiate during the first gestational trimester by passing through the thymus, which maintains control of the T cells, whereas the B cells are subject to the influence of a human analogue of the bursa of Fabricius in an animal. If this analogue is present in the human subject, it is believed likely that it is located either in the gastrointestinal tract or close to Peyer's patches, the oval elevated areas of lymphoid tissue on the mucosa of the small intestine.

In general, T cells have a longer life than do B cells. They recirculate through the thoracic duct and systemic circulation and have been found to possess a susceptivity to irradiation. The proliferation of the shorter-lived B cells has been found to be controlled effectively by immunosuppressive agents. Researchers believe the approximate ratio of T and B cells circulating at any one time to be 4 : 1.

THE IMMUNOGLOBULINS

Serum proteins are included among the humoral immunologic factors. It has been generally accepted that they separate as gamma globulins when they are subjected to electrophoresis. Antibodies that can directly interact with antigens, they are included in the serum proteins categorized as immunoglobulins. There are five classes of immunoglobulins: IgG, IgA, IgM, IgD, and IgE.

Whereas virtually no maternal IgA or IgM crosses the placental barrier, the fetus does receive maternal IgG. Cord serum IgG concentration at birth very closely approximates the mother's. In the fourth gestational month, gamma globulin begins its passage, and it is generally believed that an active transport system is initiated. In varying concentrations, IgM antibodies are synthesized by the fetus in utero. Ordinarily, levels increase quickly after birth, approximating 75 percent of the adult level by the end of the first year of life. Initial IgA synthesis occurs a few weeks after birth and reaches 75 percent of adult level by the end of the second year.

Rapidly catabolized, the newborn's maternal IgG establishes a period of physiologic hypogammaglobulinemia by the third month of life. Infantile production of IgG rises rapidly, so much so that the rate reaches adult levels by the end of the first year.

B lymphocytes differentiated into plasma cells are assigned the chore of synthesizing the immunoglobulins. Currently, investigators postulate that a single cell makes but one type of antibody with one specificity. Although usually the newborn has been found to have not more than a few plasma cells, if any, the situation changes during the baby's third month; the infant has matured immunologically. Lymphoid tissue has matured, accompanied by organization of follicles. Plasma cells appear.

CELL-MEDIATED MECHANISMS IN IMMUNOLOGY

Antigen fixed in tissue brings delayed hypersensitivity skin test responses. This is true, for example, in the case of a solid tissue homograft or if the skin is treated with a sensitizing agent such as 2,4 dinitrofluorobenzene (2,4 DNFB). Thus is cellular immunity manifested in vivo.

As they pass through tissue, lymphocytes are sensitized in the periphery and pass on to the local lymph nodes' paracortical area. Differentiated into large cells, these sensitized cells reach a peak concentration within three to four days. They then divide, forming a new population of lymphocytes. Some of these leave the local lymphatic tissue and pass on to other lymph nodes.

It should be noted that the cell-mediated response depends upon the soundness of the thymus in embryonic and early neonatal life. A fact to remember is that cellular immunity will be unable to develop if the thymus is removed in animals in their early neonatal period.

IMMUNOLOGIC DEFICIENCY

If either cellular or humoral immunity fails to properly develop, the physician is confronted with deficiency diseases that are not only rare and disabling, but frequently fatal.

Defects in both cell-mediated immunity and immunoglobulin synthesis are typical of the combined—or Swiss—type of immune deficiency disease. Responsibility for this dual disease is attributed to either a defective immunoblast cell line or the absence of this cell. The disease is autosomal recessive, or X-linked. Striking in early life, the disease is frequently fatal during the first two years of life.

Some of the signals include a lymphocyte count of frequently less than 1,500 cells per cubic millimeter, absence of all immunoglobulins, all but absent lymphoid tissue, and an undeveloped thymus that is difficult to find at postmortem examination because it usually weighs less than 1 gram. The young patients readily accept skin grafts and cannot produce contact sensitivity to 2,4 DNFB. There are repeated infections—bacterial, viral, and fungal. These children are in far more dangerous condition than young patients with defective immunoglobulin synthesis. The latter are able to battle viral infection and their defenses can be improved to near normal when replacement gamma globulin treatment is employed. Frequent clinical manifestations include intractable diarrhea with *Salmonella* and pathogenic *Escherichia coli* strains together with thrush and pyoderma. Death often is caused by infections from *Pseudomonas* and pneumonia from *Pneumocystis carinii.*

Young male children inherit defective immunoglobulin synthesis as an X-linked recessive characteristic in agammaglobulinemia [1]. In the presence of maternal immunoglobulin, these symptoms begin during the second year of life when the levels of IgG are generally below 100 mg/100 ml. Frequently occurring have been pyogenic infections with staphylococci, streptococci, pneumococci, and *Hemophilus influenzae.* Responses are lacking to tetanus toxoid, pertussis, and diphtheria. The ability to reject homografts is maintained.

Either low or absent entirely are anti-A and anti-B isohemagglutinins. Also apparent is the inability of antigenic stimulation of lymph nodes to produce plasma cells. Presenting frequently are such collagen disorders as dermatomyositis and rheumatoid arthritis. The indicated treatment here is regular and sufficient doses of gamma globulin. These patients have presented with delayed reactions to *Candida,* mumps, streptokinase-streptodornase, and 2,4 DNFB.

There have been occasional reports of congenital deficiency limited to cell-mediated immunity. Found in these cases have been lymphopenia, lymphoid tissue depletion, and thymic aplasia. It is not unexpected when these patients can neither reject homografts nor become sensitized to 2,4 DNFB. Characterized by absence of parathyroid glands and by defect in the third bronchial arch, a variant of this disease is DiGeorge's syndrome.

Statistically, secretory and serum IgA are lacking in approximately 80 percent of patients with hereditary ataxia-telangiectasia. Choreoathetoid movements in infancy may be the earliest signs of this disease. Attacking the conjunctivae and exposed areas of the body (face, arms, eyelids), telangiectasia usually begins between the ages of 6 and 14 years. As it progresses, severe infections of the middle ear, sinuses, and lungs occur frequently. Pervasive infection or lymphoreticular malignancy are the usual causes of death. Remaining unclear is the relationship between low IgA levels and infection of the respiratory tract.

Acquired Hypogammaglobulinemia
Proceeding from the congenital deficiencies to the acquired states, one is confronted with a multitude of varieties of acquired hypogammaglobulinemia. Reclassified by the World Health Organization in 1970 as *idiopathic hypogammaglobulinemia of variable duration,* this is the commonest immune deficiency disease, more often found in adult than in pediatric patients. Levels of IgG usually are less than 500 mg/100 ml. Both sexes are affected, and patient histories reveal a high percentage with systemic lupus erythematosis, thrombocytopenia, and hemolytic anemia.

Incidence of secondary acquired hypogammaglobulinemia occurs with excessive loss of protein (e.g., exfoliative dermatitis and renal gastrointestinal disorders). A large number of cases involve reticuloendothelial diseases (Hodgkin's chronic lymphatic leukemia, lymphosarcoma).

Because the immunoglobulin level usually decreases in inverse proportion to the severity of the disease, the varying levels in certain diseases are prognostically valuable. Infection by some organisms occurs more often in specific deficiency states. Just as levels of immunoglobulin may be influenced in certain neoplasms, so may be the cell-mediated response's intensity. In cases of Hodgkin's disease, for example, the span can be as far apart as anergy and normal response. It should be noted, nevertheless, that during remissions, prior anergy can be overcome. A patient's loss of cellular immunity is reversible. In the end stage of the disease, however, it is usually irreversible.

DIAGNOSIS
In fathoming these puzzling tricks of nature, a physician's best tool is his own suspicious nature, the diagnostician's warmest friend. Unlike a mother hen fretting over a sick chick, the doctor has to do more than emit clucking sounds when he is confronted by an infant who is not thriving and who has frequent infections and bouts with diarrhea. A good beginning is a Schick test, which measures IgG-neutralizing antibody to diphtheria toxin, and which should provide negative results after one or two diphtheria immunizations. Paper electrophoresis is a way of learning total gamma globulin levels (the value should be more than 400 mg/100 ml). A gauge of IgM antibodies would be saline solution titers of anti-A or anti-B isoagglutinin, or both. At 6 months of age, titers certainly should exceed 1 to 4 to A or B erythrocytes, or both, depending upon the ABO group. They should be higher at age 1 year. Absent or lowered isoagglutinin titers would indicate IgM malfunction.

Agar radial diffusion kits are commercially available to measure IgA, IgG, and IgM when any of the aforementioned test results are abnormal. Quantitative immunoglobulin levels should be determined in milligrams per 100 ml and compared with age-matched control subjects.

In the diagnosis or prognosis of a congenital problem or of a tumor-related deficiency, evaluation of cell-mediated deficiency is necessary. Tuberculin, histoplasmin, blastomycin, coccidioidin, mumps, streptokinase-streptodornase, and *Candida* skin tests should be performed. Delayed skin reactions are usually absent. The direct lymphocyte count usually is less than 1,500 cells per cubic millimeter. Response of peripheral lymphocytes to stimulation with phytohemagglutinin ordinarily has been absent or diminished. Poor or no sensitization to 2,4 DNFB is seen.

TREATMENT

In acquired or congenital hypogammaglobulinemia, gamma globulin has saved lives. It is not useful, however, in treating the combined form of deficiency, for which bone marrow or thymic transplants sometimes have proved beneficial.

Prevention of bacterial infection usually can be achieved by raising the gamma globulin level to 200 mg/100 ml. (The customary loading dose is 1.8 ml per kilogram of body weight.) The loading dose is administered in three divided doses of 0.6 ml or 100 mg per kilogram. Thereafter, a monthly injection of 0.6 ml per kilogram is given to maintain a serum level of approximately 200 mer/100 ml. This is because the gamma globulin's half-life is 25 to 30 days. Antibiotic therapy is employed only for specific infections.

It is highly important here to caution against intravenously administered gamma globulin, a possible cause of severe pyrogenic and cardiovascular difficulties.

Likely villains to blame for severe reactions to intravenous gamma globulin are the small masses of globulin formed during preparation of the blood serum fraction. Commercial gamma globulin is made from a pool of donor plasmas and contains very small amounts of IgA and IgM. Commercial globulin contains antibodies to a variety of infectious diseases. These antibodies will be present in adequate strengths.

Two of the diseases possessing immunologic disorder and associated with cutaneous or mucocutaneous disarray are the Wiskott-Aldrich syndrome and mucocutaneous candidiasis. Typically concomitant with the former are eczema, thrombocytopenia, and recurring cutaneous and respiratory infections. Patients often are insensitive to 2,4 DNFB. The principal immunoglobulin deficiency is of IgM. Presenting early in life, the Wiskott-Aldrich syndrome usually is fatal, death being caused by hemorrhage or sepsis. Antibiotic agents are the indicated therapy. There have been recent successes reported employing transfer factor, bone marrow transplants, and thymic transplants.

As for mucocutaneous candidiasis, it occurs when *Candida albicans* is pathogenic.

It appears as a rare infection in children with an endocrine system disorder or an immunologic deficiency. Severe, sometimes fatal, systemic candidiasis occurs when the cell-mediated immune system is defectively functioning or when the opsonins are not effectively facilitating phagocytosis.

From 5 to 10 percent of clinical infections in normal children during the neonatal period can be attributed to *Candida*. By the end of the first year of life, 80 percent have positive delayed hypersensitivity reactions to challenge. Eighty to 90 percent of children older than 6 months have immunofluorescent antibody titers of greater than 1 to 16.

Appropriate doses of amphotericin B for longer than a month have been found to be successful therapy. The successful use of transfer factor also has been reported.

THE COMPLEMENT SYSTEM

There are nine serum proteins in the complement system [2] that produce a variety of biologic effects by sequential reaction with each other. The interaction of the components in a cascading type sequence is similar to that of the mechanism of blood coagulation. There are a number of biologic effects of the intermediate stages, but the end product of the complement system's activation is cell membrane damage. An alternate pathway, which bypasses the initial three reactions but which activates the final six, is the properdin system. If there is a congenital lack of control of these proteins, clinical disease can result such as hereditary angioneurotic edema and a marked increase in susceptibility to infection. In the inflammatory processes, the levels of some of the proteins are lowered, e.g., C3. A measurement useful in following the course of clinical disease is CH50, which is the sum of the components of hemolytic complement.

Activation of the complement system takes place when a specific antigen unites with an antibody possessing complement-fixing properties (IgG and IgM), and

1. the C1 complex (C1qrs) attaches to the Fc fragment;
2. C1q possesses the binding site for antibody;
3. by the actions of C1r, C1s is activated, forming C1 esterase;
4. the activated C1 in turn activates C4 and C2, forming C3 convertase, an enzyme which then splits C3 into two fragments;
5. C3 engenders an anaphylatoxic and chemotactic activity;
6. C3b stays on the cell surface, which permits the interaction of the next three components;
7. complexes of C5, C6, and C7 possess chemotactic activity for polymorphonuclear leukocytes;
8. the addition of C8 results in a partially damaged cell;
9. with the addition of C9, membrane lysis occurs.

Powerful biologic effects in the complement system are not without their natural controls; ordinarily, there is a rapid deterioration and loss of their binding capacity. Loss of enzyme activity also controls the system.

Transmitted as a genetic dominant, hereditary angioneurotic edema is a rare disease presenting as intestinal mucosa and localized, transient swelling of the skin and mucous membrane. Frequently, severe and sudden abdominal pain and swelling of any part of the skin are associated with the disorder. Symptoms usually are present in the first 20 years, but they may occur later. Measuring the fourth complement component is considered a helpful diagnostic technique.

Other inherited deficiencies of the complement system are C3 deficiency associated with decreased resistance to pyogenic infection, C5 deficiency with accompanying impaired phagocytosis, and decreased C1q manifested by IgG synthesis.

IMMUNE REACTIONS
Four types of potentially injurious immune reactions are type I, immediate hypersensitivity, such as anaphylaxis; type II, cytolysis; type III, soluble antigen-antibody complexes; and type IV, delayed hypersensitivity [3].

Type I: Immediate Hypersensitivity
Anaphylaxis may be either an acute or a subacute hypersensitivity state, the one a response within seconds, the other a response within hours, both marked by an antigen-antibody reaction. When exposed to antigen, mast cells release histamine and such vasoactive peptides as bradykinin, serotonin, eosinophilic chemotactic factor of anaphylaxis, and slow-reacting substance of anaphylaxis (SRS-A), a lipoprotein believed by some investigators to be the product of the polymorphonuclear leukocyte. SRS-A is an acidic lipid the structure of which is not known.

The varied clinical manifestations of this syndrome, which characteristically affects smooth muscle fibers and small blood vessels, include both asthma and hay fever. Characteristics of the offending antibody — reagin, immunoglobulin IgE — are small concentration in serum, existence of up to six weeks at skin site, cannot be transferred across the placenta, inactivated by heat and sulfapyridine, moves as slow beta globulin electrophoretically, and does not sensitize guinea pigs. The complement system is not involved.

Everyone can produce IgE antibodies; the allergic patient cannot turn off IgE production at a specific level. Not all asthma or hay fever is mediated by IgE antibody-antigen reactions. The process involved in IgE production in allergic disease is not altogether clear. Evidence suggests that immunogens interface with plasma cells in the mucosa in the respiratory tract, but in the allergic patient, the reaction is prolific. So much IgE is formed that not all can be bound by mast cells, and thus free IgE can be detected and measured in the serum. Radioimmunoassay (RIST, or radioimmunoadsorbent test) is useful for assay of IgE.

Assays Detecting IgE to Specific Allergies
Commercially available RAST (radioallergosorbent test), still experimental, relies on the antiglobulin principle to delineate specific IgE antibody to specific allergens in the patient's serum. In the Rast test, an excess of allergen is coupled to cyanogen bromide-activated Sephodex or cellulose particles on filter paper discs. After suit-

able incubation with reaginic serum, and subsequent washing, radiolabeled and anti-IgE antibodies are added and react with IgE directed to the allergens in the particles. The amount of radioactivity on the washed particles is directly related to IgE antibody concentrations in the serum. As yet, Rast assays are not as reliable as direct skin tests.

Immunotherapy

Immunotherapy, a term applied to repeated injection of gradually increasing doses of extracts of allergenic substances, has been known for many years, but the rationale and efficacy of such therapy has been clarified only in recent years. Although precise mechanisms are not altogether clear, there is sufficient data gained by newer techniques in both immunology and pharmacology to justify use of immunotherapy in specific instances of allergic disease. For ragweed, hay fever, and probably slightly less so for other instances of pollenosis from pollens of both trees and grasses, symptoms are considerably lessened after prolonged treatment with adequate doses of potent extracts. For seasonal asthma, sufficient data from controlled studies are available to support the efficacy of immunotherapy. Injection treatment with dust and molds has aroused controversy—some studies support its efficacy and others question its value.

The immunologic phenomenon associated with immunotherapy is the noticeable increase of IgG antibodies, which can block histamine release by coupling with antigen before it interfaces with IgE antibodies fixed to the surface of basophils and mast cells. There is suggestive evidence that serum and locally produced IgA may block IgE-mediated reactions. In the unprotected patient, antigens react with IgE antibody on the surface of the tissue mast cell, and symptoms result in large measure from degranulation of mast cells with concomitant release of pharmacologically active substances—vasoactive amines such as histamine and SRS-A.

Type II: Cytolysis

Injury or death of a cell usually stems from complement. Disintegration (lysis), however, can occur following the reaction of cytophilic anaphylactic antibodies with extrinsic antigen—within the cell, or at the surface. With the exception of IgM agglutinins requiring complement, the cytolytic antibodies usually are IgG. Penicillin-induced immunohemolytic anemia is an example of complement-associated cytolysis. IgG apparently imparts to the coated cells a susceptibility to damage by macrophages and mononuclear cells.

Type III: Soluble Antigen-Antibody Complexes

A quiescent period for the connection of antibody to the cell receptors is required by cytotrophic anaphylaxis. The reaction in aggregate anaphylaxis, however, takes place within minutes of the injection of the antigen. The reticuloendothelial system removes and renders harmless the insoluble immune aggregates. However, the soluble immune complexes, persisting intravascularly, permeate the vascular system.

Inasmuch as the blood is filtered by the kidneys, it can be surmised that the complexes will be deposited in the basement membrane.

With the genesis of the chemotactic product, the complement system becomes activated and polymorphonuclear cells make their appearance and phagocytize the deposits. Lytic enzymes are released as the lysosomal granules of this cell rupture. The antigen's ratio to antibody at the region of the reaction needs to be slightly to moderately greater, the severity depending upon the concentration of the precipitating antibody. The amount of soluble immune complexes produced, and their duration, are what govern the type of disease, the prognosis, and the lesion possibly developed in the kidney.

If it is transient, acute serum sickness or acute poststreptococcal glomerulonephritis can occur and subsequently heal. In the wake of continuously forming complexes, deposits of antigen, antibody, and complement in the subepithelial area of the glomerulus can result in a membranous glomerulonephritis. Lupus nephritis can follow the renal deposits of soluble complexes of DNA and anti-DNA. Bacterial antigenic and antibacterial antibodies have been found in the diseased glomerulus of individuals with poststreptococcal glomerulonephritis.

The Arthus phenomenon in animals is a good example of an experimentally induced local, immediate hypersensitivity brought on by soluble immune antigen complexes and partially mediated by complement. Necrosis, hemorrhage, and capillary thrombosis are found by biopsy at the injection site. Man's skin and muscle have shown a wide presence of localized necrosis following cutaneous injection of various sera, vaccine, and antibodies—mild and severe examples of the Arthus phenomenon, which also probably causes vasculitides associated with the administration of drugs and foreign sera.

Serum Sickness

Urticarial rash, splenomegaly, fever, arthralgias or arthritis, nephritis — these are the characteristics of the serum sickness syndrome, which presents 8 to 12 days after foreign serum protein, usually horse antitoxin, is administered therapeutically. Unbound protein can be found in the serum before the symptoms appear. Presenting symptoms are leukopenia, albuminuria, and hypocomplementemia. Unidentified are the immunologic mechanisms, the syndrome appearing to be a product of the Arthus phenomenon and anaphylactic responses. Suggesting that serum sickness is a dispersion of some form of Arthus phenomenon reaction is the presence of antigen-antibody aggregates, focal vascular lesions, and hypocomplementemia. It is believed that the skin eruption probably is the result of antibodies of the IgE type. Anaphylaxis and immediate serum sickness upon exposure can result if a patient has become sensitized to horse serum by contact with horse dander or by the previous administration of horse antiserum.

Type IV: Delayed Hypersensitivity

Delayed hypersensitivity is an immunologic reaction occurring on exposure to an antigen and it results in an inflammatory reaction becoming apparent within a few hours of exposure, said reaction becoming normally appreciable within 24 to 48 hours.

Transferable to sensitized subjects with cells, but not with serum, the tuberculin reaction is a dermal hypersensitivity reaction in human or animal subjects that occurs within 12 to 48 hours after intradermal injection of tuberculin protein.

Histamine and kinins, the important mediators in immediate hypersensitivity, are unnecessary for delayed hypersensitivity, which can be induced with infectious agents, some chemicals, and foreign animal cells. Such agents as Freund's adjuvants favor the induction of delayed hypersensitivity.

An increasing role in biologic phenomena and the pathogenesis of a number of diseases is being filled by cellular immunity: defense against bacterial and viral infections, allograft rejections, immunologic responses against malignant diseases, graft versus host reactions, and the pathogenesis of some autoimmune diseases. Diseases without delayed hypersensitivity are congenital thymic dysplasia and the Swiss type agammaglobulinemia.

Hodgkin's disease, the Wiskott-Aldrich syndrome, chronic lymphatic leukemia, ataxia-telangiectasis, sarcoidosis, viral infections such as measles and influenza, chronic mucocutaneous candidiasis, and lepromatous leprosy are diseases in which depressed delayed hypersensitivity occurs.

Mixed Allergic Reactions
Specific disease states often involve components of the characteristic four types of reactions described above. For purposes of minimizing confusion, these diseases will be designated by the arbitrary classification of *mixed allergic reactions.*

Allergic Bronchopulmonary Aspergillosis
One such example is allergic bronchopulmonary aspergillosis (ABA), representing a combination of types I and III hypersensitivity reactions. Type I, IgE-mediated response, augments the tissue-damaging effects of the type III, soluble antigen-antibody complex process. Clinical and laboratory correlates are well defined. Wheezing, productive cough, pulmonary infiltrates, eosinophilia, and sputum loaded with mycelia and eosinophils are the cardinal features of ABA. Laboratory tests that assist in diagnosis include: (1) intradermal skin tests for *Aspergillus fumigatus* provoke an immediate wheal-and-flare (type I IgE) response, and a late 6- to 8-hour skin reaction (probable Arthus type III); (2) sputum culture for *A. fumigatus* is positive; (3) gel diffusing testing for precipitating antibody to *A. fumigatus*-soluble antigens is positive; (4) bronchial challenge with soluble antigen induces both immediate and late bronchospasm. Early recognition and treatment usually prevents the severe parenchymal destruction eventuating in bronchiectasis. Thus, atopic patients (asthma and hay fever) with pulmonary infiltrates and eosinophilia must be considered as potential victims of ABA until proved otherwise.

Extrinsic Allergic Alveolitis
Another disorder—extrinsic allergic alveolitis (hypersensitivity pneumonia)—originates from inhalation of inhaled organic antigens, and clinical reactions probably

derive from a mix of type III soluble antigen-antibody complex disease and type IV delayed hypersensitivity responses. Inhalation of such organic antigens as avian protein, the source being pigeon, parakeet, or parrot droppings, results in bird fanciers' lung disease; excessive exposure to *Thermoactinomyces vulgaris* or *Micropolyspora faeni* results in farmers' lung (moldy hay), bagassosis (moldy sugar cane), mushroom workers' disease (moldy compost), and home humidifier disease (home humidifiers and air conditioning systems). The mechanisms resulting in extrinsic allergic alveolitis have yet to be precisely defined, but the present state of the art indicates that the majority of patients are nonatopic; that sensitization results from intensive and excessive exposure; that the reactions are type III and possibly type IV; that the antibody is a precipitating one which combines with antigens in moderate excess; that severe edema begins within 4 hours, peaks at 8 hours, and generally resolves within 24 hours; that the site of the reaction is the peripheral gas-exchanging tissues, usually the alveoli and respiratory bronchioles; that after bronchial challenge, systemic and pulmonary reactions occur within 4 to 6 hours, mainly in the alveoli, although asthma may infrequently occur; and that the clinical aspects include cough and dyspnea markedly out of proportion to the benign findings on physical examination. Fever, chills, weight loss, malaise, and rales are the outstanding clinical features; x-ray studies reveal miliary infiltrates that, over a protracted period of time, can lead to diffuse fibrosis, particularly of the upper lobes.

Similar clinical response associated with sensitization to organic dusts, whose sources are multiple and often occupationally related, includes malt workers' lung, maple bark strippers' disease, and pituitary snuff-takers' lung. The list of these disease states will undoubtedly expand and parallel the development of precise laboratory techniques necessary for diagnosis.

CHEMICAL MEDIATORS

It has been postulated of late that the inefficacy of an antihistamine drug in relieving all of the symptoms of an allergic reaction can be ascribed to the multiplicity of substances involved in the reactions. It is currently believed that antigen-antibody reactions involve several chemical substances, e.g., histamine, bradykinin, serotonin, SRS-A, and the newly reported eosinophilic chemotactic factor of anaphylaxis (ECF-A). Each, it has been said, has the power to mediate the responses of smooth muscle contraction or increasing vascular permeability, both distinguishing characteristics of immediate hypersensitivity.

Histamine has been studied more extensively than all of the mediators. It is found chiefly in the granules of mammalian mast cells of perivascular connective tissue. Stored by electrostatic binding to a heparin-protein complex, histamine is released by the interaction at cell surfaces of human reaginic antibody with its specific antigen. It should be noted that this kind of immunologic release of histamine (from either the rat mast cell or the human polymorphonuclear leukocyte) does not involve the discharge of other intracellular molecules.

Convincing evidence is lacking that serotonin, also found in rat mast cells, is a contributor to man's immediate hypersensitivity reaction. Found abundantly in the platelets of some animal species, serotonin, like histamine, exists in its final form in the primary target cell and is released as a result of a relevant immunologic event.

Peptides formed by enzymatic action of kallikrein on the alpha globulin plasma substrate, kininogen, are called *kinins.* The plasma kallikrein builds up bradykinin (the nonapeptide) and tissue kallikrein elaborates kallidin (the decapeptide). Kallidin's complexity is rapidly reduced by plasma aminopeptidase. Enzyme activation, therefore, is necessary to the operation of the kinin system.

Any change in surface charge will start the enzyme system because the first protein to trigger the pathway is the Hageman factor, which also sets off the clotting sequence. Once the kinin cascade has begun, it is necessary to learn whether the activity is primary or secondary: the result of an immunologic event or secondary to nonspecific tissue injury. Either way, it is possible for the activation to aggravate the response and cause further tissue injury. Perhaps the future development of improved bradykinin-kallikrein assay methods will provide more definitive answers as to whether kinin in an anaphylactic reaction is caused by a specific immunoglobulin or results from some secondary response.

SRS-A is an acidic lipid whose structure is not known. Among the known facts are these: (1) It is released from the lungs of allergic human subjects upon challenge with specific pollen antigen. (2) Bronchiolar smooth muscle is highly sensitive to the contracting features of preparations containing SRS-A. (3) In controlling allergic bronchospasm, antihistamines are of limited value. (4) The antifilarial agent diethylcarbamazine can reduce the severity of asthma. It has been found to produce active inhibition of the immunologic release of SRS-A in the rat, this without being an end organ antagonist of SRS-A.

Altounyan, an allergic British pharmacologist, inspired a hunt for substances that would block the release of SRS-A. He was challenged with antigen, histamine, and methacholine; he noted that khellin was a safeguard against antigen, but not against the other two substances. He urged his colleagues to synthesize structurally related compounds of khellin. Thus was developed the drug we know in America as cromolyn sodium (Aarane, Intal) and abroad as disodium cromoglycate. Cromolyn sodium, proved effective against aerosol challenge tests, apparently by the stabilization of the mast cell wall membrane and by inhibiting the release of SRS-A and histamine, is now available as a unique pharmacologic agent for the prevention of asthma.

Studies demonstrate that the direct release of SRS-A and of histamine is mediated by IgE, and that diethylcarbamazine blocks the pathways leading to the release of both.

Cyclic AMP

The action of adenylcyclase on adenosine triphosphate (ATP) forms cyclic AMP, or adenosine 3':5'-cyclic monophosphate. Although the effects of cyclic AMP occur without its destruction, it is quickly inactivated by a phosphodiesterase, which opens the phosphate-ribose ring, yielding 5'-AMP. Either by increasing or decreasing cyclic AMP, an extensive number of hormones have been found in recent years to have important effects on target organs. These hormones have included ACTH, thyroxine, and glucagon among others. For example, increased cyclic AMP levels in the liver, reacting to glucagon, have been found to increase glycogenolysis and gluconeogenesis; the effect on the heart of catecholamine with elevated cyclic AMP brings about an increased ionotropic reaction. On the other hand, decreased lipolysis results when decreased cyclic AMP levels in fatty tissue are acted upon by insulin. There is evidence, also, that agents increasing intracellular levels of cyclic AMP also inhibit histamine and SRS-A release. Thus, methylxanthine derivatives such as theophylline, synergistic with beta adrenergic compounds (epinephrine, metaproterenol, ephedrine, terbutaline), benefit asthmatic patients because both beta adrenergic agents and theophyllines enhance the accumulation of cyclic AMP.

The Prostaglandins

The prostaglandins constitute another category of substances, knowledge of the action of which is currently limited. It is postulated that these agents have a probable role in anaphylaxis. Chemically, we know that they are two hydrocarbon chains connected by a cyclopentane ring. Their synthesis is attributed principally to essential fatty acids, both lipid and water soluble. Variations in the pentane ring determine the identity of four prostaglandin groups—PGI, PGF, PGA, and PGB. Differences in the biologic properties are related to the structure and include vasodilation and vasoconstriction, contraction or relaxation of smooth and cardiac muscle, water and salt diuresis, fever, and wheal-and-flare skin reactions. The complex mechanism of action and release of these compounds is believed to involve adenylcyclase and the membrane binding of calcium. Many prostaglandin properties and their formation from precursor substances are capable of inhibition by indomethacin and salicylates. That they may have a role in immediate hypersensitivity and the pathophysiology of asthma is suggested by their probable relationship to adenylcyclase and to certain biologic properties.

INFLAMMATION

Inflammation is the response of nature to cell injury or destruction by viral and bacterial causes. It also can result from provocation by heat, cold, radiation, chemicals, or mechanical trauma. Necrotic products of dead cells also can cause the response. The specific involved area or injurious agent notwithstanding, there occur tissue adjustments involving blood vessels and fluid and other cellular constituents of the blood as well as surrounding connective tissue. Increased permeability enhances the outpouring of inflammatory fluid into the injured tissue.

Blood flow slows, and often stops, with the concentration of red cells in the capillaries. Ultimately, the migration of white blood cells from vessel walls to the inflammatory focus results from peripheral movement of capillary white cells. It is conjectured that polymorphonuclear leukocytes are the first to migrate, followed by mononuclear cells—monocytes, lymphocytes, and plasma cells. Vascular dilatation, fluid exudation, and an accumulation of inflammatory white cells are necessary features of a true acute inflammatory reaction.

The result of increased vascularity in the injured areas, redness is the signal of inflammation. The production of exudative fluid causes localized swelling. Further current opinion has it that, following an injury, cells react by discharging their components or manufacturing during their dissolution endogenous substances guiding the events of inflammatory origin. In certain regions of the cells, particularly the mitochondrial lysosomes, it is possible to locate such chemical mediators as histamine and serotonin. Histamine is generally accepted as the principal chemical mediator. It does not sustain vascular response, but it probably does initiate it. Histamine is found in two types of cells, the mast cells and the basophilic leukocytes. Following injury, two states of changes in permeability occur: an early stage caused by the liberation of histamine, and a later sustained stage independent of histamine action.

There are inflammations that are completed within hours or days; others remain for weeks. Kinins and polypeptides are some of the chemicals held responsible for sustained vascular reaction. Bradykinin is one of the more active agents for dilating human blood vessels. The action of plasma kinin-forming enzymes—kallikrein—on plasma globulins forms the bradykinin, the reaction probably occurring in the interstitial tissue spaces. Believed to exert its effect on the closest blood vessels, cellular injury also takes place. Following the inactivation of the epinephrine precursors by enzymatic mechanisms (especially of monamine oxidase), the vessels dilate, the increased hydrostatic capillary pressure resulting from increased blood flow through their distended lumina leading to exudation of plasma. It has appeared likely that the destruction of leukocytes at the injury site may yield other substances to help maintain altered permeability.

Leukocytes proceed from the smallest vessels to tissue spaces during normal cellular life. Such migration, however, is greatly accelerated during injury. Microscopic investigation reveals large numbers of leukocytes at the injury site, particularly following necrosis. Because these cells are phagocytic, it is currently believed that migration and the tendency toward aggregation are defense mechanisms whose role is the destruction and neutralization of the injury-related agents. When circulation slows in the injured area, leukocytes cling to the endothelial lining, soon attaching themselves firmly. Transport from the small blood vessels is then provided for the leukocytes by pseudopods protruding into the endothelial cells and wriggling through the wall by ameboid movement.

Chemotaxis is said to be a positive directional response to a chemical stimulus, the latter appearing to direct leukocytes and monocytes toward the guilty agent and the damaged cells. Stimuli may emanate from the agents themselves or may be produced by the injured cells. Prevalence of polymorphonuclear leukocytes marks the early stage of nearly all inflammation. This is especially true if bacterial infection is the source. Mononuclear cells predominate over the polymorphonuclear leukocytes when the response subsides. There are some bacterial infections, however, in which monocytes have the primary contact, polymorphonuclear leukocytes appearing to be transiently present in the infection's early stages. This is especially true in brucellosis, typhoid fever, and tuberculosis.

PHAGOCYTOSIS

With the support of monocytes and mononuclear phagocytes, marshaling the polymorphonuclear leukocytes is the initial defensive phenomenon in pyogenic infection. Phagocytosis is defined as the ingestion and resultant immobilization of
foreign material including bacterial, parasitic, or necrotic tissue from such material.

Phagocytosis is accomplished chiefly by the polymorphonuclear leukocytes.
Opsonification of microbes by gamma globulin and complement C3 make these
microbes more susceptible to phagocytes. The opsonized microorganism is ingested
by the phagocyte. Degranulation follows and hydrogen peroxide generated by the
phagocytes brings microbial death. The failure of any of the foregoing steps subjects
the patient to increased frequency of severe pyogenic infections.

Chronic Granulomatous Disease in Children
(Chediak-Higashi Syndrome)

It would be well to interject here some comments on a disease with defective phagocytosis and dermatologic manifestations, chronic granulomatous disease of children.
This disease is X-linked, inherited, fatal, and characterized by frequent infections
and septic granulomatous lesions in skin, lymph nodes, and lungs. To identify defective cellular functions leading to low hydrogen peroxide production levels, the
nitroblue tetrazolium test (NBT) is suggested.

IMMUNOLOGIC PROCESSES IN INFECTION

Much immunity against infection is, of course, innate. Immunity to certain microorganisms and toxins, however, occurs following contact with the antigens in the
microorganism. At any given time, immunity will depend on environmental factors.

Demonstrating that innate resistance varies among races and species are genetic
traits associated with resistance to malaria, such as those of sickle cell anemia,
hemoglobin C, glucose-6-phosphate, dehydrogenase deficiency, and thalassemia.
Natural immunity to certain organisms as a result of their transplacental passage
from the mother is present at birth. Immunity occurring after infection may be
temporary or permanent.

By influencing phagocytosis, neutralizing toxins, or inhibiting the organism,
immunoglobulin antibodies play a major role in the body's defense against bacteria.
Antibodies against viruses are effective by means of neutralization of the virus-
infecting cells. Antibody cannot interfere with intracellular duplication. It can be
effective only outside the cell. Almost always, immunity to viruses is lasting. Present
in most helminthic infections is peripheral eosinophilia. One important feature of
these infections is the increased frequency of IgE antibodies against parasites, which
can be demonstrated by immediate wheal-and-flare reactions to intradermal extracts
of worms.

Cellular and humoral immunity interaction is demonstrated by the various stages
of leprosy. Cellular immune mechanisms, not antibodies, eliminate the leprosy
bacillus. Although this bacillus is not killed by antibody, it can stimulate that antibody against its constituent antigens. Leprosy bacillus growth and proliferation are

controlled in tuberculous leprosy because there is considerable specific cell-mediated immune activity to the bacillus during this phase of the disease; but in the downgrading to the lepromatous stage, there is a total failure of this specific cell-mediated immune reaction. Skin biopsy shows uncontrolled bacillus proliferation. There is no failure of antibody production. Divided tolerance is achieved because the patient now is specifically responsive to antibody production, but unresponsive to cell-mediated immune responses. The test indicated is the intradermal injection of killed whole leprosy bacilli; the reaction is negative in lepromatous leprosy, possessing as it does an immunologic lack of response.

The status of host and the strength of the noxious agent have their impact on the modification of the inflammatory reaction. Relevant to the reaction's severity are both the strength and amount of the noxious agent and the duration of exposure to the attacking agent. Whether or not an infection will occur is generally determined by the amount of bacteria involved, some bacterial and chemical agents being more virulent than others. Rarely is focal necrosis of tissue caused by viruses. Rather, there is an interstitial reaction evidenced by edema with a mononuclear infiltrate as opposed to polymorphonuclear response characteristic of pyogenic bacteria. A hemorrhagic inflammation is produced by rickettsiae.

Lowering of the mechanical barriers enhances the spread of infection. An offending agent's ability to invade the tissue depends upon a number of factors. One is lymphatic blockage, characteristic of staphylococcal infections, that elicits fibrin thrombus formation. In streptococcal infections the reverse is true, enzymes producing lysin, which dissolves ground substances and fibrin and which prevents organisms from entrapment.

Caused by clot formation, blood vessel blockage is another of nature's attempts to minimize the dissemination of infectious agents. Enzymes such as the hyaluronidases have been found to hydrolize mucopolysaccharides of connective tissue ground substance, thus rendering it more fluid and permeable. They are elaborated by staphylococci, streptococci, and clostridia.

The Host's Defense

The age, general health, and nutrition of the host are very important to its ability to counter the invading organism and to determine the extent of inflammation. Generally, the younger patient's ability to withstand injuries and reduce damage is greater than an older person's, in whom preexisting blood vessel diseases and dietary deficiencies are greatly significant. Protein-depleted cells are more vulnerable to noxious agents. Naturally occurring and acquired antibodies will modify the host's resistance to infection. Antibodies coat bacteria, making them more susceptible to phagocytosis. Diabetes mellitus and certain other metabolic diseases increase the susceptibility of older persons to severe inflammatory reactions. Hormones, such as glucocorticoids, influence inflammatory reactions by their effect on lymphocyte response. An adequate supply of blood increases the patient's resistance to infection and gives him greater ability to contain offending agents.

Inflammation may be significantly modified by the location of the injury because compact tissues have a tendency to resist the spread of infection. Lungs, subcutaneous fibrous tissues, and other loose tissues permit the spread of invasive agents because of their cleavage planes.

In patients with leukemia, lymphoreticular malignancies, or neoplasms in general, the increased use of immunosuppressive agents and steroids has increased opportunistic infections. Many of the opportunistic pathogens are known to normally inhabit humans. In the immunologically incompetent patient, however, severe — even fatal — infections can occur.

The reader is referred to Chapter 9 for a detailed discussion of the bacteriologic and antibiotic considerations in pulmonary disease.

SUMMARY

In this chapter, attempts have been made to focus on some of the experiments of nature; an understanding of the mechanisms of allergy-immunology is central to the treatment of the sick patient, pulmonary or otherwise. We have touched only briefly on the fundamental considerations of the nature of antibodies, the humoral and cellular bases of immunity, and the applications of this information for the prevention and management of human disease states. Good and Fisher placed all of this information in perspective when they stated, "The very existence of man as a consequence of our development in a veritable sea of potentially hostile fungi, bacteria, and viruses is necessarily dependent on a recognition of foreignness. Our heritage . . . demanded . . . a vital need for powerful mechanisms of homeostasis. The requirement for containment and management of these two powerful countercurrents places immunobiology in the center of all biology. This, in turn, assures its significance for student and practitioner alike" [4, p. 137].

REFERENCES

1. Bruton, O. D. Agammaglobulinemia. *Pediatrics* 9, 1952, p. 722.
2. Cooper, H. R., Polley, M. J., and Muller-Everhard, H. J. Biology of Complement. In M. Samter et al. (eds.), *Immunological Diseases* (2nd ed.), Vol. I. Boston: Little, Brown, 1971.
3. Gell, P. G. H., and Coombs, R. R. A. *Clinical Aspects of Immunology* (2nd ed.). Philadelphia: Davis, 1968.
4. Good, R. A., and Fisher, D. W. *Immunology*. Stamford, Conn.: Sinauer, 1971.

SELECTED BIBLIOGRAPHY
Bellanti, J. A. *Immunology*. Philadelphia: Saunders, 1971.
Fudenberg, H. H., et al. *Primary Immunodeficiencies*. Report of a World Health Organization Committee. *Pediatrics,* 47, 1971, p. 927.
Stiehm, E. R., and Fulginiti, V. A. *Immunologic Disorders in Infants and Children*. Philadelphia: Saunders, 1973.

Terrence Murphy

Microbiology: Epidemiology, Diagnosis, and Therapeutics as Applied to Respiratory Therapy

9

The patient with significant pulmonary disease is at high risk of contracting infection while in the hospital. To understand the reasons for this, in overview, one can represent man's defenses against infection by barriers (Table 9-1). Our outermost and most clearly delineated barriers to intruders from the outside world are the skin and mucous membranes. Hospitalized patients tend to have major breaches in this line of defense in the form of intravenous lines, urinary catheters, and surgical wounds; the lung disease patient is also likely to have a tracheostomy or endotracheal tube in place. In addition, there is a less definite but vastly important inner barrier that is composed of constitutional factors affected by underlying illness, debilitation, and drugs administered to the patient.

This chapter will discuss the factors that make the pulmonary disease patient susceptible to infection, the bacteriology of infective agents to which he is most susceptible, and the method of spread of these agents. Environmental sources of infection will be reviewed, and steps to minimize such threats will be outlined. Finally, prevention and treatment of specific infections frequently encountered in this group of patients will be discussed.

MECHANICAL DEFENSE MECHANISMS: THE BREACH OF NATURAL BARRIERS

The skin (integument) and specialized anatomy of the various orifices (e.g., nose, mouth, urethra) provide an effective barrier between one's internal and external environments. The patient with lung disease usually has multiple breaches in this barrier.

Table 9-1. Infectious Risks in Patients with Lung Disease

Mechanical: Breach of Natural Barriers
  Tracheostomy
  Endotracheal tube
  Intravenous and intraarterial lines
  Urinary catheter
  Surgical wounds

Constitutional Factors: Impairment of Host Defenses
  Inactivity
  Pain
  Hypoxia
  Chronic pulmonary disease
  Heart disease
  Malignancy
  Immunodeficiency

Drugs
  Sedative } Inactivity
  Analgesic
  Immunosuppressive agents
  Antimicrobial agents

Infectious Agents in the Environment
  Contaminated equipment and furnishings
  Personnel
  Patient crowding
  Patient's normal flora

Intravenous lines are so common that they are often taken for granted, but improper insertion or maintenance may lead to bacteremia. Long central intravenous catheters have been especially troublesome and require careful aseptic technique. Total parenteral nutrition (TPN) lines have been the source of major infectious complications. Fungemia, often fatal, is common in this setting and may be due to three collaborative factors: breaks in aseptic technique, a solution hospitable to fungal growth, and the development of metabolic changes that adversely affect host defenses (hypophosphatemia and metabolic acidosis have been demonstrated). A sporadic but life-threatening complication of intravenous therapy is bacterial contamination of the solution. This source should be considered in the patient who suddenly develops high fever without obvious cause.

The same fundamental principles apply to urinary catheters. Like the skin, the normal urethra with its closely apposed mucous membrane walls provides an effective barrier to the outside world. Catheter-associated infection and subsequent bacteremia correlate with improper insertion and maintenance, and the infectious risks are directly proportional to the length of time the catheter is in place. Frequently, the catheter is unnecessary. Indications for its insertion or continued use should be routinely reviewed.

Because alterations of the normal anatomy of the respiratory tract are necessary with mechanical ventilation, a brief review of the defensive anatomy and physiology of this organ system is in order (Figure 9-1). The nose and nasopharynx create a

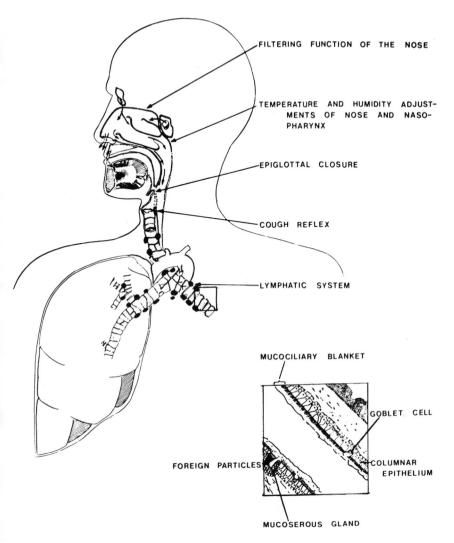

FILTERING FUNCTION OF THE NOSE

TEMPERATURE AND HUMIDITY ADJUST-
MENTS OF NOSE AND NASO-
PHARYNX

EPIGLOTTAL CLOSURE

COUGH REFLEX

LYMPHATIC SYSTEM

MUCOCILIARY BLANKET

GOBLET CELL

COLUMNAR
EPITHELIUM

FOREIGN PARTICLES

MUCOSEROUS GLAND

Figure 9-1. Defensive anatomy and physiology of the respiratory tract.

semipermeable barrier between the tracheobronchial tree and the ambient air. Particles greater than 10 μ (or one one-hundredth of a millimeter), such as dusts or pollen, are filtered out at this point. Furthermore, major adjustments in the temperature and humidity of inspired air are made here by the large surface area and rich blood supply of the mucosal surfaces of the nose and nasopharynx. One need only venture outside on a cold winter's day to know that these adjustments can be made over a wide range of environmental extremes. The relatively small surface area and scant blood supply of the tracheobronchial tree do not allow anything but the smallest of temperature or humidity adjustments once inspired air has reached it.

Particulate matter that does reach the tracheobronchial tree must be less than 10μ in diameter. Particles between 2 and 10 μ are deposited in the bronchi or bronchioles; those less than 2 μ usually reach the alveoli. Particles reaching the tracheobronchial tree are normally ejected by a highly efficient cleansing mechanism. Initially, they become trapped in a blanket of mucus secreted by goblet cells and the submucosal glands (see Chapter 5). The cilia (hair-like structures) of the epithelium project through the mucous layer and sweep foreign material upward to the subglottic space, from which they are expelled by coughing.

The endotracheal tube breaches many of these anatomic barriers and paralyzes others. Inspired air is no longer filtered or adjusted to proper temperature or humidity because the nose and nasopharynx are bypassed. In addition, the protective mechanism of epiglottic closure is lost. In spite of the most careful artificial adjustments by humidifiers and heaters, some drying and increased viscosity of the mucociliary blanket may occur, and particles are swept upward less effectively. Increased concentrations of inspired oxygen aggravate this drying effect. Finally, the cough reflex is lost.

Tracheostomy exposes the patient to all the infectious hazards seen with endotracheal intubation. Even though the epiglottis is not kept mechanically open, it becomes functionally impaired, allowing communication between the oropharynx and the trachea. On top of all this, the tracheostomy patient also faces the risk of wound infection.

Because of his illness, the patient is susceptible to multiple assaults on his integumentary barrier. In addition, such assaults are frequently in an emergency setting where appropriate aseptic technique must be sacrificed in order to save his life. In such a setting, the potential for infectious complications is greater than ever.

CONSTITUTIONAL FACTORS PREDISPOSING TO INFECTION

Inactivity is the rule in the seriously ill patient. We begin here in the discussion of constitutional factors because inactivity is common to virtually all patients, and it can indirectly affect the course of many infectious processes. Its major cause is, of course, the underlying conditions being treated. It is aggravated, however, by factors often within control of the therapist. Pain will limit movement and requires the judicious use of analgesic agents. On the other hand, excessive analgesia and/or sedation will promote equally serious inactivity. The postoperative patient with, let us say, a laparotomy can illustrate both situations. Incisional pain prevents him from turning, sighing, and coughing. The addition of excessive amounts of analgesic agents will make this patient sleepy and even less active. In addition, opiates directly decrease ventilatory drive.

The infectious complications of inactivity are numerous and include the breakdown of skin with development of decubiti, with risk of subsequent bacteremia or osteomyelitis, as well as the deposition of calcium from bone in the urinary tract causing obstruction and infection. Pulmonary complications include venous stasis and thrombosis with subsequent pulmonary embolism. Although not as a rule infectious, such emboli can frequently mimic pulmonary infection and be followed by pneumonitis. The most common pulmonary complication of inactivity is atelectasis, in which segmental collapse is caused by the inability to clear mucus from the tracheobronchial tree. The atelectatic segment is hospitable territory for infection to begin, because clearance mechanisms are inoperative.

Chronic cardiopulmonary disease, present in the majority of the patients under discussion, predisposes to infection in a fashion analogous to atelectasis. Architectural alterations caused by pulmonary diseases such as bronchiectasis, emphysema, tumor, and various pneumoconioses can prevent adequate clearance from affected areas. Likewise, the pulmonary vascular changes associated with certain cardiac diseases predispose to infection. These include congenital types with left-to-right shunts and rheumatic disease with mitral stenosis, but pulmonary vascular changes caused by left ventricular failure of any etiology are all that is needed.

The patient frequently has impairment of the immunologic systems that makes him susceptible to certain types of infection. An antigen is a substance foreign to the host that is capable of stimulating the development of specific antibody. Antigens may be soluble substances (toxins, proteins) or particulate (microorganisms, tissue-cells). Antibody is an immunoglobulin with a specific amino acid sequence that allows it to recognize and attach to a specific antigen. There are five antibody classes known in man, and they are classified as immunoglobulins IgG, IgM, IgA, IgE, and IgD. IgG is most abundant in the serum and is the major immunoglobulin. IgA is known principally as a surface immunoglobulin, being found in highest concentration in the mucosa of the tracheobronchial tree and the gastrointestinal tract. IgM, among other functions, probably helps agglutinate particulate matter. IgE is intimately involved in allergic conditions such as asthma (see Chapters 8 and 14). The function of IgD in man is unknown. Antibodies are produced by plasma cells which in turn develop from so-called B lymphocytes. This entire system is referred to as the humoral or B cell system. A typical sequence of events occurs as follows: An antigen, in this case a bacterium, is able to overcome the physical barriers of the nasal turbinates, mucociliary blanket, and cough mechanism and impacts on the bronchial mucosa. IgA, there in abundance, recognizes the antigen and complexes with it. The microorganism is then destroyed by phagocytic ("cell eating") cells such as polymorphonuclear cells, histiocytes, and (if it reaches the alveolus) alveolar macrophages.

Some invaders are handled by a different immunologic system called the cellular or T cell system. Here, the response is not as immediate as in the humoral system (hence, the old term "delayed hypersensitivity"). Upon initial encounter with the invader, specific lymphocytes derived from the thymus gland (hence, T lymphocytes) are programmed to recognize it and continue to reproduce for years. These are known as *memory cells*. Upon subsequent encounter, the invader is recognized, and rapid proliferation of specific T cells is initiated. This is called *blast transformation.* These activated lymphocytes migrate to the point of entry and attack the invader with secreted substances (lymphokines) that paralyze the invader and stimulate phagocytic cells and cytotoxic substances (such as complement) which then kill the invader.

Most bacteria are processed by the humoral system and most viruses, fungi, and *Mycobacterium tuberculosis* are processed by the cellular system. The final, phagocytic step is common to both systems.

Impairment of humoral immunity, or selective absence or abnormality of immunoglobulins, increases the risk of bacterial infection (Table 9–2). Selective IgA deficiency is associated with pulmonary bacterial infection; its cause is unknown. Liver disease and plasma cell malignancy (such as multiple myeloma) are both associated with decreased immunoglobulin production and bacterial infection. On the other hand, the link between protein-wasting syndromes (nephrotic syndrome and protein-losing enteropathy) and bacterial infection is immunoglobulin loss.

Defects in cellular immunity are apparent in many neoplastic diseases, but especially the lymphoma group (Hodgkin's disease). In such diseases, the patient is more susceptible to viral, fungal, and tubercular infection. Likewise, certain immunosuppressive drugs frequently used in organ transplantation, in cancer chemotherapy, and in the management of certain connective tissue diseases (lupus erythematosis) affect the cellular system. These drugs include cyclophosphamide, azothioprine, antithymocyte globulin, and probably corticosteroids.

Phagocytic dysfunction, when it occurs, affects both systems. Disorders such as aplastic anemia and leukemias and exposure to excessive ionizing radiation and cytotoxic drugs (alkalating agents) can drastically reduce the level of polymorphonuclear leukocytes and inhibit phagocytosis. For a detailed discussion of immunology, see Chapter 8.

MICROBIOLOGY

Appropriate treatment of infection requires identification of the infecting agent. Definitive identification is usually made by culture, but the therapist frequently must make a treatment decision long before culture results are available from the laboratory. Relevant infectious agents may be classified as bacteria, viruses, fungi, and protozoa (Table 9–3).

Gram staining of sputum (Table 9–4) is the cornerstone of early bacterial diagnosis. Combined with clinical, radiologic, and (occasionally) histologic information, this procedure provides valuable early bacteriologic diagnosis in most cases. Gram's stain provides information about both the morphology and the staining characteristics of bacteria. With this information, basic classification can be carried out. H. C. J. Gram discovered the technique that bears his name almost a century ago, and although the empirical distinction between the two groups has proved very useful, only recently has the mechanism of this procedure begun to be understood. Gram positive organisms, which take up and keep the original violet stain, and gram negative organisms, which lose the original stain when washed with acid alcohol and take up the pink counterstain, appear to have differing permeability

Table 9-2. Abnormalities Causing Immunologic Dysfunction

Humoral Immunity (B cell)	Cellular Immunity (T cell)	Phagocytic Action
Agammaglobulinemia	Lymphomas	Aplastic anemia
Bacterial infection (except agent of tuberculosis and other rarer intracellular bacteria)	Drugs used in organ transplants, cancer chemotherapy, and connective tissue diseases	Leukemia
IgA deficiency	Azothioprine	Ionizing irradiation
Liver disease	Cyclophosphamide	Cytotoxic drugs
Plasma cell malignancy	Antilymphocyte globulin	
Nephrotic syndrome	(?) Corticosteroids	
Protein-losing enteropathy	Viruses	
Splenectomy	Fungi	
Sickle cell disease	*Mycobacterium tuberculosis*	
	Nocardia species	

Table 9–3. Common Respiratory Pathogens in Approximate Order of Frequency

	Gram Positive	Gram Negative	Cell Wall–Deficient
Bacteria	*Streptococcus pneumoniae*	*Hemophilus influenzae*	*Mycoplasma pneumoniae*
	Staphylococcus aureus *	*Klebsiella pneumoniae*	Acid-Fast
	Streptococcus faecalis	*Pseudomonas aeruginosa* *	*Mycobacterium tuberculosis* *
	(enterococcus)	*Serratia* species*	*Nocardia asteroides* *
Viruses		Rhinovirus	Varicella virus*
		Adenovirus	Herpes simplex virus*
		Respiratory syncytial virus	Cytomegalovirus*
Fungi		*Candida albicans* *	*Histoplasma capsulatum* (Ohio Valley)
		Aspergillus species*	*Coccidioides immitis* (Southwest U.S.A.)
Protozoa		*Pneumocystis carinii* *	

*Seen most frequently in debilitated or immunosuppressed hosts.

Table 9-4. Sputum Stain for Microbiologic Diagnosis

Diagnosis	Gram's Stain	Other Stains
Bacteria	Gram positive or gram negative cocci, rods, or intermediate forms	Acid-fast stain for *Mycobacterium tuberculosis* and *Nocardia* species
Mycoplasma	No predominant organism; polymorphonuclear cells abundant	
Virus	No predominant organism	Giemsa stain may demonstrate giant cells (mumps, cytomegalovirus)
Fungus	Gram stain usually of little benefit; yeast and hyphal forms usually stain deeply gram positive	

characteristics in the cell wall. These cell wall differences help determine the microorganism's virulence and susceptibility to antibiotic agents.

There are two major morphologic types of bacteria: spherical cocci and rodlike bacilli. Some organisms are intermediate and are called coccobacillary or pleomorphic. Certain cocci aggregate in characteristic fashion—in pairs, chains, or clumps—and this aids in identification. Likewise, the distinction between plump and thin bacilli can be valuable.

At this point, one can make an initial bacteriologic classification (Table 9–5).

Acid-fast stains of sputum should be routinely performed in the investigation of pulmonary infection, because tuberculosis must always be tested for.

When, in the investigation of a patient with an apparent pulmonary infection, the stained sputum shows no predominant organism but shows many polymorpho-

Table 9–5. Initial Classification of Bacteria from Gram's Stain, with Some Characteristics

---

Gram Positive
  Cocci: Common causes of pulmonary infection
    S. pneumoniae (agent of pneumococcal pneumonia): usually in pairs; capsule (nonstaining rim) often seen
    Other streptococci: often in chains of various lengths
    Staphylococci: often in clumps, like grape clusters
  Bacilli: Rare causes of pulmonary infection
    Corynebacterium (agent of diphtheria)
    Bacillus anthracis (agent of anthrax)
    Listeria monocytogenes: rare cause of pulmonary infection
    Bacillus species: as a rule nonvirulent

Gram Negative
  Cocci: Rare causes of pulmonary infection
    Neisseria species ("biscuit-shaped," in pairs): normal mouth flora
    Yersinia pestis (agent of plague): rare cause of pneumonia
  Coccobacilli (pleomorphic): Common causes of pulmonary infection
    Hemophilus influenzae: considerable variation in shape
  Bacilli: Common causes of pulmonary infection; "rods" that all look much the same:
    Escherichia coli, Pseudomonas, Klebsiella (large, nonstaining capsule often seen),
    Proteus, Serratia

---

nuclear leukocytes, chances are strong that one is dealing with *Mycoplasma pneumoniae* infection. These bacteria possess no cell wall, pick up no stain, and hence remain invisible with routine techniques.

The sputum from a patient with viral infection is helpful in ruling out a superimposed bacterial process. The sputum usually contains lymphocytes and/or mononuclear cells in contrast to the polymorphonuclear leukocytes seen with *Mycoplasma* infection. Sometimes one can find virus-associated giant cells with Giemsa staining, but this procedure is not done routinely.

One should not attempt to diagnose fungal infection of the lung on the basis of Gram's stain alone. Frequently, fungal pneumonia is accompanied by a negative sputum; moreover, demonstration of yeast forms in the sputum may not be clinically significant. Yeast forms, especially those of *Candida* species, are coccal in shape, two to three times larger than coccal forms of bacteria, and stain a very deep violet. Frequently, budding can be demonstrated.

Nocardia, long thought to be a fungus but now classified as a bacterium, has a distinct appearance with Gram's stain. It consists of varying length chains of gram positive rods. The chains may be long and folded over each other, and individual cells may be seen alone. Additional help in identification is the fact that this organism is somewhat acid-fast, the younger cells holding the dye more tenaciously than the older ones.

ENVIRONMENTAL SOURCES OF INFECTION

In addition to the numerous external and internal threats already discussed, the hospitalized patient is surrounded by many potential sources of infection in his en-

Table 9-6. Modes of Spread of Infectious Agents

Source	Principal Infectious Agents
Hands	Staphylococci, especially when paronychia or other infection is present Gram negative enteric organisms (fecal-oral route) — diarrheal illness Hepatitis A virus (fecal-oral route)
Nose	Staphylococci (usually no clinical infection)
Human droplet aerosols	Respiratory viruses *Mycoplasma pneumoniae* *Mycobacterium tuberculosis* *Staphylococcus aureus* (?)
Blood and blood products	Hepatitis B virus Cytomegalovirus
Water-containing equipment (including ventilators, humidifiers, sinks)	Gram negative rods, especially *Pseudomonas aeruginosa* and other species, *Serratia,* and *Alcaligenes*

vironment (Table 9-6). Personnel, equipment, and often unsuspected materials may be sources or transmittors of infection.

As hospital medicine has become more sophisticated, the number of personnel who come in contact with the patient has multiplied. This is especially true in special care units or areas that adopt a team approach, inevitably exposing the patient to a large number of specialized personnel. Personnel infect patients, often carrying a microorganism from one patient to another, most often with their hands. All sorts of microorganisms can be transmitted in this fashion, but most frequently bacteria are implicated, and staphylococci are the most common organism. Paronychia, abscess, or cellulitis are particularly infectious. Diarrheal outbreaks and miniepidemics of hepatitis have been caused by the fecal contamination of hands. Nasal carriage is also a problem, the usual organism being *Staphylococcus aureus.* Contamination by droplet aerosol is a major mode of spread of respiratory viruses, *Mycoplasma pneumoniae* infections, tuberculosis, and probably *Staphylococcus aureus.*

Another mode of transmission is by way of fomites, inert objects that may harbor microorganisms. Instruments and material coming in contact with multiple patients fall into this group. Multiple-dose vials have been the source of bacteremia, and occasionally a carelessly used stethoscope may act as a fome.

Respiratory equipment has been repeatedly implicated as a source of infection. In fact, the dramatic change over the past decade in the nature of the infecting organism is due in large measure to the machinery. Virtually every known bacterium of clinical significance has been implicated in ventilator-induced infection, but for some very good reasons, certain gram-negative rods have become dominant. These organisms, *Pseudomonas, Serratia*, and *Alcaligenes*, thrive in a warm, moist environment. Humidifiers and nebulizers are common sources of cross-infection with such organisms because the water and other liquids in them are contaminated from the

Table 9-7. Infectiousness of Various Pneumonias

	Infectiousness	Precautions*
Bacteria		
Streptococcus pneumoniae	-	-
Staphylococcus aureus	+	Mask, gown, gloves
Hemophilus influenzae	-	-
Klebsiella pneumoniae	-	-
Pseudomonas aeruginosa	-	-
Serratia marcescens	-	-
Mycoplasma pneumoniae	+	Mask
Mycobacterium tuberculosis	+	Mask, gown, gloves
Nocardia asteroides	-	-
Viruses		
Influenza virus	+	Vaccine
Varicella virus	-	-
Herpesvirus	-	-
Cytomegalovirus	-	-
Fungi		
Candida albicans	-	-
Aspergillus species	-	-
Histoplasma capsulatum	-	-
Coccidioides immitis	-	-
Protozoa		
Pneumocystis carinii	-	-

*Beyond those taken routinely (see section, Prophylaxis).

environment or another patient, and they multiply rapidly in this hospitable environment. Room humidifiers have a comparable infectious potential.

Ventilators and intermittent positive pressure devices in themselves do not produce an aerosol and thereby do not pose as dramatic an infectious threat. However, condensation of the patient's expired gas does cause pooling in the tubing of the equipment and predisposes to the same infectious complications.

Gas pipelines have been documented as sources of infection. Here the number of organisms is usually small, and the infection threat is minimal. Heating and air-conditioning ducts have been likewise incriminated. Other aqueous environments that are potential infectious sources include sinks, whose traps may become contaminated, typically by *Pseudomonas*. Also implicated are soap dispensers, aqueous disinfectants, and jellies and creams, even those containing antibiotic agents. Blood and blood products may transmit hepatitis B virus or cytomegalovirus.

In considering environmental sources of infection for the hospitalized patient, one should remember that the distinction between pathogenic and nonpathogenic agents is blurred because of alterations in host defenses. Therefore, scrupulous attention to all environmental sources is mandatory.

A final environmental source that is especially relevant to the debilitated patient is the patient's own flora. Gram-negative rods, anaerobic bacteria, and *Candida* normally inhabit the bowel. In the setting of impaired host defenses, these microorganisms may invade the urinary tract, blood, lungs, or central nervous system and cause overwhelming infection (Table 9-7).

CLINICAL ASPECTS OF PULMONARY INFECTION

The importance of early diagnosis of infection has already been stressed. In order to facilitate this, prompt recognition of characteristic clinical signs and symptoms is crucial. This section deals with the clinical and radiologic presentation of commonly encountered bacterial, viral, and fungal pneumonias. Unfortunately, a clinical presentation that is perfectly diagnostic of a specific agent is rare. Even when clinical, radiologic, and laboratory data are considered together, a specific etiologic diagnosis is not always possible.

Classic clinical signs are frequently obscured by underlying diseases and/or defects in host defense. Radiologic signs may be obscured for the same reasons: a pneumonic infiltrate may be drastically altered by underlying obstructive changes. In addition, radiologic interpretation is often hampered because these patients are too ill to have a standard chest x-ray, and a portable x-ray, which is not as good technically, is substituted. The overinflation of the lung seen in some ventilated patients also can hamper radiologic interpretation.

Therefore, it is not surprising that the first hint that something is wrong often comes from the bacteriology laboratory, where the patient's sputum is growing out a pathogen. When this happens, one must make the distinction between colonization and infection. *Colonization* means asymptomatic carriage of an organism abnormal to a particular site. The colonization of the nasopharynx with *Staphylococcus aureus* is a common example. The distinction between colonization and infection is made by clinical, radiologic, and additional laboratory data. Clinically, infection is suggested by fever, malaise, and more specific symptoms such as cough, pleuritic pain, and signs such as rales on examination of the chest. Radiologic confirmation of pneumonia is the presence of an infiltrate. Additional laboratory data supporting infection include elevated white cell count and rises in specific antibody titers.

The distinction between colonization and infection is relevant because infection should be vigorously treated whereas colonization does not respond well to antimicrobial therapy. In the case of nasal carriers of *Staphylococcus aureus,* for instance, systemic antibiotics usually have a transient effect, and topical antibiotics (creams and ointments) seem to do little but select out resistant strains of the organism.

Before turning to specific clinical entities, an introductory word about the radiologic patterns seen in pneumonias is needed (Table 9–8). Lobar consolidation means exactly that: one or more of the five lobes of the lungs becomes radiopaque (or "white"). A bronchopneumonic infiltrate, on the other hand, refers to patchy areas of radiodensity involving one or more lobes. Still another pattern is interstitial, where there is diffuse thickening of the tissue separating alveoli causing a rather subtle increase in radiodensity.

The classic clinical picture of streptococcal or pneumococcal pneumonias is of sore throat and/or rhinorrhea for several days followed by the abrupt appearance of rigor (shaking chill) lasting upward to half an hour with fever and pleuritic pain.

Table 9-8. Common Radiologic Patterns in Specific Infections

Organism	X-ray
Streptococcus pneumoniae	Lobar; patchy with chronic obstructive pulmonary disease
Staphylococcus aureus	Patchy (or bronchopneumonic) with later coalescence and abscess formation; pyopneumothorax
Hemophilus influenzae	Patchy
Klebsiella pneumoniae	Lobar, favoring upper lobes; cavitation and empyema common; bulging interlobar fissure; rarely patchy
Pseudomonas and other gram negative rods	Patchy with coalescence and later cavitation common
Fungi, *Nocardia*	Patchy or diffuse; with or without cavitation
Herpes simplex virus, varicella virus, cytomegalovirus	Usually diffuse without cavitation
Pneumocystis carinii	Usually diffuse without cavitation; nodular densities and opacification late in disease course

Typically, there are no subsequent rigors. The sputum may be rust-colored or yellow-green. Certain types having a large capsule (e.g., type III) tend to produce a mucoid or jelly-like sputum. The x-ray picture is commonly lobar, but bronchopneumonic patterns are seen frequently in patients with underlying obstructive pulmonary disease. The infection is probably initiated by aspiration of the pneumococci from the nasopharynx into the alveoli.

Staphylococcal pneumonia, in contrast, does not readily invade the healthy lung. Previous viral injury to the respiratory epithelium appears necessary for the organism to take hold. This is reflected in the clinical observation of staphylococcal pneumonia complicating influenza and, less frequently, measles. This disease may be acquired by aspiration of organisms from the nasopharynx, inhalation of droplets from another person, or spread by means of bacteremia from a distant septic focus (e.g., a furuncle) or in right-sided endocarditis. The onset is usually sudden, with fever, cough, and pleuritic pain. Marked cyanosis is seen with severe infection. The x-ray pattern is initially bronchopneumonic (often affecting both lower lobes) but often progressing rapidly to abscess formation. The later development of pyopneumothorax is characteristic.

Hemophilus influenzae produces bronchitis more frequently than pneumonia in the adult patient. The pneumonia appears to favor lungs previously injured by viral or bacterial agents and is seen frequently in patients with chronic obstructive pulmonary disease. There are no unique clinical features to the pneumonia, which produces a bronchopneumonic x-ray pattern. Rigors are typically absent.

Klebsiella pneumoniae, or Friedländer, pneumonia, on the other hand, often provides specific clinical clues. Patients at risk for this disease are those with diabetes, alcoholism, and poor oral hygiene, but any chronic, debilitating illness may be in the background. The initial event appears to be aspiration of the organism from the mouth to the alveoli, and the characteristic supine posture of these patients seems to account for aspiration-induced involvement of the posterior segments of the upper lobes. The onset is abrupt, with multiple rigors, fever, malaise, dyspnea, and cough productive of copious greenish or blood-streaked sputum. The organism's large capsule accounts for a mucoid, tenacious sputum which, when bloody, is said to resemble currant jelly. Cyanosis and jaundice are common in severe cases. The x-ray pattern is usually lobar, favoring the upper lobes, but a bronchopneumonic pattern is occasionally seen. Infiltrates tend to break down to produce large, thick-walled cavities. Empyema is common, but the pyopneumothorax seen in staphylococcal pneumonia is distinctly uncommon. Person-to-person spread by aerosolized droplets is unusual; therefore, extraordinary respiratory precautions are not necessary.

Pseudomonas aeruginosa, Escherichia coli, Proteus species, *Serratia marcescens,* and other gram-negative bacilli may all produce pneumonia. They are discussed together because they share many characteristics. These organisms produce pneumonias in primarily the debilitated or immunosuppressed patient, and they all usually make their way to the alveoli through aspiration of previously colonized nasopharyngeal secretions. They are frequently secondary invaders, following earlier bacterial or viral respiratory infection. The radiologic pattern consists of bronchopneumonic infiltrates that tend to coalesce and eventually cavitate. Some characteristic features of the specific pneumonias are helpful but rarely diagnostic. *E. coli* pneumonia is more common in patients with diabetes mellitus, and especially in those with preexisting *E. coli* urinary tract infection. The sputum is usually yellow and not blood-tinged. *Pseudomonas aeruginosa* is now a major cause of pneumonia in the ventilated patient; as noted earlier, it thrives in aqueous solutions. The sputum is frequently green and sweet-smelling. In the presence of bacteremia, ecthyma gangrenosa with necrotizing lesions of the distal extremities is sometimes seen. A minority of strains of *Serratia marcescens* produces red pigment: when the patient's sputum is red but hematest negative, *Serratia* is probably present.

Mycoplasma pneumoniae infection usually follows a few days of upper respiratory symptoms with fever, malaise, and cough productive of yellowish sputum. X-ray studies typically show perihilar bronchopneumonic infiltrates; lobar consolidation and pleural effusion are rare. This is predominantly a disease of young adults, but the elderly can occasionally be affected.

Silent foci of tuberculosis may be reactivated by the stress of surgery, neoplastic disease, intercurrent infection, or immunosuppressive drugs. Preliminary evaluation of all patients should include careful inquiry about past exposure, skin test positivity, or active infection; and x-ray pictures should be examined for evidence of inactive disease. Tuberculous infection in the hospitalized patient is often subtle, and classic symptoms such as weight loss, night sweats, cough, and hemoptysis are frequently obscured by other complex medical problems. Immunosuppression and underlying architectural alterations in the lung (as in chronic obstructive disease) often totally obscure the classic radiologic picture of reactivation, with upper lobe infiltrates and cavity formation.

The key to the recognition of tuberculosis is awareness of the patients at high risk, including those with evidence of old infection or exposure and those currently suffering from alterations of the cellular immunologic system. These groups should have careful sputum stains for acid-fast bacilli on a regular basis. Special criteria for chemoprophylaxis and treatment are listed below (see the following two sections, Prophylaxis and Antimicrobial Treatment). Miliary or disseminated disease often occurs with reactivation, but the snowstorm effect on chest x-ray is a late event. Unexplained fever, a leukemoid or leukoerythroblastic reaction (indicating bone marrow involvement), the sudden elevation of the alkaline phosphatase (caused by multiple hepatic lesions), or a lymphocytic meningitis should suggest tuberculosis. The finding of liver and/or bone-marrow granulomas, often noncaseating, would be confirmatory. Suspected or confirmed tuberculous infection demands patient isolation and mask, gown, and glove precautions.

The last group of pneumonias to be considered include *Nocardia,* various fungi and viruses that cause disseminated disease, and *Pneumocystis carinii,* a protozoan. They are considered together because they share many common characteristics. In spite of their similarities, careful distinction among them is mandatory, for specific chemotherapy may be effective against one agent but not another. This group of organisms produces pulmonary infection, often as a part of disseminated disease, in the patient with impairment of the cellular immunologic system.

Of the fungi, *Histoplasma capsulatum* and *Coccidioides immitis* rarely cause disseminated disease; primary pulmonary involvement is restricted to the Ohio Valley and southwestern United States, respectively. The disseminated form occurs in previously exposed individuals with cellular immunologic defects and acts much like miliary tuberculosis. *Aspergillus fumagatus* and *Candida albicans* often cause fever, patchy pulmonary infiltrates that tend to coalesce and cavitate, and progressive respiratory difficulty. The allergic and mycetoma forms of aspergillosis will not be discussed. *Candida* and *Aspergillus* are not often seen in sputum smears, and diagnosis is made by lung biopsy. *Nocardia asteroides* pneumonia has similar clinical and radiologic features, but on occasion it can present as a coin lesion on x-ray. This infection is seen most frequently in renal transplant recipients and in association with alveolar proteinosis. The sputum is positive about 50 percent of the time. Here, too, lung biopsy often makes the diagnosis.

Herpesvirus, varicella virus, and cytomegalovirus may all produce severe pulmonary infection in the T cell-compromised patient. Clinically, one is often struck by the disparity between severe respiratory embarrassment with marked hypoxemia and the paucity of auscultatory and radiologic signs. The x-ray pattern is interstitial in most cases and can be quite subtle. Diagnosis may be aided by the typical skin lesions of varicella and the presence of giant cells in the Giemsa stain of the urinary sediment with cytomegalovirus, but lung biopsy is usually necessary to rule out other, more treatable lesions. A frequent accompaniment of these infections may be marked alterations of hepatocellular function as reflected by elevated transaminase levels.

Pneumocystis carinii also causes pneumonia primarily in the T cell-deficient patient, and exposure to corticosteroids appears to be an additional predisposing factor. The onset may be gradual or abrupt, with tachypnea and respiratory distress being the most common clinical findings. Fever is inconstant. The radiologic picture is of an interstitial infiltrate with later appearance of nodular densities and ultimate opacification of the lung. Sputum is rarely helpful, but in experienced hands the organism can be demonstrated by means of methenamine silver staining in specimens obtained by bronchial brushings. Otherwise, lung biopsy is necessary for diagnosis.

Because the fungal, viral, and protozoan diseases of this group are rarely seen in immunocompetent individuals, no extraordinary precautions are needed to protect the therapist.

PROPHYLAXIS

Prophylaxis, or preventive treatment of infection, is probably more important than treatment after the fact, because many of the commonly encountered organisms display variable resistance to antimicrobial agents. A common source of pulmonary infection is aspiration of pathogens from the nasopharynx. Initial steps should then be diverted toward prevention of upper airway colonization. Earlier discussion of mechanical, constitutional, and environmental factors again become relevant, and measures taken in these areas can help prevent colonization from taking place.

A major mechanical factor is the endotracheal tube or tracheostomy. Warm humidification of air to prevent drying and impairment of clearing mechanisms is important. With an open communication between the outside world and the lower respiratory tract, direct infection of the lungs may easily occur if strict aseptic technique is not followed.

A major source of contamination is improper suctioning. When caring for a tracheostomy, the tube should be changed about once a week. The inner cannula should be removed every 8 hours and cleaned by washing in glutaraldehyde or a phenolic compound. The skin around the tube should be cleaned thoroughly at least twice a day, and antibacterial ointment (such as that containing bacitracin) should be applied.

Other areas of potential mechanical breakdowns include vascular lines and urinary catheters. All lines and catheters require aseptic technique with insertion. Intravenous lines pose less infectious threat if they are superficial. The use of butterfly type devices is desirable when possible. They may be rotated frequently (every 2 to 3 days) because vascular damage is minimal and veins may be reused. Central venous catheters and other long lines should remain closed. They should not be used to administer drugs or obtain blood samples because such use maximizes infectious risks. There are strict regulations regarding total parenteral nutrition lines, preventing their use for other purposes. When these lines are being used, the risk of fungemia should be kept in mind. At the first sign of redness, tenderness, or pain in the area of a vascular line, this line should be removed immediately and cultures taken from the tip.

The longer a urinary catheter is in place, the greater is the probability of infection. Because such infection can lead to life-threatening bacteremia, avoidance of unnecessary catheterization and constant reevaluation of the utility of unavoidable catheterization should be routine precautions. In addition, periodic surveillance — every 2 to 3 days—of urine cultures should be performed. Irrigants such as neomycin and acetic acid may retard infection with short-term catheterization.

Constitutional factors may be modified to reduce the development of infection. Inactivity is a major determinant of pulmonary infection, especially in the debilitated patient. Deep breathing exercises and encouragement to cough are helpful, as is the use of intermittent positive pressure breathing, blow bottles, pulmonary physiotherapy, and postural drainage when indicated. Arm and leg exercises and the use of a footboard help maintain muscle tone and may inhibit venous thrombosis. Special care should be directed to the skin of the debilitated patient to avoid decubitus ulcers with subsequent risk of deep tissue infection and bacteremia. Frequent turning and the use of an air mattress and heat lamp are helpful. Because pain in itself may cause secondary inactivity, the judicious use of analgesic and narcotic agents is indicated. At the same time, oversedation and respiratory depression must be avoided.

Underlying conditions that may directly or indirectly alter the course of infection should be treated vigorously. Aggressive treatment of left ventricular failure may help to clarify a confusing pulmonary picture as well as to allow more rapid clearing of a pneumonia. The removal of a foreign body or tumor by bronchoscopy, surgery, or radiotherapy will allow relief of obstruction and clearing of a distal infection. Useful management of conditions such as diabetes mellitus and hypothyroidism probably reduces the incidence of infectious complications.

Some progress has been made in altering immunologic factors predisposing to infection, and current research interest holds promise for major advances in the near future. At present, immunization against respiratory pathogens is very limited. Influenza vaccine is widely used and probably helpful. Pneumococcal vaccines, first used in the 1930s and reintroduced periodically, are probably helpful, but they are rarely used. BCG, an attenuated strain of the tubercle bacillus, is controversial and rarely used in the United States. Zoster immune globulin (ZIG) is undergoing trial as prophylaxis for the immunocompromised patient exposed to varicella, and it may be effective. Less convincing are the results of trials of anti-*Pseudomonas* vaccines, but work continues.

Successful alteration of specific immunologic defects has been successful with the periodic administration of gamma globulin to patients with hypogammaglobulinemia or agammaglobulinemia. More controversial have been the results with transfer factor, a serum fraction thought to have T cell effects in the treatment of T cell deficiency diseases such as mucocutaneous candidiasis and states of T cell failure as in disseminated tuberculosis.

Quantitative white cell defects have been treated with some success by white cell transfusion, allowing the patient to mount an adequate response to infection.

Drug-induced immunosuppression has been discussed. When faced with the potentiality or actuality of infection, one must reduce or discontinue such agents as rapidly as possible.

The patient faces numerous environmental hazards which must be controlled. These include personnel, respiratory equipment, other inanimate objects in his environment, other patients, and his own flora, as discussed in the section Environmental Sources of Infection (p. 177).

The majority of infectious threats in personnel can be controlled by hand washing with soap both before and after coming in contact with each patient. Personnel with skin lesions, especially of the hands, should be prohibited from patient contact until successfully treated, as should also anyone with a diarrheal illness. Less clear is the approach to the problem of chronic hepatitis-associated antigen (HAA) positivity in patient care personnel; they should probably retain their clinical duties, using extra care in hand washing and in avoiding contamination of others with their blood. Equally difficult is the worker with persistent nasal carriage of *Staphylococcus aureus.* Focal or systemic antibiotic treatment is not successful, but eradication has been accomplished by experimentally inoculating a nonpathogenic strain of *Staphylococcus* into the nose, where it replaces the pathogen. Because the clinical effect of such *Staphylococcus* carriers is not clear, these people should probably continue patient care activities under close observation.

The role of contaminated respiratory equipment in hospital-acquired infection is widely known, and when recommended steps are followed, this source of infection can be drastically reduced. Tubing and humidifiers are the major sources of infection and should be changed routinely at least every 24 hours. For the patient with respiratory infection we change the equipment every 8 hours. Various decontamination procedures are available for respiratory equipment, the pros and cons of which are outlined in Table 9–9. Before any procedure is undertaken, one must first clean and dry the equipment thoroughly, because organisms, especially spores, can survive in dried sputum, blood, or other debris if not cleaned away. We are presently using pasteurization for most materials; the remainder are treated with gas sterilization.

Another approach has been the insertion of various filters into the tubing to trap bacteria and protect the equipment from contamination. Copper mesh has been successfully used and is thought to be effective in part because of copper's antibacterial effect. More recently HEPA filters (see Chapter 3) have been introduced for this purpose.

Patient-to-patient transmission of infection is drastically reduced by adequate hand washing, except in cases of tuberculosis and staphylococcal pneumonia, where aerosol droplet spread is common. With these diseases, complete isolation of the patient is mandatory.

In the case of the immunosuppressed patient, especially with marked granulo-

Table 9-9. Decontamination Methods: Pros and Cons

Method	Advantages	Disadvantages
Steam autoclaving (saturated steam under pressure, 121° C for 30 min)	Thorough (kills spores); rapid; nontoxic; inexpensive; allows prepackaging	Too small for some equipment; harms plastic and rubber; cannot penetrate oils, closed liquids; dulls sharp edges
Pasteurization (160° C water bath for 30 min)	Effective (but not sporicidal); rapid; nontoxic; inexpensive	Too small for some equipment; must dry afterward—danger of contamination; no prepackaging
Ethylene oxide gas sterilization	Effective; low corrosion potential (may harm some acrylic and polystyrene plastics); allows prepackaging	Relatively expensive; fire and explosion risk with CO_2 or from mixture; time-consuming (materials must be aerated after exposure)
Glutaraldehyde washing	Rapid; inexpensive	Not as effective as other agents; may damage rubber and plastic; must rinse and dry afterward; no prepackaging

cytopenia, reverse isolation is often advocated. In our experience, segregation in a private room without strict gown-and-glove precautions is adequate. Otherwise, the need for precautions reduces patient-personnel relations almost to the point of neglect. In such patients, the risks of infection from within (usually from the gastrointestinal tract) pose as great a threat as those from the environment. Attempts to sterilize the bowel in such situations have been unsuccessful. It should be kept in mind that bowel flora and aerobic and anaerobic bacteria, as well as *Candida,* pose a threat of dissemination in these patients.

The role of prophylactic antibiotics is very restricted. In fact, they are really indicated only for tuberculosis. Our present criteria for chemotherapy for tuberculosis are (1) household members and other close contacts of patients with active tuberculosis, (2) individuals under 35 with a positive tuberculin skin test, (3) patients with newly converted PPD, from negative to positive, and (4) patients with special clinical circumstances such as those receiving immunosuppressive therapy. The criteria for chemoprophylaxis require continual reassessment. INH (isoniazid) is given 300 mg/day for one year. Pyridoxine (vitamin B_6), 50 to 100 mg/day, is added because it apparently prevents the appearance of peripheral neuropathy and rarer central venous system side effects of INH. Because INH can be hepatotoxic, we use it only when the criteria are met. Periodic tests of liver function are appropriate, especially in older women and individuals with underlying liver disease, because they are at highest risk for this complication.

Prophylactic systemic antibiotics in other situations appear to do no good and in fact may do the patient real harm by allowing alterations of normal flora and overgrowth of resistant organisms. Awareness of the key role of upper airway colonization in the development of pneumonia has prompted trials of locally admini-stered antibiotics, especially by aerosol. Unfortunately, these efforts have not met with success.

The effectiveness of prophylactic measures is best gauged by a program of bac-teriologic monitoring. In addition, such surveillance cultures can provide crucial data for intertreatment decisions. The acutely ill patient with endotracheal tube or tracheostomy should have daily culture of the tracheal aspirate. Furthermore, areas of potential danger, such as the urine in the catheterized patient and the stool in the immunosuppressed patient, should be cultured every few days. Colonization of the upper airway of the pulmonary patient should be monitored by nasopharyngeal cultures every few days.

Personnel should have monthly nasopharyngeal cultures. In the event of an out-break of staphylococcal infection, all positive staphylococcal cultures from patients, staff, and equipment should be macrophage-typed, allowing for more specific iden-tification of the causative organism and its source.

Random surveillance cultures of respiratory equipment after decontamination may be performed by swabbing, but air trap cultures from ventilators should also be done. Bacteriologic sampling from equipment and surroundings such as sinks, walls, and furniture should be carried out on a routine basis, especially in high den-sity areas such as intensive care units.

ANTIMICROBIAL TREATMENT

Once a specific organism is identified as being apparently responsible for an infec-tious process, the choice of an appropriate antibiotic agent remains. In order to make such a choice with skill, certain basic criteria should be met. A careful allergy history is crucial, for often there is confusion between an idiosyncratic or "allergic" reaction to a drug and an expected side effect or even an independent but unrelated event.

In choosing an antimicrobial agent for a specific infection one should also choose a drug with the narrowest effective spectrum. In doing so, one avoids wide spec-trum agents that tend to wipe out normal flora and make the patient susceptible to suprainfection.

If the drug one chooses has significant toxic effects—and most do—one must de-termine whether there is any impairment of the system or systems most often affected. For instance, one should check the patient's renal function prior to ad-ministering a potentially nephrotoxic drug.

Major antimicrobial agents are listed and appropriate chemotherapy for specific infections is outlined in Table 9–10. Doses are omitted because this table (and in-deed this whole chapter) should be used only as a general reference, not as a spe-cific treatment guide.

SELECTED BIBLIOGRAPHY

American Hospital Association. *Infection Control in the Hospital (3rd ed.)*. Chicago: American Hospital Association, 1974.

Table 9-10. Classification of Antimicrobial Agents Commonly Used for Pulmonary Infection

Class or Group	Agents	Spectrum	Major Toxicity
Penicillin	Penicillin	Gram-positive organisms; *staphylococcus aureus* often resistant	Allergy
Semisynthetic penicillins	Ampicillin	Gram-positive *Hemophilus influenzae*; variable against gram-negative rods	Diarrhea and rash, especially with viral disease (mononucleosis)
	Oxacillin, Nafcillin	Like penicillin, with antistaphylococcal effects	Allergy
	Carbenicillin	Like penicillin, with anti-*Pseudomonas* effects	Sodium overload-congestive failure
Cephalosporins	Cephalothin, Cephalexin, Cefazolin	Like penicillin, with antistaphylococcal effects	Renal (usually not severe)
Aminoglycosides	Streptomycin	Primarily tuberculostatic	Vestibular, renal
	Kanamycin	Gram-negative rods except *Pseudomonas* and some *Proteus*	Auditory, renal
	Gentamicin, Tobramycin	Gram-negative rods, including *Pseudomonas* and *Proteus*	Vestibular, renal
Macrolide	Erythromycin	Like penicillin (used in penicillin allergy); drug of choice for *Mycoplasma*	Gastrointestinal
Tetracyclines	Tetracycline, Minocycline, Doxycycline	Broad spectrum—useful against *Hemophilus* and *Mycoplasma* infections	Fungal overgrowth in bowel or vagina; hepatic with large IV doses
	Chloramphenicol	Broad spectrum—used for *Hemophilus* if it is ampicillin-resistant or if patient is allergic	Bone marrow
Tuberculostatic agents	Isoniazid	Used for both prophylaxis and treatment	Hepatic
	Ethambutol, Rifampin	Used for tuberculostatic therapy	Retinal (maculopathy), hepatic
Antifungal agents	Amphotericin B	Major agent for systemic fungal disease	Renal, gastrointestinal
	5-fluorocyosine	Usually used in combination with amphotericin B	Bone marrow
Sulfonamides	Sulfisoxazole	Broad spectrum—primary drug for *Nocardia*	Allergy
	Pentamidine	Specific for *Pneumocystis carinii*	Anemia

Feingold, D. S. Hospital-acquired infections. *N. Engl. J. Med.* 283, 1970, p. 1384.

Jawetz, E., et al. *Review of Medical Microbiology (11th ed.),* Los Altos, Calif.: Lange, 1974.

Johanson, W. G., et al. Nosocomial respiratory infections with Gram-negative bacilli. The significance of colonization of the respiratory tract. *Ann. Intern. Med.* 77, 1972, p. 701.

Reinarz, J. A., et al. The potential role of inhalation therapy equipment in nosocomial pulmonary infection. *J. Clin. Invest.* 44, 1965, p. 831.

Grace R. Baldwin

Oxygen: Therapeutics, Toxicity, Advances

10

We have reached a point in the evolutionary continuum when sufficient free oxygen exists in the atmosphere to support life. Furthermore, this is accomplished without that life succumbing to the toxicity of oxygen. The existence of free oxygen and the defense mechanisms requisite for its utilization as an energy source are taken for granted. However, there was a time when free oxygen was virtually nonexistent. Indeed, it has been a long and gradual process to reach a point when life can generate, utilize, and tolerate oxygen.

The first atmosphere was a hydrogen-dependent (reducing) atmosphere. In this phase, water was split and the oxygen from it was combined with methane to form carbohydrate compounds. In this process ($H_2O + CH_4 \rightarrow CHO + H_2$), hydrogen was liberated. This was first accomplished nonbiologically and then later by primitive organisms. Primitive biological reductions reversed this process by combining CHO and H_2 to regenerate methane and water.

Nonbiological   Biological   Biological

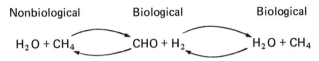

$$H_2O + CH_4 \qquad CHO + H_2 \qquad H_2O + CH_4$$

Because H^+ is light, its escape from the atmosphere resulted in a continuous loss of hydrogen. Most free H^+ was generated from bound sources such as H_2O. Photo-dissociation (splitting by light energy) of water liberated oxygen as well as hydrogen. The hydrogen would drift away from the atmosphere and leave behind oxygen, giving rise to the transition from a reducing (hydrogen) to an oxidizing atmosphere. Because this source of oxygen was limited, the concentration of oxygen remained low. Then organisms learned to photodissociate water in the presence of carbon dioxide to produce CHO and O_2 ($H_2O + CO_2 \rightarrow CHO + O_2$). Thus photosynthesis was born. It was then that the concentration of atmospheric oxygen rose significantly. Oxygen became a new energy source possessing many of the properties requisite for a good source of energy: it was plentiful and not too reactive, and it had the potential to release much energy.

This state of affairs created a dilemma. On the one hand, oxygen provided a new, better energy source. On the other hand, it liberated into the atmosphere a toxic gas. As the concentration of free oxygen increased, organisms displayed different methods of coping with this new adversity, oxygen toxicity. Some organisms retreated to parts of the planet where oxygen remained scarce. Thus anaerobic organisms, exquisitely sensitive to oxygen, exist today as evolutionary remnants of an oxygen-free environment. Other organisms chose to carry on oxidative metabolism by hydrogen removal (fermentation) rather than by oxygen addition. However, this solution to oxygen toxicity is inefficient. Fermentative organisms are parasites using up high-energy compounds and giving off low-energy compounds as end products. A third possible solution was to develop defense mechanisms so that oxygen could be tapped as an energy source. Only this solution could pave the way for the development of oxidative metabolism, which alone can generate enough energy to meet the demands of multicellular organisms.

Through the process of oxidative metabolism (respiration), organisms trap the energy liberated by burning organic compounds in the presence of oxygen (CHO + $O_2 \rightarrow CO_2 + H_2O$ + energy). The supply of oxygen and carbon compounds is continuously replenished by photosynthesis ($CO_2 + H_2O$ + sunlight $\rightarrow CHO + O_2$). Thus photosynthesizing and oxidizing organisms are mutually dependent on each other for fuel. The cycle is complete: there is no net production of oxygen.

Photosynthesis   Respiration

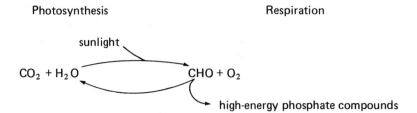

Aerobic oxidative metabolism proceeds in three phases. First, six carbon sugars are broken down anaerobically to three carbon compounds (pyruvate) by a process of glycolysis. Further utilization of pyruvate requires oxygen to metabolize it to its components, CO_2 and H_2O. This is accomplished by the Krebs (tricarboxylic acid) cycle, in which CO_2 is liberated. Finally, H_2O is produced by the joining of O_2 and H^+ at the end of a chain of oxidation-reduction reactions where H^+ electrons are passed bucket brigade fashion by a group of iron- and copper-containing enzymes known as the cytochrome system.

The single most important aspect of this process is the liberation and the harnessing of energy in the form of high-energy phosphate compounds (such as adenosine triphosphate, or ATP). These high energy compounds serve as the primary energy source of all multicellular organisms. Oxygen acts as the final H^+ electron recipient in the bucket brigade, carrying off H^+ in the form of H_2O, thus driving the reaction to continue producing fuel at a rapid rate. In the absence of oxygen the sequence of reactions stops at glycolysis. Pyruvate, instead of entering the Krebs cycle, is converted to lactate, and few high energy bonds are generated. When the supply of energy is cut off, ultimately all cellular functions cease.

The process of oxidation takes place in specialized cell organelles (mitochondria). For small organisms, diffusion of oxygen across cell membranes can adequately maintain the supply of oxygen. However, in higher forms, the mitochondrial demand far exceeds what could be supplied by diffusion alone. The delivery of oxygen and the removal of carbon dioxide require efficient transport mechanisms to handle the high turnover rate of these compounds. The large surface areas of the capillary beds in the lung and in the tissue provide for adequate gas exchange. Once in the blood, adequate gas transport is mediated by hemoglobin and the cardiovascular system.

OXYGEN TRANSPORT

Man consumes about 250 ml of oxygen per minute at rest, and with exercise he can increase this consumption more than tenfold. How is this amount of oxygen transported from the atmosphere to the mitochondria, its ultimate destination? The journey is accomplished through the integrated efforts of the pulmonary, cardiovascular, hematologic, and nervous systems (Table 10-1). If the oxygen tensions along its course are plotted, it can be seen that oxygen flows "downhill" from the atmosphere to the mitochondria (Figure 10-1).

Gas Phase

Gas flows first through the conducting airways, which branch dichotomously into progressively smaller airways. The size of the branches and the angles of branching are expertly engineered to provide a system offering a minimum of resistance to the flow of gases. Moreover, resistance is further diminished by the rapid increase in the total cross-sectional area of the airways. The conducting airways terminate at the alveoli, the actual site of gas exchange. The alveoli are surrounded by a pool of blood, the pulmonary capillary bed. The immense area of the blood-air interface allows rapid, full equilibration between alveolar and blood gas tensions. At rest, the system is not taxed. It possesses a tremendous reserve capacity to increase gas exchange many times over.

Blood Phase

Once in the blood, oxygen rapidly diffuses into the red blood cells, where it combines reversibly with hemoglobin. The oxygenated blood is then transported to the

Table 10-1. Factors Influencing Oxygen Transport

Factors	Requirements
Gas Phase	
Inspired air	Adequate partial pressure of oxygen
Airways	Unobstructed, offering low resistance
Lungs	Normal volumes and capacities; normal compliance
Alveolar ventilation	Adjusted to maintain arterial carbon dioxide tension in normal range; evenly distributed for geographic matching with capillary perfusion
Blood Phase	
Arterial oxygen tension	Sufficient to utilize fully the oxygen-carrying capacity of blood
Arterial oxygen content	Normal hemoglobin content and arterial oxygen tension
Cardiac output	Normal volume and appropriate distribution
Pulmonary circulation	Normal volume and distribution, permitting geographic matching of alveolar ventilation and pulmonary capillary perfusion
Chemical environment	Normal pH, temperature, buffer and electrolyte content, DPG concentration
Tissue Phase	
Capillaries and tissues	Normal membrane permeability and tissue metabolism

Source: Bendixen, H. H., et al. *Respiratory Care.* St. Louis: The C. V. Mosby Co., 1965. Table 3, p. 5.

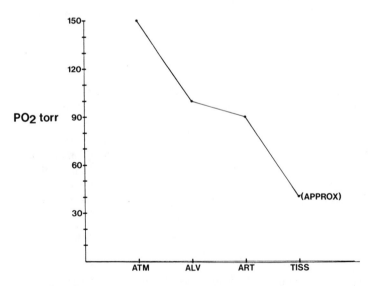

Figure 10-1. Oxygen tensions from the atmosphere to the tissues.

tissues by the cardiovascular system. The amount and distribution of blood flow (and therefore the rate at which oxygen arrives at the tissues) is determined by a series of complex physiologic adjustments requiring the integration of neurologic and hemodynamic controls. Once the oxygenated blood arrives at the tissues, the amount of oxygen removed (the arterial minus the venous oxygen content) is dependent on two determinants: (1) the concentration and affinity characteristics of hemoglobin (arterial oxygen content), and (2) the oxygen extraction properties of the tissues (venous oxygen content). Thus, tissue oxygenation is determined by the rate at which blood reaches the tissues. Tissue extraction characteristics can be established by analyzing the difference in the arterial and venous oxygen contents. This relationship can be expressed as the Fick equation:

O_2 consumption = $(A\text{-}VO_2) \times COP$.

Analysis of the Fick equation, under a variety of physiologic stresses, reveals a number of adjustments that are employed to assure adequate tissue oxygenation. For example, if increased oxygen requirements (fever, exercise) are to be met, the cardiac output (COP) and/or the arteriovenous oxygen $(A\text{-}VO_2)$ difference must increase.

$\uparrow O_2$ consumption = $\uparrow (A\text{-}VO_2) \times \uparrow COP$

     primary   compensatory

Similarly, a fall in cardiac output must be accompanied by an augmented arteriovenous difference in oxygen content if the oxygen consumption is to remain normal.

(normal) O_2 consumption = $\uparrow (A\text{-}VO_2) \times \downarrow COP$

               compensation   defect

Likewise, a decrease in the arteriovenous difference in oxygen content necessitates an increased cardiac output to maintain a normal oxygen consumption.

(normal) O_2 consumption = $\downarrow (A\text{-}VO_2) \times \uparrow COP$

               defect   compensation

Thus, arterial oxygenation, tissue extraction of oxygen, hemoglobin affinity, cardiac output, and regional perfusion are all intimately interrelated in the transport of oxygen to the tissues. If the oxygen deficit at the time is not too severe, then the various previously described compensatory responses maintain normal oxygenation (oxygen consumption). However, if the abnormality is extreme, or if it involves more than one parameter of oxygen transport, compensation will not be complete and oxygen consumption will fall. Then, cellular metabolism will proceed anaerobically, arrested at glycolysis. Pyruvate will be converted to lactate and hydrogen ions instead of entering the Krebs cycle. Lactic acidosis will result.

That which determines the arterial and venous oxygen content determines the magnitude of the arteriovenous oxygen difference. Under normobaric conditions (1 atmosphere), because the dissolved fraction of oxygen does not contribute significantly to the overall oxygen content, the arterial oxygen content depends on the number of grams of saturated hemoglobin. The amount of saturated hemoglobin depends in turn on hemoglobin's affinity for oxygen and the plasma oxygen tension.

Tissue oxygen extraction and the affinity characteristics of hemoglobin set the venous oxygen content. Alterations in these parameters give rise to changes in the arteriovenous oxygen content. A narrow arteriovenous oxygen difference more often results from a decrease in the arterial oxygen content (anemia, abnormal hemoglobin saturation secondary to low oxygen tension) than from an elevation in the venous oxygen content (defect in oxygen release from hemoglobin secondary to its increased affinity for oxygen).

A widened arteriovenous oxygen difference can result from increased tissue oxygen extraction and/or decreased hemoglobin affinity for oxygen. Tissues extract oxygen according to their needs. When cellular metabolism exceeds its oxygen supply, then tissue oxygen tension falls. The resultant increase in the blood-tissue oxygen gradient facilitates the diffusion of oxygen into the cells, thus lowering the venous oxygen content (indicated by a fall in the venous oxygen tension). The diminished venous oxygen content expands the arteriovenous difference. This extra oxygen that is released can be used to meet increased cellular needs or to compensate for any decrease in arterial oxygen content or to provide more oxygen in the instance of decreased tissue perfusion.

The inverse relationship between perfusion and oxygen extraction is operative in the normal resting state as well as in a compensatory capacity. Furthermore, this relationship applies to local differences in perfusion and organ variation in oxygen extraction. In the normal, resting state, not all organs have the same oxygen extraction capacities, as evidenced by local variation in arteriovenous oxygen content. High-extracting tissues (e.g., brain and heart) are more efficient because more oxygen is obtained per unit of blood flow, whereas low-extracting tissues (kidney, muscle) require more blood flow to achieve an equivalent supply of oxygen. In tissues with maximal extraction at rest, only increased perfusion, accomplished by diverting flow from low-extracting tissues, will bring more oxygen. Low extraction tissues now compensate for the decrease in perfusion by increasing oxygen extraction (lowering partial venous oxygen). However, if the disturbances are severe, then the diminution in blood supply may result in ischemic injury. Teleologically, there are established priorities: the kidneys and muscles are sacrificed for the welfare of the brain and the heart. This phenomenon of redistribution of blood flow can be used clinically to monitor adequate tissue oxygenation by means of measurement of the muscle pH (see Chapter 2).

HEMOGLOBIN AFFINITY FOR OXYGEN

The body has yet another way to enhance tissue oxygenation that does not necessitate an augmented cardiac output, regional perfusion, arterial oxygen content, or
tissue oxygen extraction. This mechanism, contained within the red blood cell, is
the ability of this cell to reduce the affinity of hemoglobin for oxygen. At the tissue
level, a diminished affinity results in the release of more molecules of oxygen (a
lower hemoglobin saturation), without a lowered venous oxygen tension. This phenomenon is mediated by alterations in temperature, and in red blood cell concentrations of hydrogen, carbon dioxide, and, most importantly, the organic phosphate,
diphosphoglycerate (DPG). The recent discovery that DPG profoundly affects the
hemoglobin-oxygen interaction produced a burst of interest in this field. The clinical significance of this most fascinating physiologic observation has not been
established. If the controversy is settled in favor of altered hemoglobin affinity
(especially that mediated by DPG), then therapeutic manipulations of DPG, or even
of synthetic substances capable of altering affinity, could have sweeping clinical
consequences. In order to grasp the issues surrounding the clinical significance of
hemoglobin affinity, it is necessary to understand the physiology of hemoglobin
structure as it relates to oxygen binding and the factors that influence this union.

Structure of Hemoglobin

Each giant molecule of hemoglobin is composed of four subunits. Each subunit consists of one polypeptide chain (globin portion) and one heme group (the site of
oxygen binding). Therefore, the hemoglobin molecule, containing four polypeptide-
heme groups, is capable of carrying four molecules of oxygen. A polypeptide chain
consists of a long amino acid sequence (primary structure) twisted on its longitudinal
axis to form a helix (secondary structure). Each molecule contains two types of
polypeptide chains (two chains of each type). The types of chains are designated
by the Greek letters α, β, γ, δ. Normally, more than 90 percent of adult hemoglobin
is HgbA (two alpha and two beta chains) with a small percentage of $HgbA_2$ (two
alpha and two delta chains). Fetal hemoglobin (hemoglobin F) consists of two alpha
and two gamma chains. The amino acid helix is then folded on itself, giving the
appearance of a tangled, random structure. Just the opposite is the case, however,
for the three-dimensional arrangement (tertiary structure) is one of the critical
determinants in the oxygen-hemoglobin interaction. The folds in the helix create
divisions (segments) in the chains. The polarity (charge) dictates the positioning of
the segments. The polar environment bathing the surface of the molecule on the one
hand forces the nonpolar (uncharged) segments into the interior, and on the other
hand draws the polar (charged) segments to the surface of the molecule. This positioning is important because it forms a cleft for the heme moiety. The center of
each heme group contains one iron atom, the actual site of oxygen binding [38] .

Hemoglobin-Oxygen Binding

Hemoglobin transports oxygen by combining with it in the lungs and releasing it to
the tissues. The critical aspect of the interaction is its reversibility, which is governed

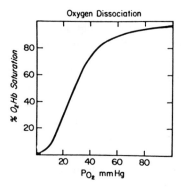

Figure 10–2. The oxyhemoglobin dissociation curve.

by the affinity properties of hemoglobin. If it were not for the nature of hemoglobin affinity for oxygen, tissue oxygenation could not be achieved within the
physiologic range of oxygen tensions. The two main determinants of hemoglobin
affinity are the inherent ability of hemoglobin to alter its own affinity and the
presence of erythrocyte DPG. The saturation of hemoglobin with oxygen is directly
related to its affinity and to the oxygen tension. If the affinity of hemoglobin for
oxygen were fixed, the relationship would be linear. Instead, a sigmoid curve known
as the *oxyhemoglobin dissociation curve* is formed when the percent saturation is
plotted against the oxygen tension. The shape of the curve indicates that, as oxygen
molecules are added to hemoglobin, the remaining binding sites have an increased
affinity for oxygen. It is presumed that the change occurs after three sites are
saturated, then the affinity of the fourth is so great that it is immediately saturated
[36]. Conversely, as the hemoglobin saturation falls, so does the affinity for the
remaining oxygen, which is thus more readily surrendered to the tissues. The ability
of hemoglobin to alter its affinity greatly facilitates the loading of oxygen in the
lung and the unloading of oxygen in the tissues (Figure 10–2).

   A change in the structure of the hemoglobin molecule is responsible for this
phenomenon. The change in structure occurs in the position of the beta subunits,
which move back and forth depending on their state of oxygenation. They slide together when oxygenated and apart when deoxygenated, leaving a gap between them
[36] (Figure 10–3). These changes in the spatial relationships in the two beta
chains alter the affinity characteristics of hemoglobin. When the beta chains are
apart, the atomic arrangements that must precede oxygenation are prevented. The
exact mechanism is unknown, but the changes are thought to originate in the iron
atom [36]. The shape of the curve remains relatively fixed, not altered significantly
by any substance or condition. However, the curve itself often shifts its position
(secondary to change in the relationship between percentage of saturated hemoglobin and the oxygen tension) (Figure 10–4). A curve that is shifted to the right
indicates that hemoglobin affinity for oxygen is less than normal, and a left-shifted
curve corresponds to hemoglobin with an elevated affinity. For simplicity, hemo-

Hgb–DPG BINDING

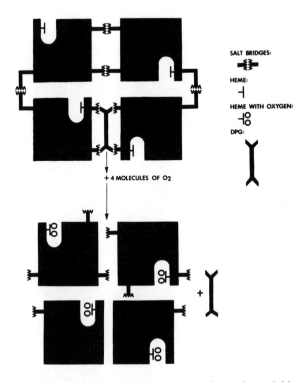

Figure 10–3. The hemoglobin molecule in the oxyhemoglobin and the deoxyhemoglobin states.

globin affinity (position of the curve) is expressed in terms of P50 (the oxygen required to achieve saturation of 50 percent of the hemoglobin with oxygen). The normal P50 is 27 torr, which means that when the arterial oxygen tension is 27 torr the hemoglobin is 50 percent saturated with oxygen. Inspection of the oxyhemoglobin dissociation curve reveals that if the affinity of hemoglobin is higher than normal, half of the hemoglobin will be saturated at an oxygen tension of less than 27 (P50 < 27 torr) and the curve will be shifted to the left (Figure 10–4, curve A). Likewise, a hemoglobin of decreased affinity will require an oxygen tension of greater than 27 torr to saturate half of the binding sites (P50 > 27 torr) and the curve (curve C) will be located to the right of the normal curve (Figure 10–4).

Many factors affect the hemoglobin affinity for oxygen, including temperature and substances that bind to hemoglobin, called *ligands*. The most important ligands are hydrogen, carbon dioxide, and organic phosphates (ATP and especially DPG). Each ligand binds preferentially either to deoxyhemoglobin or oxyhemoglobin. The ligands hydrogen, carbon dioxide, and DPG decrease affinity (increase P50, shift curve to right) because they bind preferentially to the deoxyhemoglobin form,

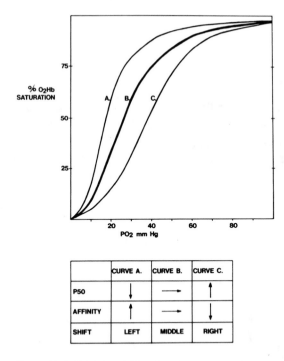

	CURVE A.	CURVE B.	CURVE C.
P50	↓	→	↑
AFFINITY	↑	→	↓
SHIFT	LEFT	MIDDLE	RIGHT

Figure 10–4. Oxyhemoglobin dissociation curves demonstrating the relationships among the position of the curve, P50, affinity, and direction of the shift. Curve B is the normal condition.

stabilize it, and in doing so, interfere with oxygenation [36] . Ligands such as carbon monoxide bind to oxyhemoglobin and thereby increase its affinity for oxygen (shift the curve to the left, decrease P50).

Temperature
Because the dissociation of oxyhemoglobin is an endothermic reaction (absorbs heat), temperature and affinity are inversely related [42] . Teleologically, when there is fever, there is increased oxygen need, and the decreased affinity promotes oxygen release to the tissues.

Bohr Effect (pH)
By combining preferentially with deoxyhemoglobin, H^+ decreases hemoglobin's affinity for oxygen. It is thought that the hydrogen ions, by preventing the breaking of salt bridges [37] , stabilize the deoxyhemoglobin form so that more energy is required to carry out the chemical changes in structure that must precede oxygenation. Thus an increase in hydrogen ion concentration (acidosis, decreased pH) causes an immediate decrease in affinity, whereas a decrease in the hydrogen ion concentration (alkalosis, increased pH) causes an immediate increase in hemoglobin

Table 10–2. Factors that Alter Hemoglobin Affinity for Oxygen

	Right-Shift Oxyhemoglobin Dissociation Curve (increased P50, decreased affinity)	Left-Shift Oxyhemoglobin Dissociation Curve (decreased P50, increased affinity)
Direct		
Major	Decreased pH	Increased pH
	Increased temperature	Decreased temperature
	Increased PCO_2 (Haldane)	Decreased PCO_2
	Increased diphosphoglycerate (DPG)	Decreased DPG
Minor	(?) Decreased hemoglobin concentration	Carbon monoxide
	Hemoglobins of abnormal affinity	Methemoglobin
	Aldosterone	
	Exercise	
	(?) Zinc	
	Inorganic ions	
Indirect		
	(*through increased DPG*)	(*through decreased DPG*)
	Hypoxia: lung disease, congestive heart failure	Acidosis
	Alkalosis	Bank blood
	Increased inorganic phosphate	Fetal hemoglobin
	Anemia	Decreased inorganic phosphate
	Increased thyroxine	Old erythrocytes
	Pyruvate kinase deficiency	Sex (male)
	Young erythrocytes	Hexokinase deficiency
	Cortisone	
	Sex (female)	
	Down's syndrome	
	High altitude, through respiratory alkalosis	
	Angina (local change in DPG)	

affinity. Furthermore, deoxyhemoglobin combines more readily with hydrogen than oxyhemoglobin. In other words, deoxyhemoglobin is a weaker acid and therefore a better buffer. The interrelationship of hydrogen, hemoglobin affinity, and its buffer capacity have an interesting physiologic effect at the tissues (Figure 10–5). Normally, higher hydrogen concentration at the tissues, generated by tissue metabolism, promotes oxygen release through the Bohr effect. At the same time, the increased proportion of deoxyhemoglobin buffers the hydrogen produced by the tissues [37]. These two mutually advantageous effects further complement each other in times of stress (increased oxygen requirements or decreased oxygen supply). Under such conditions, there are further increases in the proportion of deoxyhemoglobin in the hydrogen ion concentration. The drop in pH results from the anaerobically generated lactic acid. The further decrease in pH promotes more oxygen release; the increased proportion of deoxyhemoglobin helps to neutralize some of the excess acid production.

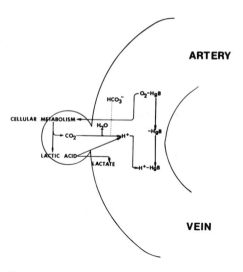

Figure 10–5. The interrelationship among hydrogen, hemoglobin affinity, and hemoglobin buffer capacity.

Carbon Dioxide

Carbon dioxide lowers hemoglobin's affinity for oxygen by two mechanisms. First, it decreases affinity through the Bohr effect because CO_2 combines with H_2O to form $HCO_3^- + H^+$. Second, carbon dioxide binds preferentially with deoxyhemoglobin to form carbaminohemoglobin [37]. The lowering of affinity of this mechanism is analogous to the effect of hydrogen on affinity.

Diphosphoglycerate

Of all these factors, DPG has the most profound effect on hemoglobin affinity. It was observed for many years that isolated hemoglobin exhibited an unphysiologically high affinity for oxygen (isolated hemoglobin's P50 = 5 versus intraerythrocytic hemoglobin's P50 = 27). At this high affinity, isolated hemoglobin cannot effectively transport oxygen within the physiologic range of oxygen tension required in the body, because hemoglobin would return from the tissues still nearly saturated. Furthermore, it had been known for decades that in hypoxic states, hemoglobin decreases its affinity for oxygen, seemingly in an attempt to compensate for the oxygen deficiencies in tissue oxygenation. It was noted only that the organic phosphate DPG existed in much higher concentrations in the red blood cell than anywhere else in the body, but no function could be assigned to this substance.

These phenomena remained unexplained until 1967, when Benesch and Benesch [6] and Chanutin and Curnish [11] independently linked the decreased affinity to the presence of red blood cell DPG. They also demonstrated that DPG combines with hemoglobin in equimolar proportions (one molecule of DPG combines with one molecule of hemoglobin). Furthermore, DPG does not combine with isolated monomers (single chains) of hemoglobin or with tetramers of alpha chains (hemo-globin molecules consisting of four alpha chains). However, DPG does combine with tetramers of beta chains and with hemoglobin A (two alpha, two beta) and weakly with fetal hemoglobin (two alpha, two gamma). Thus it was proposed [36] that its binding site was located in the central cavity of the hemoglobin molecule between the two beta chains (see Figure 10-3). DPG binds only to deoxyhemo-globin, presumably because the space between the two beta chains in the oxyhemo-globin is too narrow to admit a molecule of DPG. Similarly, when DPG is located between the beta chains, the structural changes that must precede oxygenation are hindered. Thus, a higher oxygen tension is required to force oxygenation.

DPG alters affinity in two ways. First, DPG binds reversibly with deoxyhemo-globin which impairs oxygenation by stabilizing the deoxyhemoglobin form [37]. Second, DPG decreases oxygen affinity indirectly through the Bohr effect [18]. Nondiffusible anions (negatively charged), such as DPG, located on one side of a semipermeable membrane (e.g., red blood cell wall) cause a redistribution of smaller positively charged molecules (e.g., hydrogen) across the membrane to maintain electrochemical neutrality (the Gibbs-Donnan effect). The net result is the influx of hydrogen into the cell, which lowers the intraerythrocytic pH. By lowering the pH, affinity decreases. At low levels of DPG, the direct effect (chemical combination) is thought to play the dominant role, whereas at high DPG concentrations the indirect (Bohr) effect becomes increasingly significant, perhaps surpassing the other in importance [18]. DPG binding is not autonomous. It depends not only on the concentrations of oxygen and hemoglobin, but also on pH, carbon dioxide pressure, and temperature. These complex interactions make the in vivo quantitating of the relationship between DPG and hemoglobin affinity difficult, if not impossible. In vitro, an 8 percent change in the DPG concentration corresponds to a P50 change of approximately 1.0 torr [34].

DPG is produced in the red blood cell by anaerobic glycolysis (Figure 10-6). In nonerythrocytic glycolysis, 1,3-DPG is converted directly to 3-phosphoglycerate. In the red blood cell, a side reaction takes place that generates the high concentra-tions of 2,3-DPG found there. 1,3-DPG is first converted to 2,3-DPG, which is then metabolized to 3-DPG. The rate of DPG generation is governed by pH, the overall rate of the pathway's reaction (here, anaerobic glycolysis), the concentrations of the intermediate compounds, and the activity of the specific enzymes that catalyze the various steps in the pathway [2]. The factors that govern the synthesis of DPG are many, and their relative importance remains controversial. The critical enzym-atic steps appear to be at hexokinase, phosphofructokinase, and pyruvate kinase. Other enzymatic steps have varying importance depending on the conditions within the red blood cell.

DISEASES ASSOCIATED WITH ALTERATIONS IN DPG
Discrepancies between tissue oxygen supply and need are often associated with decreased hemoglobin affinity for oxygen, presumably a compensatory mechanism

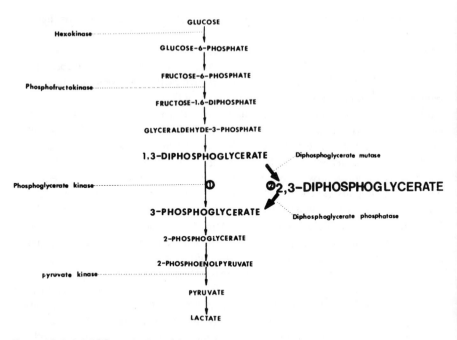

Figure 10-6. 2,3-DPG synthesis and degradation.

to facilitate tissue oxygenation. It is usually advantageous that increased temperature, carbon dioxide tension, and hydrogen ion concentration decrease hemoglobin affinity because fever, hypercapnia, and acidosis often occur in disease states that would benefit from enhanced oxygen transport. Likewise, in many conditions associated with hypoxia, there is an increase in the red blood cell DPG concentration and a resultant decrease in the hemoglobin affinity, apparently to augment oxygen unloading at the tissues. Theoretically, if the oxyhemoglobin dissociation curve is shifted to the right, the arteriovenous difference will be greater for any given venous oxygen tension as long as the arterial oxygen content is not too severely reduced (Figure 10-7). This theoretical model demonstrates that a right-shifted curve expands the arteriovenous difference by 60 percent, so that tissue oxygenation is enhanced without a change in any other parameter of oxygen transport.

Examples of altered affinity secondary to changes in DPG levels are numerous and include anemia, congestive heart failure, cyanotic heart disease, cirrhosis, endocrinopathies, bank blood, metabolic disturbances, carboxyhemoglobinemia, hypoxic pulmonary disease, and high altitude adaptation. In anemic patients, the magnitude of the increased DPG levels correlated well with the severity of the anemia [47]. Whether control of DPG synthesis is directly or indirectly mediated by hemoglobin remains controversial. One recent study demonstrated that decreased hemoglobin concentrations alone does not result in increased DPG production [31].

Congestive heart failure is also associated with decreased hemoglobin affinity

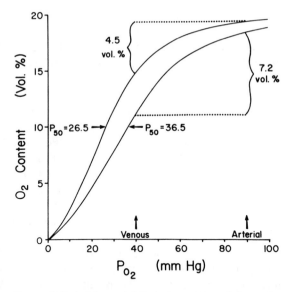

Figure 10-7. A rightward shift in the position of the oxyhemoglobin dissociation curve results in an augmented arteriovenous oxygen difference (more oxygen released to the tissues) when the arterial and venous oxygen tensions are normal. (Reproduced with permission from Klocke, R. A. Oxygen transport and 2,3-diphosphoglycerate. *Chest* 62, 1972, p. 79S. Fig. 1.)

secondary to increased DPG levels. The magnitude of DPG elevation correlates with the level of venous oxygen content and the severity of the process. One study demonstrated that oxygen consumption remained normal, which would indicate that perhaps the DPG-mediated compensation may have been complete [52].

In cyanotic heart disease, there is a close correlation between the severity of the shunt and the level of DPG. Acute changes in the P50 of coronary sinus blood of patients during acute angina attacks occur, but there is no accompanying change in the DPG, pH, or ATP. The mechanism of this immediate alteration in hemoglobin affinity is unknown [43].

The elevated DPG levels that occur in cirrhosis are partly secondary to the anemia that often accompanies cirrhosis, but the DPG levels exceed those expected for the severity of the anemia. Possible mechanisms include the respiratory alkalosis (a potent stimulus of DPG synthesis) and the right-to-left shunts that are seen with cirrhosis [1]. DPG levels vary directly with the level of thyroid hormone. That is, deficiency of thyroid hormone is associated with a decreased DPG concentration that rises to normal with replacement therapy. Whether this is related primarily to increased oxygen consumption or to a direct effect of thyroid hormone on glycolysis and the DPG pathway has not been established [40]. The administration of steroids has been shown to induce DPG synthesis by a mechanism yet unknown [44].

Metabolic disturbances that demonstrate abnormal DPG levels include hypophosphatemia and diabetes. Inorganic phosphate has been shown to be a potent regulator of DPG synthesis. Increased DPG levels have been induced with phosphate infusions [20] and decreased DPG levels have been noted in hypophosphatemic patients [48]. Nonacidotic diabetic patients were found to have significantly increased DPG concentrations in the presence of increased rather than decreased affinity, a finding that remains unexplained [17].

It is now known that the progressive increase in the hemoglobin affinity of stored blood is secondary to the decreased DPG concentration. Furthermore, the preservative citrate-phosphate-dextrose (CPD) maintains higher levels of DPG than blood stored in acid-citrate-dextrose (ACD). Studies indicate that the improved DPG levels are probably related to the increase in the pH of CPD (alkalosis stimulates DPG synthesis) [41]. In patients receiving small amounts of bank blood or those without precarious oxygen transport, a difference in the DPG concentration in the transfusions may not be clinically significant. However, in situations where blood loss is massive or where oxygen transport is already disturbed, the preservation of adequate levels of DPG becomes increasingly important.

Abnormal hemoglobin structure can result in an increased, decreased, or normal affinity for oxygen. In general, hemoglobins with increased affinity are associated with polycythemia [50], indicating that the increase in the affinity alters tissue oxygenation. Hemoglobin Seattle is interesting in that, although patients with it have low hemoglobin concentrations, they do not appear to be physiologically anemic.

The low affinity of hemoglobin Seattle (P50 = 40) probably is responsible for maintaining normal oxygen transport in spite of a decreased hemoglobin content [46]. Because hemoglobin Seattle is unstable, some hemolysis occurs. It is interesting to surmise whether the "anemia" is primarily secondary to hemolysis or to negative feedback (increased ability to transport oxygen-inhibiting erythropoiesis). There is evidence that erythropoietin is not increased, which would favor the "negative feedback" theory [46]. Defects in the enzymes of the glycolytic pathway can give rise to abnormal concentrations of DPG. Enzyme defects that occur proximal to DPG (e.g., hexokinase deficiency) result in decreased DPG and increased affinity; those that occur distal to the DPG shunt (e.g., pyruvate kinase deficiency) give rise to increased DPG and decreased affinity. The physiologic effect of this was demonstrated by comparing the exercise tolerance of two patients, one with pyruvate kinase deficiency and one with hexokinase deficiency. The increased tolerance of the pyruvate kinase-deficient patient suggests that this patient's increased DPG resulted in enhanced oxygen transport [35].

The foregoing discussion of the effects of increased DPG emphasizes its ability to increase oxygen transport through increasing oxygen release at the tissues. However, a right-shifted curve is not always advantageous. When the arterial oxygen content is normal, or nearly normal, then a decreased affinity will increase unloading (decrease the saturation of the blood leaving the tissue capillaries) but will not significantly lower the arterial oxygen content because of the shape of the oxyhemoglobin dissociation curve. However, if the arterial oxygen tension is very low (on the steep portion of the oxyhemoglobin dissociation curve), then an increased P50 will significantly impair arterial oxygen-loading in the lungs. In other words, the arterial saturation as well as the venous saturation can decrease with a right-shifted curve. As the arterial hypoxemia worsens, so does the arterial saturation. Eventually the amount of saturation "lost" on the arterial side will approach, and even exceed, the amount of desaturation "gained" on the venous side, resulting in an equivalent or a decreased arteriovenous difference. Although the arterial oxygen content and the P50 can be determined, the venous oxygen content and perfusion of individual organs is not taken into consideration. Therefore, hemoglobin affinity cannot be predicted from this insufficient data. Furthermore, because of individual variation in organ perfusion and oxygen-extracting properties, the direction of the most beneficial shift may not be the same for all organs (Figure 10-8).

Extreme high altitude, severe hypoxemia secondary to pulmonary disease, and the properties of fetal hemoglobin illustrate that increased hemoglobin affinity for oxygen facilitates tissue oxygenation. Moderately high altitudes (moderate decrease in inspired oxygen tension) is associated with increased DPG levels [8, 30]. However, at extreme altitudes (severely decreased inspired oxygen tension), a left-shifted curve appears to be more physiologic [19, 21]. The high affinity of fetal hemoglobin presumably is better suited for intrauterine life.

In severe hypoxia associated with pulmonary disease, the P50 and the DPG level are variable [22]. This is not surprising considering the complexities in the severely hypoxic patient that determine hemoglobin affinity, DPG level, and ideal P50. In pulmonary patients, the situation is even more complex, probably because of the

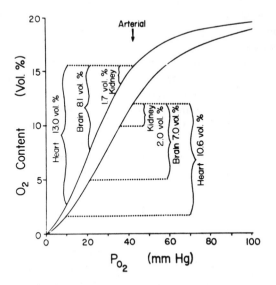

Figure 10-8. Oxygen release (arteriovenous difference) to various tissues of different extraction properties. Comparison of the effect of a rightward shift on the arteriovenous differences in high versus low extraction tissues under hypoxic conditions. A rightward shift can have a deleterious effect on oxygen delivery to the brain and the heart. (Reproduced with permission from Klocke, R. A. Oxygen transport and 2,3-diphosphoglycerate. *Chest* 62, 1972, p. 81S. Fig. 4.)

variations in arterial oxygen tension, hemoglobin concentrations, cardiovascular status, and acid-base balance. These factors are all known to have potent effects on P50 and DPG synthesis. One study showed considerable variability in the P50 and DPG level but remarkably consistent venous oxygen tension. From this, it was concluded that the discrepancies in the hemoglobin affinity and DPG level "had little effect on oxygen delivery to the tissues" [22]. However, without direct measurement of tissue oxygenation this statement cannot be absolutely substantiated.

The exact mechanism by which hypoxia mediates increased DPG synthesis is unknown. Several factors are considered to be involved: excess deoxyhemoglobin, systemic pH, and intraerythrocytic pH. Initially, it was proposed that the excess deoxyhemoglobin in hypoxia was the main mechanism of increased DPG production. This assumption stemmed from the observation that DPG itself modifies its own rate of synthesis by exerting negative feedback (product inhibition) on the rate-limiting enzymes of glycolysis. Under hypoxic conditions, there is more deoxyhemoglobin available to combine with DPG. Thus, by lowering the concentration of "free" DPG and by releasing the pathway from product inhibition, deoxyhemoglobin promotes the generation of yet more DPG [34].

A more favored explanation centers around changes in pH as the mediator of hypoxia-induced increased DPG. Alkalosis is a potent stimulator of DPG synthesis [5]. In hypoxia, there are two factors that tend to produce alkalosis. First, many types of hypoxia are accompanied by respiratory alkalosis. Acute alkalosis raises the hemoglobin affinity (Bohr effect). The sustained effect of alkalosis on hemoglobin affinity (decrease) occurs over several hours.

To test the hypothesis that hypoxia alters hemoglobin affinity through pH changes, subjects were given carbonic anhydrase inhibitor (to prevent alkalosis) and then exposed to low inspired oxygen tensions. The DPG response was diminished in one study [30] and abolished in another. The second way proposed for alkalosis-mediated increased DPG is an increase in the intraerythrocytic, rather than systemic, pH [2]. Deoxyhemoglobin, which is increased in hypoxia, combines with hydrogen more readily than oxyhemoglobin. As a result, increasing the proportion of hemoglobin in the deoxyhemoglobin form causes a rise in the intraerythrocytic pH. This is a more inviting proposal because it does not necessitate the presence of a systemic alkalosis. However, it is a difficult hypothesis to test because the measurement of intraerythrocytic pH is indirect at best.

MECHANISMS OF HYPOXIA

When the various components of oxygen transport fail, tissues suffer from inadequate oxygen supply. The underlying pathophysiologic mechanisms of hypoxia can be classified as follows: hypoventilation, decreased inspired oxygen tension from high altitude, ventilation-perfusion mismatch, right-to-left shunt, diffusion defects, hypoperfusion (local or general), and abnormal blood-oxygen transport. In most cases of clinically encountered hypoxia, more than one mechanism is active (Table 10–3).

Table 10-3. Mechanisms of Hypoxia

Inadequate arterial oxygen tension
  Decreased inspired oxygen tension (high altitude)
    Hypoventilation
    Right-to-left shunt
    Diffusion defects
    Ventilation-perfusion mismatch
Inadequate blood oxygen content
  Inadequate arterial oxygen tension
  Anemia
  Abnormal hemoglobin affinity
Inadequate transport of blood to tissues
  General
    Congestive heart failure
    Vasomotor collapse
    Hypovolemia
  Local
    Vascular occlusions

High Altitude

High altitude causes hypoxia because the inspired oxygen tension (PI_{O_2}) is inversely related to the elevation above sea level. At sea level, where the barometric pressure is about 760 torr, the corresponding PI_{O_2} is about 150 torr. With ascent, the inspired oxygen tension drops. In Leadville, Colorado, with an altitude of 10,200 feet, the PI_{O_2} is only 101 torr. It can be seen that above a certain altitude, life cannot exist. Even before these altitudes are reached, compensatory mechanisms come into play to aid the high-altitude dweller adapt to his environment. Certain elevations are tolerated if the ascent is gradual; rapid ascent is not tolerated. Hyperventilation, polycythemia, and decreased density of gases aid in tolerance to high altitudes.

Hypoventilation

Hypoventilation refers to abnormal *alveolar* ventilation. When the amount of ventilation reaching the alveoli is inadequate, alveolar carbon dioxide accumulates and alveolar oxygen is depleted. Alveolar carbon dioxide tension reflects the balance between the rate of carbon dioxide removal by ventilation and the rate of carbon dioxide production. Likewise, alveolar oxygen tension reflects the balance between the rate of oxygen addition by ventilation and the rate of oxygen removal by the blood. Because the blood is in equilibrium with the disturbed alveolar gas tensions, the arterial blood demonstrates a low oxygen tension, an elevated carbon dioxide tension, and a low pH (secondary to the elevated carbon dioxide tension). Because carbon dioxide is inversely proportional to alveolar ventilation, the carbon dioxide tension must be abnormal relative to the amount of alveolar ventilation to make the diagnosis of disturbed ventilation. Because the relationship between the carbon dioxide tension and ventilation is linear, the carbon dioxide tension level correlates with the severity of the process.

There are two types of hypoventilation: absolute or global (decreased minute ventilation) and relative or regional (increased minute ventilation). In absolute hypoventilation, the overall ventilation (minute ventilation = tidal volume × respiratory rate) is decreased. Here, the abnormality of depth and rate of respiration is secondary to abnormal regulatory mechanisms or to the inability of the chest wall to respond to the regulatory center's signals. In the first case, the respiratory center does not respond to elevations in carbon dioxide tension. Drug overdose is the most common clinical example of this condition. A decreased overall ventilation can also occur when the chest wall cannot respond to the respiratory center (e.g., chest wall trauma, skeletal muscle paralysis, abdominal distention).

In relative hypoventilation, the respiratory center appropriately responds to an elevated carbon dioxide tension by stimulating an increase in the overall ventilation. But if the underlying pulmonary process is extensive, the increase in minute ventilation may not compensate for the markedly disturbed alveolar ventilation. Alveolar ventilation = (tidal volume – dead space) × respiratory rate. If the dead space (wasted ventilation) is very high, it can be seen that the alveolar ventilation may not be significantly improved by increasing the rate and depth of respiration.

Ventilation-Perfusion Imbalance

Ventilation-perfusion imbalance is the most common cause of hypoxia. It arises when ventilation and perfusion are not equally matched throughout the lung. The effects of underventilation and underperfusion differ.

Consider first underventilation with normal perfusion. Blood passing through underventilated but normally perfused lung is not fully oxygenated. It mixes with fully oxygenated blood from normally ventilated regions, causing a fall in the arterial oxygen tension. Underventilation causes the net accumulation of alveolar carbon dioxide and the net loss of alveolar oxygen, which is reflected in the blood gas tensions of these regions. The extent and degree of underventilation will determine the severity of the overall disturbance in blood gases. The initial elevation in carbon dioxide tension caused by underventilation will stimulate an increase in ventilation. The overventilation of the other regions will result in excretion of the carbon dioxide retained by the underventilated areas. However, if the underlying lung disease is so extensive that further increase in ventilation is impossible, the arterial carbon dioxide tension will rise. Because the relationship between blood oxygen content and ventilation is not linear, the increase in oxygen content of blood from overventilated regions is insufficient to compensate for the decrease in blood oxygen content from the underventilated lung. Therefore, hypoxia secondary to ventilation-perfusion imbalances is not usually associated with hypercapnia.

The other type of ventilation-perfusion imbalance, abnormal perfusion with normal ventilation, does not cause hypoxia or hypercapnia. Here, alveolar oxygen accumulates and alveolar carbon dioxide is depleted. Therefore, the blood perfusing these regions has a higher oxygen tension and a lower carbon dioxide tension than normal. The adverse effect of this disturbance causes an increase in "wasted" ventilation. In order to maintain a normal alveolar ventilation, the overall ventilation must be increased, because alveolar ventilation = (tidal volume – dead space) × respiratory rate. This increases the work of breathing. If extensive, then the volume of dead space is very high, and alveolar ventilation will fall because the increase in minute ventilation will be insufficient to compensate for the increased wasted ventilation. Then the oxygen tension will fall and the carbon dioxide tension will rise.

Right-to-Left Shunt
When blood reaches the arterial circulation without passing through the lung, hypoxia results. This condition can occur with anomalous connections anywhere along the circulatory system as long as a fraction of the blood bypasses the alveoli. Physiologically, as far as gas exchange is concerned, a right-to-left shunt is equivalent to a ventilation-perfusion imbalance where the ventilation is zero. The degree of hypoxia is proportional to the size of the shunt (see Chapter 4). As with ventilation-perfusion abnormalities, the hypoxia is not accompanied by hypercapnia unless it is massive and cannot be eradicated by hyperventilation.

Diffusion Defects
Hypoxemia is associated with diseases characterized by an increase in the blood-air barrier. The mechanism of hypoxemia in these diseases remains controversial. The most popular view is that ventilation-perfusion imbalance is responsible. However, according to the alveolar-capillary block theory, it is the increased barrier, a result of a thickened alveolar-capillary membrane, that impedes diffusion and gives rise to hypoxia. Normally, the diffusion time of carbon dioxide and oxygen is sufficiently short to allow full equilibration between alveolar and blood gas tensions. Even with exercise, when the blood spends less time in the capillary, there is still time for equilibration to occur.

In diffusion defects, it is postulated that the time required for equilibration between alveoli and blood is increased and the time spent by the blood in the capillary is insufficient for normal gas exchange. Therefore, the oxygen tension of the blood leaving the capillary is less than that of the alveoli. It is also postulated that the arterial carbon dioxide tension is normal because the carbon dioxide diffusion is so rapid that, even with the increased distance it has to traverse, full equilibration of carbon dioxide occurs. However, the supporters of the ventilation-perfusion mechanism maintain that the diffusion time of oxygen is not sufficiently prolonged to prevent equilibration.

DIFFERENTIAL DIAGNOSIS OF HYPOXIA
On exposure to 100% oxygen, the characteristic pattern of arterial oxygen tension response can serve as a point of differentiating the various mechanisms of hypoxia. Normally, the arterial oxygen tension rises rapidly to about 600 torr. In diffusion defects and shunts, the arterial oxygen tension also rises rapidly. However, in diffusion defects the rise, although slightly delayed, will equal the normal maximal

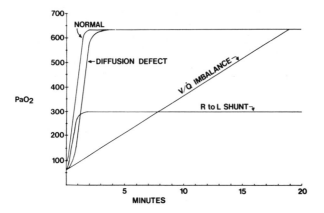

Figure 10–9. Characteristic patterns of Pa_{O_2} response with change of FI_{O_2} from 0.21 to 1.0.

level, whereas in shunts the rate of rise is normal but the maximal level attained will be abnormally low. With ventilation-perfusion imbalances, the oxygen tension rises slowly but will eventually attain the normal level because the alveolar oxygen tension rises slowly in the poorly ventilated areas. Because it is always associated with hypercapnia, hypoventilation is usually easily differentiated from the other mechanisms (hypercapnia will occur with massive shunts). In the individual patient, more than one mechanism is usually active so that these distinctions will not be as clear-cut as outlined above (Figure 10–9).

Hypoxia Secondary to Inadequate Cardiac Output

Hypoxia can result from an abnormally low cardiac output. Here, because the gas exchange is normal, the arterial blood gases are normal. The disturbance is in the rate at which oxygenated blood reaches the tissues. The tissues compensate by increasing oxygen extraction, thus lowering the venous oxygen tension. A low central venous oxygen tension (less than 40 torr) is the hallmark of this mechanism of hypoxia.

Hypoxia Secondary to Abnormalities of the Blood

Hypoxia can be caused by disturbances in the blood's ability to carry or release oxygen. Examples of this condition include hemoglobins with high affinities for oxygen, low levels of red blood cell 2,3-DPG levels, and carbon monoxide poisoning.

OXYGEN TOXICITY

That oxygen is universally poisonous to life presents the student of oxygen toxicity with the seemingly paradoxical and ambivalent relationship between the aerobic organism and its environment. However, on further consideration, one realizes that all forms of life exist in systems where all physical parameters must be maintained within certain bounds in order to sustain them. If the tolerance limits are exceeded, life forms must either develop new adaptive mechanisms or become extinct. Therefore, just as man cannot tolerate abnormally low concentrations of oxygen, so he suffers from high concentrations of oxygen.

Throughout the history of the earth, maximum and minimum tolerance limits have not remained static. It appears that at the time of the origin of life, free oxygen was virtually nonexistent. The main source of free oxygen was nonbiological, primarily from photodissociation (the splitting of water by radiation energy). As photosynthesis evolved, its breakdown product, free oxygen, began to accumulate. This gave rise to two opposing forces. On the one hand it provided another source of energy to support life, and on the other hand it polluted the atmosphere with a poisonous gas. Thus the evolution of organisms that not only utilized but depended on oxygen for their existence must have paralleled the evolution of protective mechanisms against this dangerous gas. Organisms protected themselves against damaging oxidations by developing enzyme systems that metabolize oxygen to less toxic forms.

Another adaptive mechanism is hemoglobin, which through its ability to increase the blood's oxygen-carrying capacity allows adequate oxygen supply to tissues at lower, less toxic oxygen tensions. The process of photosynthesis governs its own potential to give rise to ever-increasing atmospheric concentrations of oxygen. Oxygen, through product inhibition, acts as a negative feedback mechanism on the rate of photosynthesis. This results in a balance between oxidative metabolism and photosynthesis (no net production of oxygen or carbon dioxide). If oxidative metabolism declines, then the unused oxygen accumulates. The increase in oxygen inhibits photosynthesis, which in turn brings the oxygen level back to the baseline concentration.

To what degree the present level of oxygen in the atmosphere is toxic to man poses a fascinating question. It has been proposed that the mechanism of aging is oxygen toxicity, and that the clinical entity of oxygen toxicity is simply an example of this phenomenon in an accelerated form. Antioxidant mechanisms only retard the process; they do not prevent it. When these defense mechanisms are overwhelmed by greater oxygen exposure, then clinically overt oxygen toxicity develops.

Pathology of Oxygen Toxicity
The pathologic lesion seen with pulmonary oxygen toxicity [26, 32] can be classified into two types: acute and chronic [27]. The acute type is seen with high concentrations of oxygen, whereas lower doses of oxygen produce the chronic form. The acute form has two phases, an initial exudative phase followed by a proliferative phase. The exudative phase is characterized by atelectasis, alveolar and interstitial edema, and intraalveolar hemorrhage. The edema gives rise to an increase in the blood-air barrier. There is protein and fibrin exudation along with cellular debris, which may coalesce to form prominent hyaline membranes. Accompanying

these changes there may be widespread destruction of both capillary endothelium and alveolar lining cells, especially the type I (membranous) pneumocyte [26]. Infiltration by inflammatory cells is minimal.

The proliferative phase follows the exudative phase as long as death has not intervened. There are prominent hyperplasia of type II pneumocytes, fibroplastic proliferation, scattered regions of early fibrosis, and cellular swelling that give rise to a markedly thickened blood-air barrier [26]. Again, inflammatory and type I cells may be sparse (Figure 10-10). The chronic form of oxygen toxicity resembles the proliferative phase of acute injury with hyperplasia of the type II pneumocyte and fibrosis (Figure 10-11).

There is marked species variability in the time course of oxygen toxicity. In primates, the exudative phase lasts about four days, after which the proliferative phase begins, becoming most pronounced on the twelfth day. After a recovery period lasting many days, the monkey lung shows large focal areas of fibrosis bordered by normal lung. Electron microscopy reveals a slight increase in the blood-air barrier [26, 27].

Because the various oxygen-induced changes in the lung represent a continuum, the division of these changes into distinct entities is somewhat artificial. Elements of all phases are often simultaneously present [32]. Furthermore, these pathologic

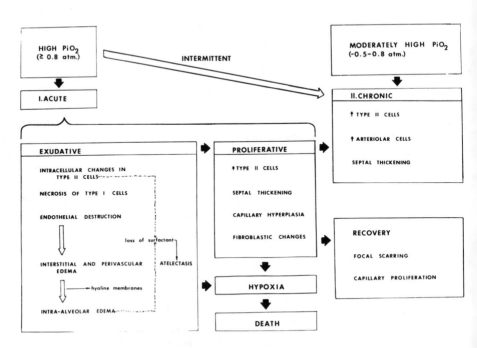

Figure 10-10. The pathological response of the mammalian lung to a toxic pressure of oxygen. (Modified with permission from Winter, P. M., and Smith, G. The toxicity of oxygen. *Anesthesiology* 37, 1972, p. 220. Fig. 5.)

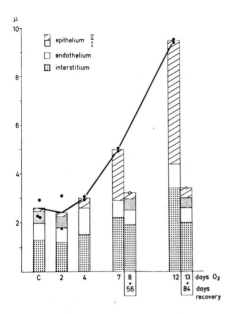

Figure 10-11. Morphometric measurements of the lungs of monkeys exposed to 100% O_2 for 2, 4, 7, 12 days, showing the change in the thickness of the air-blood barrier. C indicates control animals. (Reproduced with permission from Kapanci, Y., Weibel, E. R., Kaplan, H. P., and Robinson, F. R. Pathogenesis and reversibility of the pulmonary lesion of oxygen toxicity in monkeys. II. Ultrastructural and morphometric studies. *Laboratory Investigation* 20, 1969, p. 107. Fig. 11.)

changes (edema, hyaline membranes, fibrosis, proliferation of type II cells, and destruction of type I cells) constitute a nonspecific pulmonary reaction to many noxious stimuli and thus are not unique to oxygen toxicity.

Pulmonary Function Tests in Oxygen Toxicity

The administration of high inspired oxygen tensions is associated with abnormalities in vital capacity, compliance, diffusing capacity, alveolar-arterial gradient, and alveolar ventilation [10, 13] (Table 10-4). In general, these disturbances progress with continued exposure, and their severity is dose related. The vital capacity may not return to normal immediately upon cessation of the high oxygen pressure; in fact, the disturbance can progress before finally returning to normal [10]. Perhaps the abnormalities in vital capacity are secondary to the decrease in the inspiratory capacity; decrease in forced inspiratory volume at one second and the maximum midinspiratory flow rate have been noted experimentally. The pleuritic chest pain associated with high oxygen exposure is not a likely explanation for this defect because high oxygen exposure does in fact occur in the absence of chest pain. Unlike vital capacity and compliance, the diffusing capacity tends to fall later. Possible explanations include atelectasis, increase in the blood-air

Table 10–4. Pulmonary Oxygen Tolerance Studies in Normal Man

Oxygen Partial Pressure (atm)	Ambient Pressure (atm)	Exposure Duration (hr)	Number of Subjects	Indices of Pulmonary Oxygen Toxicity (see accompanying list of symbols and definitions)
0.23	0.25	408	8	VC, FEV, Ca_{O_2}, chest x-ray
0.23	0.25	408	2	VC, $FEV_{1.0}$, %FEV, MBC, Vt
0.24	0.26	120	2	VC
0.24	0.26	72	1	VC, FEV, ERV, IC, MVC, $\dot{V}E$, Vt, chest x-ray
0.25	0.26	336	6	VC, TLV, MBC, DL_{CO}, Pa_{O_2}, chest x-ray
0.26	0.31	72	2	VC, $\dot{V}E$, PA_{CO_2}, Ca_{CO_2}, chest x-ray
0.31	0.92	720	4	FEV, RV, MBC, DL_{CO}, Pa_{O_2}
0.32	0.34	336	3	VC, ERV, IC, FRC, RV, MBC, RL, DL_{CO}, CL, R_{aw}, $\dot{V}E$, Pa_{O_2}, Pa_{CO_2}, single-breath distribution, chest x-ray
0.32	0.34	336	4	VC, PA_{O_2}, PA_{CO_2}, Pa_{CO_2}, chest x-ray
0.33	0.34	336	6	VC, TLV, MBC, DL_{CO}, Pa_{O_2}, chest x-ray
0.33	0.34	720	4	FEV, RV, MBC, DL_{CO}, PA_{O_2}, Pa_{O_2}
0.45	1.0	168	2	$\dot{V}E$, Pa_{CO_2}
0.49	0.50	336	6	VC, TLV, MBC, DL_{CO}, Pa_{O_2}, chest x-ray
0.49	0.50	24	6	VC, f
0.51	1.0	24	10	VC, f
0.55	0.69	168	6	VC, f, chest x-ray
0.75	1.0	24*	9	VC, f
0.83	1.0	53–57	6	VC, f, chest x-ray
0.90	1.0	65	2	VC, PA_{CO_2}
0.95	1.0	42–100	12	VC, $\dot{V}E$, VT, f, pHa, O_2 sat.a, Pa_{O_2}, Pa_{CO_2}, Ca_{CO_2}
0.98	1.0	24	34	VC, f, O_2 sat.a, Pa_{O_2}, $\dot{V}E$, chest x-ray
0.98	1.0	30–74	4	VC, TLV, FEV, RV, DL_{CO}, DM, Vc, PA_{O_2}, Pa_{O_2}, Pa_{CO_2}, pHa, CL, chest x-ray
1.99	2.0	6–12	13	VC, IC, ERV, RV, FRC, FEV, %FEV, MMEF, FIV, %FIV, MMIF, f, CL, R_{aw}, RL, Vt, $\dot{Q}c$, DL_{CO}, DM, Vc, PA_{O_2}, Pa_{CO_2}, pHa, Ca_{O_2}, $Capa\,O_2$, chest x-ray
2.0	2.0	11	1	VC, FRC, f, CL, VT

Table 10-4 *(continued)*

Symbols and Definitions

Ca_{CO_2}	Arterial carbon dioxide concentration
Ca_{O_2}	Arterial oxygen concentration
$Capa\,O_2$	Arterial oxygen capacity
CL	Pulmonary lung compliance
DL_{CO}	Carbon monoxide diffusing capacity of the lung
DM	Diffusing capacity of the pulmonary alveolar membrane
ERV	Expiratory reserve volume
f	Respiratory rate
FEV	Forced expired volume
$FEV_{1.0}$	1-second forced expired volume
%FEV	Percent of forced expired volume expired in 1 sec
FIV	Forced inspired volume
$FIV_{1.0}$	1-second forced inspired volume
%FIV	Percent of forced inspired volume inspired in 1 sec
FRC	Functional residual capacity
IC	Inspiratory capacity
MBC	Maximum breathing capacity
MMEF	Maximum flow rate during midexpiration
MMIF	Maximum flow rate during midinspiration
O_2 sat.a	Arterial oxygen saturation
Pa_{CO_2}	Arterial carbon dioxide tension
PA_{CO_2}	Alveolar carbon dioxide tension
Pa_{O_2}	Arterial oxygen tension
PA_{O_2}	Alveolar oxygen tension
pHa	Arterial pH
$\dot{Q}c$	Pulmonary capillary blood flow
R_{aw}	Airway resistance
RL	Pulmonary resistance
RV	Residual volume
TLV	Total lung volume
Vc	Pulmonary capillary blood volume
VC	Vital capacity
$\dot{V}E$	Expired minute volume
Vt	Pulmonary parenchymal tissue volume
V_T	Tidal volume

*Subjects breathed room air for 15 min every 3 hours. All other exposures were continuous.
Note: Underscored indices showed a significant change during or after exposure.
Source: Reproduced with permission from Clark, J. M., and Lambertsen, C. J. Pulmonary oxygen toxicity: A review. *Pharmacological Reviews* 23, 1971, p. 37. Table 3, p. 70.

barrier (alveolar-capillary block), ventilation-perfusion mismatch, and decreased pulmonary blood flow. One study demonstrated a decrease in the pulmonary capillary volume, which could perhaps account for the decrease in diffusing capacity. An increase in the alveolar-arterial gradient, a prominent feature of overt oxygen toxicity, is not a consistent finding in early oxygen exposure [10]. However, in one clinical study, a marked increase in the alveolar-arterial gradient occurred [4], but the patients were receiving steroids, known potentiators of oxygen toxicity, rendering the interpretation of this finding difficult.

Mechanisms of Oxygen Toxicity

The precise mechanism of oxygen toxicity is unknown. Numerous enzymes and coenzymes are inactivated by oxygen, especially those containing sulf-hydryl (−SH) groups. The oxidation of the sulf-hydryl group results in a disulfide bond (−S−S−). Important sulf-hydryl−containing substances inactivated by oxygen include reduced glutathione, coenzyme A, and many dehydrogenases. Glutathione appears to function as a regulator of many oxidation-reduction reactions within the cell by regenerating reduced forms of substances, which are oxidized in the process of performing their normal biochemical functions.

Inactivation of coenzyme A interferes with the Krebs cycle and fat metabolism. Of the dehydrogenases inactivated by oxygen, glyceraldehyde-3-phosphate dehydrogenase is perhaps one of the most important because it is a key enzyme in the glycolytic pathway. Lipid peroxidation is also considered an important factor in oxygen toxicity because it leads to mitochondrial swelling and to protein and enzyme damage. Another class of compounds sensitive to oxygen are the flavoprotein enzymes, including xanthine oxidase and cytochrome c reductase. The complex, interdependent biochemical consequences of oxygen thus lead to disturbances in many of the cellular processes fundamental to cell viability and organ function [24].

The current unifying theory of oxygen toxicity is the free radical theory [23]. A free radical is a chemical species with a single unpaired electron. The superoxide radical O_2^- appears to be the common denominator of the toxic biochemical effects of oxygen. Oxygen toxicity closely resembles radiation injury to the lung. Ionizing radiation causes the formation of the cytotoxic, unstable free radicals. Biologically, the superoxide radical formed by the single electron reduction of oxygen is generated by many reactions. It is the natural byproduct of oxygen-utilizing cells. Its single, unpaired electron renders O_2^- a powerful reductant and oxidant. Even low levels are thought to be toxic. The accumulation of superoxide radical is prevented by protective enzymes, which further reduce O_2^- to hydrogen peroxide by the chemical reaction

$$O_2^- + O_2^- + 2H \rightarrow H_2O_2 + O_2.$$

The enzymes responsible for this conversion are called *superoxide dismutases* [23]. As long as the substrate (O_2^-) concentration is low, the enzyme can maintain low levels of O_2^-. However, if the system is overwhelmed by substrate, the rate of conversion of O_2^- cannot prevent accumulation of this potentially toxic substance.

There is evidence that the level of superoxide dismutase activity may be correlated with the degree of tolerance to oxygen [28]. Obligate anaerobes lack superoxide dismutase activity. Aerotolerant organisms (organisms that tolerate, but do not utilize, oxygen) have some superoxide dismutase activity. All aerobic cells contain significant superoxide dismutase activity. There is evidence that induced superoxide dismutase is responsible for the increased tolerance to oxygen displayed by organisms after a preliminary sublethal exposure [14]. Experimentally, rats first exposed to 85% and then 100% oxygen survived longer than control rats. The tolerant rats all showed increased superoxide dismutase activity. Furthermore, the loss of tolerance was temporally related to the return of superoxide dismutase activity to baseline levels. Thus, it appears that the proliferation of the type II cells is responsible for the increased superoxide dismutase activity [15]. In that case, type II cell hyperplasia is a protective response of the organism rather than a toxic effect of oxygen.

Under certain circumstances, the cytotoxicity of the superoxide radical can be advantageous to the host because the generation of this radical by leukocytes appears to be important to the killing of phagocytized bacteria [51]. In chronic granulomatous disease, a disease characterized by recurrent suppurative infections, the polymorphonuclear leukocytes do not generate O_2^- during phagocytosis [16, 51]. It has been postulated that the deficiency of oxygen accounts for the fact that chronic granulomatous disease leukocytes can phagocytize but not kill bacteria. Also, superoxide dismutase has been shown to inhibit the killing of bacteria, presumably because it converts O_2^- to a less bactericidal form (H_2O_2) (see Chapter 8).

Clinical Aspects of Oxygen Toxicity

Oxygen has the potential to damage virtually all tissues in the body, i.e., the eye of the neonate, the central nervous system, and the lung. The following discussion will be confined to the clinical aspects of pulmonary oxygen toxicity, a condition that was recognized soon after the discovery of oxygen. Its clinical importance was not fully appreciated until after the development of mechanical ventilation and oxygen delivery systems that made possible the sustained administration of high oxygen tensions. If the clinician is aware of the potential risks of oxygen toxicity, this condition is often preventable with the prudent use of oxygen therapy. If the toxic limitations of oxygen therapy were known, the task of preventing pulmonary oxygen toxicity would be even easier.

In principle, the clinical recommendation concerning oxygen therapy is simple: do not give too much for too long, and above all, do not give too little. In practice, however, this becomes a problem because the precise limits of what is "too little" and "too much" oxygen have not been established. Oxygen toxicity depends on the level of oxygen and the duration of exposure. Extensive studies on animals and on isolated enzyme, cell, and tissue preparations have been done. However, because of large species variation, this information has limited clinical applicability.

The nature of oxygen toxicity does not lend itself to study. The clinical and laboratory disturbances caused by oxygen are insidious in onset and confusingly nonspecific. Furthermore, most patients who require toxic levels of oxygen have underlying pulmonary disease that renders differentiation of that disease from oxygen toxicity difficult. Here, the pulmonary manifestations of oxygen toxicity occur on a background of already disturbed pulmonary function. The symptoms of oxygen toxicity may be masked by medication, by the patient's obtunded state, or by the symptoms of the underlying pulmonary disorder. When a patient who is receiving high levels of oxygen clinically deteriorates, it can never be established beyond doubt whether this deterioration is secondary to progression of the primary process or to oxygen. In studying healthy human volunteers, the ethical limitations are obvious—oxygen exposure must be limited and pathologic examination of the lungs is impossible. Most human studies have been confined to healthy volunteers [10], most clinical studies have been retrospective [25, 32, 33], and those which have been prospective were of limited applicability because of the inherent complexities of studying critically ill patients [4, 45].

Human volunteers can survive exposure of 1 atmosphere of pure oxygen for many hours. During exposure to high oxygen tension, subjects may develop substernal burning chest discomfort, cough, paresthesias, and conjunctival irritation [10, 29, 49]. Functionally, abnormalities in vital capacity, alveolar-arterial gradient, minute ventilation, compliance, and diffusing capacity may be seen [10]. These functional disturbances have not been detected at less than 0.5 atmosphere of pure oxygen even after prolonged exposure. There is marked individual variation in the onset and intensity of the symptoms. The nature of the underlying pathophysiology responsible for these changes remains controversial.

Exposure to 1 atmosphere of pure oxygen for 24 to 48 hours may not induce overt toxicity [10, 45]. Therefore, an exposure of this magnitude is not absolutely contraindicated. It should not be inferred, however, that this degree of exposure has no adverse consequences; rather only that it may not cause a striking deterioration in pulmonary function. Furthermore, overt toxicity has not been observed even after prolonged exposures to fractional concentrations of inspired oxygen of less than 0.4 atmosphere. However, one should not conclude that low oxygen concentrations can be administered with impunity. Long-term, low-flow oxygen therapy has been implemented in chronically hypoxic patients with severe chronic obstructive pulmonary disease. Over the course of months, these low concentrations of oxygen did not produce clinically evident toxicity. On the contrary, the clinical picture improved and survival may even have been prolonged. However, some of the patients who were autopsied demonstrated pathologic findings consistent with oxygen toxicity [39]. Because of the severity of their underlying lung disease, the interpretation of the pathology was especially difficult. Because the lowest oxygen tension that can be tolerated indefinitely without adverse consequences remains unknown, it is questionable that the quantification of man's tolerance to oxygen will ever be possible. Nevertheless, conclusions must be drawn from the scant data available in order to construct clinical guidelines.

Because there is as yet no evidence that short exposures to high concentrations of oxygen at 1 atmosphere cause irreversible pulmonary injury, there is no justification to withhold oxygen in the emergency situation (e.g., cardiopulmonary resuscitation). Even in these patients, as soon as they have been stabilized, inspired oxygen should be lowered, but only to a level proved sufficient by arterial blood gases. Overreaction to the threat of oxygen toxicity here is potentially more harmful than beneficial.

The worst clinical dilemma in oxygen therapy arises in patients with severe, prolonged respiratory failure necessitating long-term exposure to oxygen levels known to be toxic. The very therapy that is sustaining them may ultimately cause their demise. Pulmonary oxygen toxicity may constitute the limiting factor in their recovery. Here, the implementation of other therapeutic measures to improve gas exchange is especially critical, for salvaging these patients may become a race against oxygen toxicity. Because oxygen represents symptomatic, supportive therapy only, attention must be directed to correcting the underlying cause of respiratory failure and the derangement of other organ systems (e.g., congestive heart failure, uremia).

The prudent use of oxygen therapy dictates that oxygen should be administered only in those situations where a low arterial oxygen tension has been documented. An exception to this is carbon monoxide poisoning, where, in the face of a normal arterial oxygen pressure, the oxygen content of the blood may be markedly reduced. Here, high oxygen tensions aid oxygen in its competition with carbon monoxide for hemoglobin binding. Furthermore, oxygen therapy should be continued only when an ongoing need for oxygen has been established by frequent reevaluation of the patient, including repeated arterial blood gas determinations.

In general, administration of the lowest inspired oxygen tension that will result in an arterial oxygen tension of between 60 and 90 torr is recommended. The rationale behind this recommendation lies in an understanding of the oxyhemoglobin dissociation curve. Normally, an arterial oxygen tension of greater than 60 torr corresponds to a saturation of greater than 90 percent. Above an oxygen tension of 60 torr, the flat curve indicates that further increases in arterial oxygen tension will not substantially augment the blood's oxygen-carrying capacity. However, below an arterial oxygen tension of 60 torr, the steep slope indicates that small changes in the arterial oxygen tension will result in relatively large changes in blood oxygen content. Therefore, if the arterial oxygen tension is maintained between 60 and 90 torr, adequate hemoglobin saturation is achieved with the least amount of risk. It is advisable to maintain the arterial oxygen tension slightly above the theoretical minimum of 60 torr to provide a margin of safety. The choice of 60 torr as the minimally acceptable arterial oxygen tension is theoretical and does not take into consideration the many other factors that influence oxygen transport (e.g., hemoglobin concentration, cardiac output, regional perfusion, shifts in the oxyhemo-globin dissociation curve). Changing tissue needs may also dictate a different mini-mal, adequate arterial oxygen tension. To "treat" the arterial oxygen tension without considering the other parameters that affect tissue oxygenation constitutes therapeutic "tunnel vision."

In summary, there is little controversy concerning the guidelines for oxygen therapy in the extreme ranges of arterial oxygen tensions. The consequences of severe, acute hypoxia are so catastrophic that they warrant the administration of even very high oxygen concentrations. Correction of the arterial oxygen tension above "normal" is unjustified because it merely increases the risk of oxygen toxicity without any evidence that tissue oxygenation will be improved. At the two extremes, the recommendations are clear. In the middle gray area, the physician is advised to use his clinical judgment, which here amounts to making an educated guess.

Hyperbaric Oxygen Therapy

Man continuously searches for new therapeutic maneuvers that will improve tissue oxygenation. One such technique is hyperbaric oxygen therapy (oxygen adminis-tered at greater than 1 atmosphere). At 1 atmosphere, the maximum inspired oxygen tension is about 760 torr at sea level. A higher inspired oxygen tension can be achieved with hyperbaric conditions. At greater than 1 atmosphere, the increase in the plasma fraction alone accounts for the increase in the total blood oxygen content, because hemoglobin is fully saturated at much lower pressures (see Table 10–5). However, because hyperbaric oxygen therapy greatly accelerates oxygen toxicity, its clinical usefulness is limited. Hyperbaric therapy has no role in many diseases associated with abnormal tissue oxygenation, e.g., shunting, congestive heart failure, peripheral vascular disease, respiratory failure. Nonetheless, there are two specific indications for hyperbaric oxygen therapy: carbon monoxide poison-ing and anaerobic infections. Carbon monoxide has such a high affinity for hemo-globin that at physiologic oxygen tensions, oxygen cannot effectively compete with carbon monoxide for binding sites on hemoglobin. As a result, the arterial oxygen content is markedly reduced. Moreover, carbon monoxide increases the hemoglobin affinity for oxygen so that it also interferes with peripheral oxygen release. By markedly increasing the plasma fraction of oxygen (hyperbaric therapy), oxygen can better compete with carbon monoxide and force the carbon monoxide from hemoglobin. In some anaerobic infections such as clostridia [9], the very high plasma oxygen levels create a less favorable environment for the bacteria, a situa-tion that uses oxygen toxicity as an advantage.

Artificial Gas Transport Systems

Inadequate tissue oxygenation is a common and devastating clinical problem. As a result, much interest has been generated in the field of artificial gas transport sys-tems. Investigators are currently striving to develop a nontoxic, practical substance that will approach, or even exceed, the oxygen-carrying capacity of whole blood.

Table 10-5. Total Arterial Oxygen Content at Various Inspired Oxygen Tensions

Inspired O_2 Pressure (atm)	O_2 Content Dissolved in Plasma (vol %)	O_2 Content Associated with Hemoglobin (vol %)	Total Arterial O_2 Content (vol %)
0.21	0.3	20	20.3
1.0	2.0	21	23.0
2.0	4.0	21	25.0
3.0	6.0	21	27.0
4.0	8.0	21	29.0

The clinical and experimental applications of such a substance would be limitless. Most importantly, it would eliminate many of the inherent problems encountered with natural blood products such as disease transmission (e.g., hepatitis), time-consuming cross-matching, and availability of compatible donors. In general, the difficulties of natural blood products do not relate to oxygen transport, because transport is adequate as long as sufficient erythrocytic diphosphoglycerate levels are preserved.

In emergency situations such as massive hemorrhage and carbon monoxide poisoning, artificial blood would have a number of advantages. At the present time, hemorrhaging patients cannot receive blood transfusions until compatibility of bank blood can be established. This costly delay may cause hypoxic damage and could be prevented by the immediate administration of the nonantigenic blood substitutes. Synthetic blood could also be used when oxygen transport is inadequate, not because of blood loss, but because of a defect in hemoglobin's capacity to carry oxygen (e.g., carbon monoxide poisoning, methemoglobinemia). In carbon monoxide poisoning, hemoglobin-carbon monoxide complexes interfere with oxygen loading (carbon monoxide competes with it for hemoglobin-binding sites) and with oxygen release (carbon monoxide increases hemoglobin-oxygen affinity). If it were technically feasible, immediate total exchange transfusion could effectively correct this disorder by removing the lethal hemoglobin-carbon monoxide complexes. Perhaps in the future, swift total circulatory replacement with artificial blood will be possible so that these patients would be salvaged.

Three classes of substances currently under investigation are the perfluorocarbons, the free hemoglobin solutions, and chelating agents. Hemoglobin solutions and chelating agents, which carry oxygen by chemical combination, are the most promising theoretically, for it has been postulated that if the relationship between their oxygen content and their oxygen tension could simulate the oxyhemoglobin dissociation curve, then their efficiency to carry oxygen could approach that of intraerythrocytic hemoglobin [3]. Because perfluorocarbons operate on the principle of solubility, the relationship of oxygen content and oxygen tension is linear. As yet, the solubility of perfluorocarbons is too low to achieve sufficient oxygen content to sustain life without the administration of high oxygen tensions. The synthesis of perfluorocarbons with higher solubility would eliminate this disadvantage.

Experimentally, total circulatory replacement has been achieved with the perfluorocarbon, perfluorotributylamine, which can sustain life without apparent toxicity or gross physiologic disturbance. The infused solutions of perfluorocarbons contain substances to maintain normal oncotic pressure and pH. Simultaneously, all natural blood elements (red blood cells, proteins, clotting factors, antibodies, and hormones) are removed. The animals breathe 1 atmosphere of pure oxygen. The animals have been observed to exhibit normal behavior and growth. Immediately rapid erythropoeisis begins, and at the end of a week, their circulatory systems have been reconstituted with all the natural blood components. The fate of the perfluorocarbon is unknown. However, autopsied animals show increased liver and spleen weights, presumably because of sequestered perfluorocarbon. The dramatic survival of these animals demonstrates that these blood substitutes can maintain adequate gas transport [12].

Isolated hemoglobin solutions have been experimentally tested as a potential artificial gas transport system. Although free hemoglobin has a higher affinity for oxygen than intraerythrocytic hemoglobin, there is experimental evidence that free hemoglobin can still release enough oxygen at the tissue level to significantly augment oxygen transport [7]. In hypoxic situations, the increased ability of the tissues to extract oxygen makes the oxygen associated with free hemoglobin accessible to the tissues.

It will be far in the future when these compounds are available for clinical use, for tremendous technical problems remain, for example, limitations of currently available perfluorocarbons, difficulties with preparation techniques, and short duration of oxygen-carrying capacity. The search for the ideal blood substitute continues; even when these problems have been overcome, extensive testing as to the safety of this substitute will further delay its clinical application.

REFERENCES

1. Astrup, J., and Rorth, M. Oxygen affinity of hemoglobin and red cell 2,3-diphosphoglycerate in hepatic cirrhosis. *Scand. J. Clin. Lab. Invest.* 31, 1973, p. 311.
2. Astrup, P. Red-cell pH and oxygen affinity of hemoglobin. *N. Engl. J. Med.* 283, 1970, p. 202.
3. Baldwin, J. E. Chelating agents as possible artificial blood substitutes. *Fed. Proc.* 34, 1975, p. 1441.
4. Barber, R. E., Lee, J., and Hamilton, W. K. Oxygen toxicity in man. *N. Engl. J. Med.* 283, 1970, p. 1478.
5. Bellingham, A. J., Detter, J. C., and Lenfant, C. The role of hemoglobin affinity for oxygen and red-cell 2,3-diphosphoglycerate in the management of diabetic ketoacidosis. *Trans. Assoc. Am. Physicians* 83, 1970, p. 113.
6. Benesch, R. and Benesch, R. The effect of organic phosphates from the human erythrocyte on the allosteric properties of hemoglobin. *Biochem. Biophys. Res. Commun.* 26, 1967, p. 162.

7. Bonhard, K. Acute oxygen supply by infusion of hemoglobin solutions. *Fed. Proc.* 34, 1975, p. 1466.
8. Brewer, J. J., et al. Effects on hemoglobin oxygen affinity of smoking in residents of intermediate altitude. *J. Lab. Clin. Med.* 84, 1974, p. 191.
9. Brummelkamp, W. H., Boerema, I., and Hogendyk, L. Treatment of clostridial infections with hyperbaric oxygen drenching: A report on 26 cases. *Lancet* 1, 1963, p. 235.
10. Caldwell, P. R. B., et al. Changes in lung volume, diffusing capacity, and blood gases in men breathing oxygen. *J. Appl. Physiol.* 21, 1966, p. 1477.
11. Chanutin, A., and Curnish, R. R. Effect of organic and inorganic phosphates on the oxygen equilibrium of human erythrocytes. *Arch. Biochem. Biophys.* 121, 1967, p. 96.
12. Clark, L. C., Kaplan, S., and Becattini, F. The physiology of synthetic blood. *J. Thorac. Cardiovasc. Surg.* 60, 1970, p. 757.
13. Comroe, J. H., et al. Oxygen toxicity: The effect of inhalation of high concentrations of oxygen for 24 hours on normal men at sea level and at a simulated altitude of 18,000 feet. *J.A.M.A.* 128, 1945, p. 710.
14. Crapo, J. D. Superoxide dismutase and tolerance to pulmonary oxygen toxicity. *Chest* 67, 1975, p. 39S.
15. Cross, C. E. The granular type II pneumonocyte and lung antioxidant defense. *Ann. Intern. Med.* 80, 1974, p. 409.
16. Curnutte, J. T., Whitten, D. M., and Babior, B. M. Defective superoxide production by granulocytes from patients with chronic granulomatous disease. *N. Engl. J. Med.* 290, 1974, p. 593.
17. Ditzel, J., Andersen, H., and Peters, N. D. Increased hemoglobin A_{1c} and 2,3-diphosphoglycerate in diabetics and their effects on red-cell oxygen-releasing capacity. *Lancet* 2, 1973, p. 1034.
18. Duhm, J.   2,3-diphosphoglycerate-induced displacements of the oxyhemoglobin dissociation curve of blood: Mechanisms and consequences. *Adv. Exp. Med. Biol.* 37-A, 1973, p. 179. First half of the International Symposium on Oxygen Transport to Tissue, held in Charleston-Clemson, South Carolina, April 22–28, 1973.
19. Eaton, J. W., Shelton, J. D., and Berger, E. Survival at extreme altitude: Protective effect of increased hemoglobin-oxygen affinity. *Science* 183, 1974, p. 743.
20. Farber, M. O., et al. Oxygen transport during acute alkalosis and hyperphosphatemia in dogs. *Anesthesiology* 40, 1974, p. 525.
21. Filley, G. F. *Acid-Base and Blood Gas Regulation.* Philadelphia: Lea & Febiger, 1971.
22. Flenley, D. C., et al. Changes in haemoglobin binding curve and oxygen transport in chronic hypoxic lung disease. *Br. Med. J.* 1, 1975, p. 602.
23. Fridovich, I. Oxygen: Boon and bane. *Am. Sci.* 63, Jan/Feb, 1975, p. 54.
24. Haugaard, N. Cellular mechanisms of oxygen toxicity. *Physiol. Rev.* 48, 1968, p. 311.
25. Hyde, R. W., and Rawson, A. Unintentional iatrogenic oxygen pneumonitis — response to therapy. *Ann. Intern. Med.* 71, 1969, p. 517.
26. Kapanci, Y., et al. Pathogenesis and reversibility of the pulmonary lesions of

oxygen toxicity in monkeys. II. Ultrastructural and morphometric studies. *Lab. Invest.* 20, 1969, p. 101.

27. Kaplan, H. P., et al. Pathogenesis and reversibility of the pulmonary lesions of oxygen toxicity in monkeys. I. Clinical and light microscopic studies. *Lab. Invest.* 20, 1969, p. 94.

28. McCord, J. M., Keele, B. B., Jr., and Fridovich, I. Obligate anaerobiosis: An enzyme-based theory. The physiological function of superoxide dismutase. *Proc. Natl. Acad. Sci. U.S.A.* 68, 1971, p. 1024.

29. Michel, E. L., Lanevin, R. W., and Gell, C. F. Effect of continuous human exposure to oxygen tension of 418 mm Hg for 168 hours. *Aerosp. Med.* 31, 1960, p. 138.

30. Miller, M. E., et al. pH effect on erythropoietin response to hypoxia. *N. Engl. J. Med.* 288, 1973, p. 706.

31. Murphy, J. R., Wengerd, M., and Kellermeyer, R. W. Erythrocyte O_2 affinity: Influence of cell density and in vitro changes in hemoglobin concentration. *J. Lab. Clin. Med.* 84, 1974, p. 218.

32. Nash, G., Blennerhassett, J. B., and Pontoppidan, H. Pulmonary lesions associated with oxygen therapy and artificial ventilation. *N. Engl. J. Med.* 276, 1967, p. 368.

33. Northway, W. H., Rosan, R. C., and Porter, D. Y. Pulmonary disease following respirator therapy of hyaline membrane disease. Bronchopulmonary dysplasia. *N. Engl. J. Med.* 276, 1967, p. 357.

34. Oski, F. A., et al. The effects of deoxygenation of adult and fetal hemoglobin on the synthesis of red cell 2,3-dephosphoglycerate and its in vivo consequences. *J. Clin. Invest.* 49, 1970, p. 400.

35. Oski, F. A., et al. Exercise with anemia. The role of the left-shifted or right-shifted oxygen-hemoglobin equilibrium curve. *Ann. Intern. Med.* 74, 1971, p. 44.

36. Perutz, M. F. Stereochemistry of cooperative effects in haemoglobin. *Nature* 228, 1970, p. 726.

37. Perutz, M. F. The Bohr effect and combination with organic phosphates. *Nature* 228, 1970, p. 734.

38. Perutz, M. F. The hemoglobin molecule. *Sci. Am.* 211, 1974, p. 64.

39. Petty, T. L., Stanford, R. E., and Neff, T. A. Continuous oxygen therapy in chronic airway obstruction. *Ann. Intern. Med.* 75, 1971, p. 361.

40. Rodriguez, J. M., and Shahidi, N. T. Erythrocyte, 2,3-diphosphoglycerate in adaptive red-cell-volume deficiency. *N. Engl. J. Med.* 285, 1971, p. 479.

41. Schweizer, O., and Howland, W. S. 2,3-diphosphoglycerate levels in CPD-preserved bank blood. *Anesth. Analg.* 53, 1974, p. 516.

42. Severinghaus, J. W. Blood gas calculator. *J. Appl. Physiol.* 21, 1966, p. 1108.

43. Shappell, S. D., et al. Acute change in hemoglobin affinity for oxygen during angina pectoris. *N. Engl. J. Med.* 282, 1970, p. 1219.

44. Silken, A. B. The clinical significance of 2,3-diphosphoglycerate. *Conn. Med.* 38, 1974, p. 281.

45. Singer, M. M., et al. Oxygen toxicity in man. *N. Engl. J. Med.* 283, 1970, p. 1473.

46. Stamatoyannopoulos, G., Parrer, J. T., and Finch, C. A. Physiologic implica-

tions of a hemoglobin with decreased oxygen affinity (hemoglobin Seattle). *N. Engl. J. Med.* 281, 1969, p. 915.

47. Torrance, J., et al. Intraerythrocytic adaptation to anemia. *N. Engl. J. Med.* 283, 1970, p. 165.

48. Travis, S. F., et al. Alterations of red-cell glycolytic intermediates and oxygen transport as a consequence of hypophosphatemia in patients receiving intravenous hyperalimentation. *N. Engl. J. Med.* 285, 1971, p. 763.

49. Van DeWater, J. M., et al. Response of the lung to six to twelve hours of 100 percent oxygen inhalation in normal man. *N. Engl. J. Med.* 283, 1970, p. 621.

50. Weatherall, D. J. Polycythemia resulting from abnormal hemoglobins. *N. Engl. J. Med.* 280, 1969, p. 604.

51. Weening, R. S., Wever, R., and Roos, D. Quantitative aspects of the production of superoxide radicals by phagocytizing human granulocytes. *J. Lab. Clin. Med.* 85, 1975, p. 245.

52. Woodson, R. D., et al. The effect of cardiac disease on hemoglobin-oxygen binding. *J. Clin. Invest.* 49, 1970, p. 1349.

Kenneth F. MacDonnell
Bijan Sadrnoori

Positive Pressure Breathing: Physiologic Effects and Consequences*

11

Ventilation with positive pressure breathing devices results in a reversal of the usual pressure relations within the thorax. The resultant physiologic consequences are complex and diverse, affecting a number of organ systems (e.g., kidney, heart). Much of the investigative work in this field has examined the physiologic disruption caused by positive pressure breathing in normal subjects or normal laboratory animals. Thus, a good deal of caution should temper any extrapolation of such data to the clinical setting. For example, the ill patient (e.g., with stiff lung) may be insulated from some of the negative consequences of positive pressure, and may be at high risk for others (e.g., hypovolemia and decreased cardiac output).

It is clear that proper respiratory support with pressure devices such as for intermittent positive pressure breathing (IPPB), positive end expiratory pressure (PEEP), continuous positive airway pressure (CPAP), and negative end expiratory pressure (NEEP) demand an understanding and awareness of the potential for serious homeostatic disruption. The effects of pressure breathing on (1) hemodynamics, (2) bile flow and portal blood flow, (3) water retention, and (4) renal blood flow are of particular interest and will be discussed in detail.

HEMODYNAMICS

The hemodynamic effects of positive pressure have been related to the mean intrathoracic pressure of the complete respiratory cycle. Cournand and associates

*Portions of this chapter were presented at the John Hartnett Lecture, St. Michael's College, Winooski, Vermont.

[5] observed that the decline in cardiac output associated with intermittent positive pressure could be minimized by using a type 3 mask pressure cure, maintaining a peak pressure of less than 25 cm H_2O and allowing for an inspiratory-expiratory ratio of no greater than 1. Numerous reports utilizing techniques of varying sensitivities have documented these observations in man and dog [4, 12, 29].

Systems of mechanical ventilation that employ positive end expiratory pressure have an even more unfavorable effect on cardiac output. These adverse hemodynamic effects of positive pressure ventilation have been ascribed to the resultant combination of (1) decreased venous return, and (2) increased pulmonary vascular resistance.

An increase in intrathoracic and intrapleural pressure results in a decrease in peripheral venous return, along with a decrease in net right ventricular filling pressure, which in turn results in a reduced stroke volume. The net right ventricular filling pressure is equal to the right ventricular end diastolic pressure minus intrathoracic pressure.

An increase in intrathoracic pressure produces an immediate decrease in vena caval flow, resulting in decreased pulmonary arterial flow and systemic aortic flow [8]. Vena caval flow is decreased in a proportionate manner with the increase in intrapleural pressure. Conversely, as pleural pressure falls during the expiratory phase of respiration, vena caval flow increases and the previously described hemodynamic events are reversed.

The role of airway pressure changes and pulmonary vascular resistance is clarified by analysis of the interrelationships between pulmonary blood flow and arterial, venous, and alveolar pressures. West [36] notes that the distribution of blood flow in the upright individual is determined by gravity, with higher flow at the bases of the lung and less flow at the apices. The distribution of ventilation is also gravity dependent, with the upper zones of the lung (apices) more inflated than the bases. West thus divides the lung into four zones. In zone 1, which is represented by the apex of the lung, pulmonary arterial pressure is less than the amount by which alveolar pressure exceeds venous pressure. Flow will be determined by the difference between the arterial and alveolar pressures. In zone 2, pulmonary arterial pressure is greater than alveolar pressure, which in turn is greater than pulmonary venous pressure. The driving pressure in this zone is determined by the difference between the arterial pressure and the alveolar pressure. In zone 3, represented by the basal areas of the lung, flow will be determined in the classic fashion: by the pressure difference between the arterial and the venous sides of the circulation. Zone 4 is the lowest basal portion, where perfusion is relatively decreased as compared to zone 3 (Figure 11-1).

Pulmonary vascular resistance in the excised dog lung is volume (air) dependent [20]. It is lowest at 50 percent of the maximum lung volume, with the least total resistance at functional residual capacity. West also has shown that the resistance of small vessels (below 30 μ in diameter) —the ones that would be exposed to the increased alveolar pressure with IPPB or PEEP—increases with rising lung volume.

Increases in alveolar wall pressure by applying positive pressure ventilation (es-

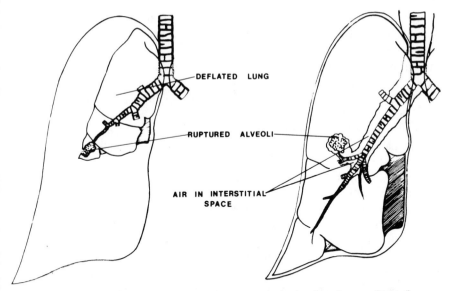

Figure 11-1. *Left*: Pneumothorax, a result of lung rupture in the pleural space. *Right:* Pneumo-mediastinum, a result of lung rupture with dissection of air along the loose peribronchial connective tissue into the mediastinum.

pecially at high pressure levels, or with positive end expiratory pressure) may result in increased pulmonary capillary resistance.

MINIMIZING THE EFFECT OF POSITIVE PRESSURE BREATHING UPON CARDIAC OUTPUT

A number of factors modify the hemodynamic response to positive pressure breathing. Among them are the following:

1. The least amount of inspiratory pressure that is consistent with adequate alveolar ventilation and arterial oxygenation should be utilized (peak pressure 25 cm H_2O if consistent with adequate ventilation) [5].

2. A shortening of the respiratory inspiratory phase may be necessary to establish a favorable [5] inspiratory-expiratory ratio and time-pressure relationship [1,5].

3. A hemodynamically advantageous respirator flow pattern utilizes a type 3 Cournand curve, an asymmetrical curve with gradually increasing pressure during inspiration and a rapid drop to atmospheric pressure during expiration.

4. If a negative expiratory phase is used, it may offset the loss of the normal thoracic pump [24, 37] and improve venous return to the right heart. This effect, even though it may be theoretically desirable, is in practice not significant in the usual clinical setting. The response of the heart to mechanical ventilation is affected not only by venous return but also by pulmonary resistance. Also, the hazard of premature airway closure, especially in the patient with chronic obstructive pulmonary disease must be kept in mind [24, 37].

5. The patient receiving respirator support must be examined closely to assure

the maintenance of a normal blood volume [22, 31]. Individuals in this group are particularly susceptible to the deleterious hemodynamic effects of positive pressure ventilation.

6. Hypoxemia and alterations in arterial carbon dioxide pressure and pH [21, 25, 27, 30] may further aggravate the hemodynamic dysfunction.

7. The prompt and vigorous treatment of any underlying heart or lung disease should be employed, accompanied by an awareness that a fall in cardiac output can be accentuated by impairment of the capacity for reconstituting the gradient from the peripheral venous system to the heart (increasing the main circulatory pressure) [8]. This may be the case with hemorrhagic shock, sympathetic blockade (high spinal anesthesia), or anesthetic depression [19].

8. Interrupted PEEP minimizes the hemodynamic effects of continuous PEEP when used experimentally in normal dogs [18].

9. Optimal PEEP [33] is that level at which alveolar recruitment is maximal, as reflected in the greatest total static compliance while being ventilated. Static compliance is calculated by recording tidal volume and airway pressure. The tidal volume is then divided by the difference between a period of no flow of 1 to 1.5 sec at the end of inspiration and the pressure at the end of expiration.

The stiff, diseased lung is somewhat insulated against the adverse hemodynamic effects of positive pressure breathing, because much of the airway pressure is dissipated and never transmitted to the alveolar and pleural spaces. Indeed, in situations complicated by left ventricular failure, cardiac output may be augmented. The positive pressure acts in these cases much like a tourniquet, decreasing the volume load to the left ventricle. Enhanced systemic oxygenation may improve left ventricular function. The crux of therapy still is systemic oxygen delivery, as illustrated by those instances in which cardiac output may be slightly reduced; but arterial oxygenation is greatly enhanced, the net result being improved oxygen delivery.

The decision for continuous intermittent positive pressure breathing with or without positive end expiratory pressure remains a clinical one, based on the total evaluation of the patient. Indeed, the selection of pressure limits and levels is a carefully titrated, well-planned maneuver, with frequent adjustments according to the patient's response.

EFFECT OF PEEP ON CHOLEDOCHODUODENAL FLOW RESISTANCE AND PORTAL BLOOD FLOW

The jaundice occasionally seen in patients receiving CPAP or PEEP is complex and poorly understood [10, 13]. A variety of mechanisms have been postulated: (1) increased intraabdominal pressure as a result of diaphragmatic depression, which may substantially decrease portal blood flow; (2) obstruction to outflow at the choledochoduodenal junction and the sphincter of Oddi [11, 13, 14, 26]; (3) intrahepatic bile duct compression; and (4) decrease in cardiac output.

Increases in intraabdominal pressure can be transmitted to the compressible liver. With compression there is a damming up or obstruction to the intrahepatic blood flow. The most commonly suggested sites for this obstruction are the portal venules and sinusoids. As a result, there is an overall decrease in portal blood flow. The liver maintains a dual blood supply; if portal blood flow is reduced, an increase in the hepatic arterial blood flow is the usual compensation. This compensatory hemodynamic adjustment may be inadequate in the face of significant hypoxemia or when cardiac output is decreased (cardiac output may be further reduced with PEEP). The resultant decrease in tissue oxygen delivery may result in hypoxic injury. Johnson and Hedley-Whyte [13, 14] have demonstrated increases in choledochoduodenal pressure of 20 percent, with the application of continuous positive pressure ventilation in anesthetized dogs, presumably the result of impaired venous drainage. Compression of the intrahepatic biliary tree secondary to increased intraabdominal pressure is an attractive postulate, but it still remains speculative.

Hyperbilirubinemia, or liver malfunction, observed in the patient receiving PEEP may be ascribed to any one or all of these mechanisms. However, it remains for the clinician to maintain a measure of suspicion as patients on respirators are just as likely to develop primary diseases of the hepatobiliary system as those without respiratory disease.

WATER RETENTION, URINE FLOW, VASOPRESSIN, AND MECHANICAL VENTILATION

Excess fluid retention is a frequently encountered problem in the setting of the respiratory intensive care unit. Increased plasma vasopressin, along with decreased urine flow, has been demonstrated in conscious man receiving IPPB [16]. To better understand the role of vasopressin with mechanical ventilation, let us first consider the normal mechanisms of vasopressin release [35].

Vasopressin Secretion

The control of vasopressin secretion is multifactual, requiring a complex interaction of the following:

1. Activation of the osmoreceptor system
2. The activation of left atrial stretch receptors and osmoreceptors   have a feedback mechanism
3. The activation of baroreceptor system
4. Release of vasopressin in response to pain   —   does not have a feedback mechanism

Other factors also may influence vasopressin release, e.g., psychogenic stress, change in position, environmental temperature, intermittent diuretic therapy, and alterations in arterial carbon dioxide pressure.

Increased plasma osmolarity stimulates osmoreceptors located in the hypothalamus, causing a release of vasopressin. The increase in vasopressin results in an augmented resorption of free water in the renal tubular cell. Further vasopressin release is inhibited once the serum osmolarity is returned to a normal level.

Left atrial osmoreceptors continuously fire the vagus nerve, which in turn stimulates the hypothalamus to secrete vasopressin. With a diminution in thoracic blood volume, the afferent impulses are less frequent and vasopressin secretion is increased. Left atrial osmoreceptors are activated by a change in thoracic blood volume, whereas baroreceptors located in the carotid and aortic bodies are activated by hypotension, once the blood pressure is restored, vasopressin release is inhibited.

In the fourth mechanism, vasopressin is released as long as the stimuli continue. Along with causing the release of vasopressin, stress may increase plasma adreno-corticotropic hormone (ACTH) levels. If such is the case, then corticotropin also may lead to water and salt retention in patients requiring mechanical ventilation.

With IPPB there is a decrease in urine flow and an increase in vasopressin secretion [16, 32]. If the intrathoracic blood volume is decreased secondary to high levels of PEEP, the left atrial osmoreceptors then decrease their activity, thereby increasing vasopressin secretion. Low $PaCO_2$ levels [27] result in decreased plasma vasopressin. This response can be blocked with the addition of carbon dioxide to the inspired gas. On the other hand, elevated $PaCO_2$, especially above 50 torr, may result in an increased level of plasma vasopressin. The addition of PEEP [17] is not associated with a consistent or significant alteration in plasma osmolarity. Thus, activation of osmoreceptors seems an unlikely mechanism for vasopressin release. An alternative explanation proposes that the increase of plasma vasopressin following the use of PEEP is the result of stimulation of baroreceptors as well as a volume receptor mechanism. Altered lymph flow secondary to PEEP [25] is the result of two possible mechanisms: (1) an increase in central venous pressure, which impedes lymphatic emptying; and (2) an increase in intrathoracic pressure acting to collapse intrathoracic lymph channels, which are returning lymph from the periphery. Discontinuance of PEEP is associated with an increase in the quantity of lymph as well as the rate of flow. Elevation of systemic venous pressure is associated with PEEP. This increase in pressure on the venous side of the capillary bed causes an increase in lymph formation and the appearance of edema. Thus, the combined effect of decreasing lymph return and increasing lymph formation contributes to a positive water balance. A decrease in lymph turnover, resulting from lymph sequestration in the peripheral tissue, causes a diminution in blood volume that can lead to a decrease in glomerular filtration rate and urinary flow. Of course, this process can be further aggravated by the release of vasopressin, a consequence of decreased blood volume.

RENAL RESPONSE TO POSITIVE PRESSURE BREATHING

Change in Intrarenal Blood Flow

Tucker and Murray [34] found no change in renal blood flow in anesthetized dogs ventilated with 10 cm H_2O of PEEP. Hall, Johnson, and Hedley-Whyte [10] found only a slight change in intrarenal blood flow with IPPB. Murdaugh, Sicker, and Manfredi [23], however, found a 30 percent decrease in effective renal plasma flow when they used 32 cm H_2O of PEEP. Baratz and Ingraham [2] found a 50 percent decrease in intrarenal blood flow in dogs ventilated with CPPB of 15 cm H_2O. These discrepancies are related, in part, to the amount of positive pressure and partly to different techniques used to measure renal blood flow.

A Decrease in Glomerular Filtration Rate

Recent studies [2, 6, 23] have shown a discrepancy between renal blood perfusion and glomerular filtration rate, in both the dog and rat [9], with continuous positive pressure ventilation. Alteration in sympathetic tone and the level of circulating vasoactive hormone with continuous positive pressure ventilation can lead to a redistribution of intrarenal blood flow and a subsequent decrease in the glomerular filtration pressure and glomerular filtration rates, without a significant change in total renal blood flow.

An increase in sodium retention has been related to a decrease in glomerular filtration rate [9] and to a redistribution of blood flow toward the juxtamedullary nephron, an area of the kidney capable of great sodium conservation. Such a flow diversion triggers the renin-angiotensin-aldosterone loop, resulting in further sodium retention and potassium loss.

PULMONARY BAROTRAUMA

Pulmonary barotrauma is most frequently observed in patients who are ventilated at large tidal volumes [3]. Tidal volume and PEEP (in Bone's patients) were 22 ± 4 ml per kilogram of body weight and 16 ± 4 cm H_2O, respectively, in those patients suffering pulmonary barotrauma. This was compared to patients without barotrauma, whose tidal volumes were 17 ± 4 ml per kilogram of body weight and PEEP levels of 12 ± 4 cm H_2O. The most commonly encountered problems are pneumothorax, pneumomediastinum (see Figure 10-1), and subcutaneous emphysema. Indeed, bilateral pneumothorax is not a rare event. This, along with the potential for a tension pneumothorax, constitutes a true medical emergency. To assure adequate hemodynamic and respiratory function, prompt evacuation of the pneumothorax by means of chest tube and underwater drainage is necessary. Figure 11-2 shows a pneumothorax with chest tube (A) in place at the apex of pleural space, allowing for more complete evacuation of pleural space air (B), collapsed lung (C), ribs (D), intercostal muscles (E), and trachea (F). The Krale Pleur-Evac (Figure 11-3) is a nonmetered water-seal suction unit designed for drainage of the pleural cavity. Suction is variable from about -10 cm H_2O to -28 cm H_2O, and is regulated by vent (A) and the height of the water added to the suction control chamber (B). The water-seal chamber (C), in conjunction with the excess vacuum safety float valve (D), acts to prevent loss of suction during patient transportation or backflow during patient inspiration. The collection chambers (E, F, G) fill sequentially and hold a maximum of 2,350 ml. The suction pathway is indicated by arrows.

The clinical diagnosis of pneumothorax should be suspected in those patients in whom unexplained deterioration in their clinical status is evident. This may be

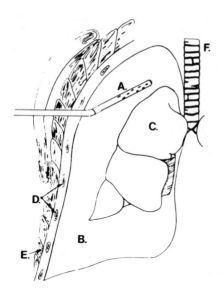

Figure 11–2. Pneumothorax.

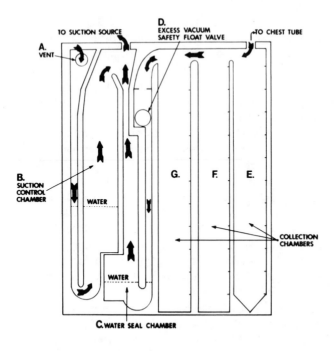

Figure 11–3. Krale Pleur-Evac.

reflected by tachycardia, hypotension, restlessness, agitation, and cyanosis.

Increased alveolar pressure per se is capable of damaging alveoli. There may be overdistention of alveoli with rupture of alveolar septa if excessive pressure and volumes are employed. Whether chronic ventilatory support with positive pressure can result in permanent injury to the alveolar lining cells has not been established. It is clear that patients who are ventilated with standard tidal volumes, 10 to 15 ml per kilogram of body weight, can tolerate prolonged periods of mechanical ventilation without any obvious untoward effects.

It has been suggested [33] that ventilation with the aid of a static compliance curve may prevent severe overinflation, thus lessening the likelihood of pulmonary barotrauma (see Chapter 12).

PEEP, CPAP, NEEP
PEEP, CPAP, and *NEEP* are commonly used terms in the jargon of the respiratory therapist; for the purpose of review each will be briefly discussed.

PEEP: Positive End Expiratory Pressure
PEEP is a system in which positive pressure is maintained throughout the entire respiratory cycle. There are various methods of delivering PEEP. The most commonly employed are depicted in Figure 11–4. The balloon system is controlled by a regulated pressure source (A), which serves to inflate the exhalation valve balloon at the prescribed level of positive pressure. The underwater drainage system (B) directs the exhalation tubing into a container with a specified amount of water. The depth of the water defines the amount of end expiratory pressure.

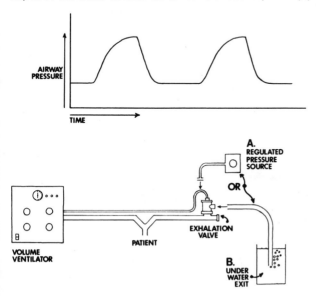

Figure 11–4. PEEP: Positive end expiratory pressure.

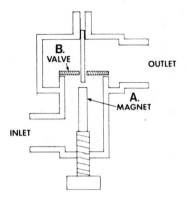

Figure 11–5. Magnetic PEEP valve III BE 142.

The magnetic PEEP valve manufactured by Instrumentation Industries, Inc. (Figure 11–5) uses a magnet (A) in conjunction with a metal disc valve (B) to provide PEEP or CPAP. The distance from the magnet to the valve disc determines the PEEP pressure, which is adjustable from 0 to 20 cm H_2O. In use, the magnetic PEEP valve is connected downstream to the exhalation valve and can be added to any closed patient circuit.

CPAP: Constant Positive Airway Pressure
Gregory et al. [7] described a system of CPAP for the treatment of infant respiratory distress syndrome (IRDS); subsequently, this type of circuit, which utilizes

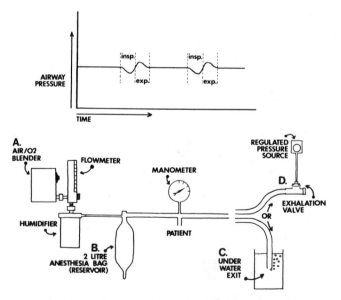

Figure 11–6. CPAP: Constant positive airway pressure.

a humidifier reservoir bag, a one-way valve, and an end expiratory pressure system, has been successfully used in treating adults (Figure 11-6). The humidifier may be replaced with a pressure ventilator.

CPAP is PEEP without the ventilator. Airway pressure is always above ambient, and the patient breathes without assistance. On this system a low flow (0 to 20 liters/min) blender (A) is used to mix air and oxygen. The flow rate must be set above the patient's minute volume. Between each breath, the mixed humidified gas is stored in a reservoir, usually a 2-liter anesthesia bag (B). The overflow is vented out the system's exhalation port. The constant system pressure is provided by either an underwater exit (C) for expired gases (wherein the depth of the water is equal to the airway pressure in cm H_2O) or through an exhalation valve balloon (D) maintained at a desired preset pressure that is greater than ambient. CPAP can also be provided by hood arrangements in which the head is enclosed by the hood.

In the alert adult with an adequate spontaneous tidal volume CPAP therapy may be administered by means of a specialized tight-fitting mask. Positive airway pressure is maintained in a mask-CPAP system by a continuous input of gas flow and, by patient exhalation, through an adjustable spring-loaded exhalation valve.

NEEP: Negative End Expiratory Pressure
NEEP is a system that maintains an airway pressure at the end expiratory point of the respiratory cycle that is below ambient (atmospheric) pressure (Figure 11-7).

A venturi is usually attached to the expiration port. The flow rate of the

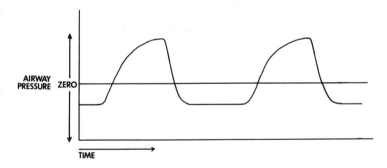

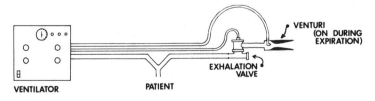

Figure 11-7. NEEP: Negative end expiratory pressure.

venturi determines the amount of negative pressure. The venturi's upstream port is attached to the exhalation valve; the downstream port opens to the atmosphere. Although it is possible to leave it on during the entire respiratory cycle, the venturi is usually cycled on only during expiration.

The Bennett PR-2, the Gill, and the Amsterdam respirators all have NEEP available.

ASSISTED PEEP

In some situations, adaptation and modification of the various available ventilators may be necessary to provide optimal care. Surely tinkering with the respirator must be discouraged. A thorough and intimate understanding of the selected ventilator is mandatory for those whose responsibility it is to maintain and operate it. It is in this setting that design alterations become useful. Such alterations allow for respiratory care to be tailored to the needs of the individual patient; for example, allowing the patient to assist while receiving PEEP is desirable. A relatively simple modification of the MA-1 or Ohio 56, described below, allows for assisted PEEP [15].

Until recently, most volume ventilator assist mechanisms (MA-1 and Ohio 560) used atmospheric pressure as a baseline. Because PEEP maintains a patient's baseline airway pressure above ambient, it is difficult to provide assisted ventilation when PEEP is used. By enclosing an assist mechanism (Figure 11-8A) in a pressure-tight chamber (B), and by ensuring that the pressure inside the chamber is essentially the same as the patient's end expiratory level, the assist mechanism will operate on the same pressure baseline as the patient and will allow the ventilator to cycle at essentially the same sensitivity as without PEEP. The begin inspiration signal (C) closes the solenoid valve (D), isolating the chamber surrounding the assist mechanism from the patient circuit. The end inspiration signal (C), after a delay (E) tailored to the patient's expiratory time, opens the solenoid valve

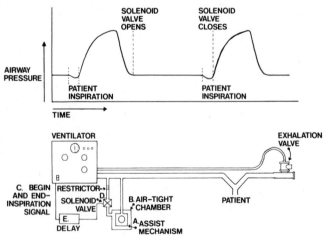

Figure 11-8. Assisted ventilation with PEEP.

to the chamber (B), reestablishing the patient's end expiratory pressure as the assist mechanism's baseline.

Variations of this principle are present on many of the most recent volume ventilators, such as Gill, Searle, and Ohio Critical Care. Although the following modification is tailored for the Bennett MA-1, the principle described can be applied to other ventilators.

First, the assist mechanism must be isolated from atmospheric pressure. A hole is drilled and a nipple attached to the casing of the MA-1 assist mechanism. The casing then can be sealed with a silicon rubber. However, the adjustment shaft protrudes from the bottom of the mechanism and must be sealed, yet still be able to turn. To accomplish this the electrical contact on the shaft side of the mechanism must be turned 90 degrees away from the shaft. Then a small container, metal or plastic, slightly longer and wider than the shaft, can be affixed with epoxy glue in a position that surrounds the shaft.

Second, a solenoid valve and a 0 to 3 second time-delay relay are used to admit only end expiratory pressure through the previously attached nipple to the chamber surrounding the assist mechanism. The leads to the main inspiration-control solenoid valve of the MA-1 are tapped into so that a begin and end inspiration signal is provided. The time delay relay is connected in parallel to these leads, and the solenoid valve is connected to the time delay relay. When inspiration is initiated, the time delay relay resets, closing the solenoid valve and isolating the pressure-tight chamber surrounding the assist mechanism from the patient circuit. At the end of inspiration, the time delay relay waits an appropriate length of time (adjustable to fit the individual needs of the patient), and then opens the solenoid valve, allowing the assist mechanism to adjust its baseline to that of the patient.

This modification automatically will follow the patient's end expiratory pressure, regardless of leaks in the patient circuit and of the actual PEEP pressure employed, with little variation in the sensitivity of the assist mechanism.

INTERRUPTED PEEP

Another example of what may prove to be a valuable machine alteration is interrupted PEEP, a system whereby intrathoracic and airway pressure return to atmospheric at a preset number (e.g., every three breaths or four breaths) (Figure 11-9). This system, which has been studied in normal dogs, reduces the negative effects of PEEP on cardiac output [18]. It should be stressed, however, that this method has not been and should not be used clinically. Before any consideration for clinical application, further laboratory investigation is required.

A Bennett MA-1 respirator may be modified in the following manner to allow the end expiratory pressure to drop to atmospheric level at every fourth breath (Figure 11-10). The MA-1 inspiration control valve (I) located on top of the MA-1 bellows toward the back of the machine, is energized during inspiration. Connected in parallel with the inspiration control valve is a SPDT relay (H). When the SPDT switch (G) is closed, the relay advances the stepping relay (E) one con-

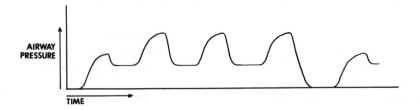

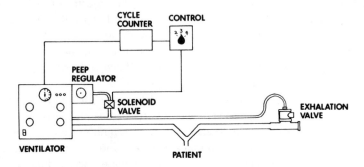

Figure 11-9. Interrupted PEEP.

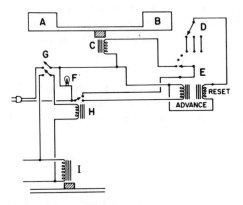

Figure 11-10. A Bennett MA-1 respirator modified to allow the end expiratory pressure to drop to atmospheric level at every fourth breath.

tact for each machine inspiration. During the expiration phase, the relay is connected to the contact arm on the stepping relay, which, depending upon its position, controls either the reset coil on the steeping relay or the solenoid valve (C). When the solenoid valve is activated, it disconnects the PEEP mechanism (B) from its pressure source (A), thereby turning off the PEEP. During the next inspiration, the stepping relay advances and the solenoid valve opens, allowing PEEP to be reestablished. The rotary switch (D) decides how many breaths on PEEP are allowed before the stepping relay resets and PEEP is shut off by the solenoid valve [18].

REFERENCES

1. Barach, A. L., et al. Studies on positive pressure respiration. *J. Aviation* 17, 1946, p. 290.
2. Baratz, R. A., and Ingraham, R. C. Renal hemodynamic and antidiuretic hormone release associated with volume regulator. *Am. J. Physiol.* 198, 1960, p. 565.
3. Bone, R. C., Francis, P. B., and Pierce, A. K. Pulmonary barotrauma complicating positive end-expiratory pressure. *Am. Rev. Respir. Dis.* 111, 1975, p. 921.
4. Colgan, F., and Marocco, P. Cardiac respiratory effects of constant and intermittent positive pressure breathing. *Anesthesiology* 36, 1972, p. 444.
5. Cournand, A., et al. Physiological studies of the effects of intermittent positive pressure breathing on cardiac output in man. *Am. J. Physiol.* 152, 1948, p. 162.
6. Drury, D. R., Henry, J. P., and Goodman, J. The effect of continuous positive pressure breathing on kidney function. *J. Clin. Invest.* 26, 1947, p. 945.
7. Gregory, G. A., et al. Treatment of the idiopathic respiratory distress syndrome with continuous positive airway pressure. *N. Engl. J. Med.* 284, 1971, p. 1333.
8. Guntheroth, W. G., et al. Hemodynamic effects of intermittent positive pressure respiration. *Anesthesiology* 27, 1966, p. 584.
9. Guyton, A. C. *Circulatory Physiology: Cardiac Output and Its Regulations.* Philadelphia: Saunders, 1963.
10. Hall, S. V., Johnson, E., and Hedley-Whyte, J. Renal hemodynamics and function with CPPV in dogs. *Anesthesiology* 41, 1974, p. 452.
11. Hess, W. *Surgery of the Biliary Passage and the Pancreas.* Princeton, N. J.: Van Nostrand, 1965.
12. Hubay, C. A., Brecher, G. A., and Clement, F. L. Etiological factors affecting pulmonary artery flow with controlled respiration. *Surgery* 38, 1955, p. 215.
13. Johnson, E. E., and Hedley-Whyte, J. Continuous positive-pressure ventilation and portal blood flow in dogs with pulmonary edema. *J. Appl. Physiol.* 33, 1972, p. 385.
14. Johnson, E. E., and Hedley-Whyte, J. Continuous positive-pressure ventilation and choledochoduodenal flow resistance. *J. Appl. Physiol.* 39, 1975, p. 937.
15. Johnston, R. P., Donovan, D. J., and MacDonnell, K. F. PEEP during assisted ventilation. *Anesthesiology* 40, 1974, p. 308.
16. Khambotta, H. J., and Baratz, R. A. IPPB and plasma ADH and urine flow in conscious man. *J. Appl. Physiol.* 33, 1972, p. 362.
17. Kumar, A., et al. Inappropriate response to increased plasma ADH during mechanical ventilation in acute respiratory failure. *Anesthesiology* 40, 1974, p. 215.
18. MacDonnell, K. F., et al. Comparative hemodynamic consequences of inflation hold, PEEP, and interrupted PEEP. An experimental study in normal dogs. *Ann. Thorac. Surg.* 19, 1975, p. 552.
19. Maloney, J. V., Jr., et al. Electrophrenic respiration. IX. Comparison of effects of positive pressure breathing and electrophonic respiration on the circulation during hemorrhagic shock and barbiturate poisoning. *Surg. Gynecol. Obstet.* 92, 1951, p. 672.

20. Mead, J., and Whittenberger, J. L. Lung Inflation and Hemodynamics. In W. O. Fenn and H. Rahn (eds.), *Handbook of Physiology*. Section 3. *Respiration*. Baltimore: Williams & Wilkins, 1964. Vol. 1, p. 477.

21. Morgan, B. C., Crawford, E. W., and Guntheroth, W. G. The hemodynamic effects of change in blood volume during intermittent positive pressure ventilation. *Anesthesiology* 30, 1969, p. 297.

22. Morgan, B. C., et al. Hemodynamic effect of changes in arterial carbon dioxide tension during IPPV. *Anesthesiology* 22, 1967, p. 866.

23. Murdaugh, H. V., Jr., Sicker, H. O., and Manfredi, F. Effect of altered intra-thoracic pressure on renal hemodynamics, electrolyte excretion, and water clearance. *J. Clin. Invest.* 38, 1959, p. 834.

24. Mushin, W. L., Rendell-Baker, L., and Thomson, P. W. *Automatic Ventilation of the Lungs*. Springfield, Ill.: Thomas, 1959.

25. Neville, W. E., et al. Tracheostomy and assisted ventilation: Use in respiratory insufficiency in the postsurgical patient. *Arch. Surg.* 89, 1964, p. 149.

26. Olerud, S. Experimental studies on portal circulation at increased intra-abdominal pressure. *Acta Physiol. Scand.* (Suppl.) 109, 1954, p. 1.

27. Philbin, O. M., Baratz, R. A., and Patterson, R. W. Influence of carbon dioxide on plasma antidiuretic hormone level during IPPB. *Anesthesiology* 33, 1970, p. 349.

28. Pilon, R. N., and Bittar, D. A. The effect of PEEP on thoracic duct lymph flow during continued ventilation in anesthetized dogs. *Anesthesiology* 39, 1973, p. 607.

29. Powers, S. R., Jr., et al. Physiologic consequences of positive end-expiratory pressure (PEEP) ventilation. *Ann. Surg.* 178, 1973, p. 265.

30. Prys-Roberts, C., and Kelman, G. R. Hemodynamic effects of graded hypercapnia in anesthetized man. *Br. J. Anaesth.* 38, 1966, p. 661.

31. Quist, J., et al. Hemodynamic response to mechanical ventilation with PEEP. The effect of hypervolemia. *Anesthesiology* 42, 1975, p. 45.

32. Sladen, A., Laver, M. B., and Pontoppidan, H. Pulmonary complication and water retention in prolonged mechanical ventilation. *N. Engl. J. Med.* 279, 1968, p. 484.

33. Suter, P. M., Fairley, H. B., and Isenberg, M. D. Optimum end-expiratory airway pressure in patients with acute pulmonary failure. *N. Engl. J. Med.* 292, 1975, p. 284.

34. Tucker, H. J., and Murray, J. F. Effect of end-expiratory pressure on organ blood flow in normal and diseased dogs. *J. Appl. Physiol.* 34, 1973, p. 573.

35. Ukai, M., Moran, W. H., Jr., and Zimmerman, B. The visceral afferent pathways of vasopressin secretion and urinary excretory patterns during surgical stress. *Ann. Surg.* 168, 1966, p. 16.

36. West, J. B. Distribution of Blood Flow and Ventilation Measurements Measured with Radioactive Gases. In M. Simon (ed.), *Frontiers of Pulmonary Radiology*. New York: Grune & Stratton, 1969.

37. Whittenberger, J. L. *Artificial Respirator*. New York: Harper & Row, 1962, Chapter 4.

Kenneth F. MacDonnell

Weaning: Criteria; Intermittent Mandatory Ventilation

12

Weaning, a phenomenon formerly restricted to the field of pediatrics, has truly become the problem child of advanced technology. Weaning a patient from mechanical ventilation is a stubborn, recurrent problem faced by those charged with the care of patients suffering from acute and chronic respiratory failure. The ability and rapidity of successful respirator weaning is related in most instances to the patient's underlying disease processes; for example, the young overdose patient generally poses no problem, depending on the overdose agent, and usually is easily extubated once conscious and alert. In contrast is the patient affected with severe chronic obstructive pulmonary lung disease (COPD) such as emphysema, who may have lost his last remaining pulmonary reserve and who may find it impossible to be without mechanical ventilation. Nonetheless, diligent, devoted effort by respiratory teams have recorded rather extraordinary examples of successful weaning, in some instances after years of mechanical support. It is important to stress the team approach to this problem, utilizing to the fullest the skills of the physician, therapist, and nurse.

Objective criteria for extubation have been developed, and in most instances they serve as reliable guides. These parameters include determinations reflective of both mechanical and gas exchange characteristics of the lung, those most commonly employed being the vital capacity (VC), inspiratory force, arterial-alveolar oxygen gradient ($AaPO_2$, dead space–tidal volume ratio (VD/VT), minute ventilation (MV), maximum voluntary ventilation (MVV), carbon dioxide tension (pCO_2), and shunt fraction. The use of such measurements clearly requires an appreciation of the patient's premorbid state; for instance, some patients with chronic lung disease even in their steady state might be unable to meet the minimum quantities necessary for extubation. Nonetheless, it is quite clear that the final decision regarding extubation must remain a composite of objective data, experience, and clinical judgment.

Generally, a VC of 10 to 15 ml per kilogram of body weight and a forced expiratory volume in 1 second (FEV_1) of 10 ml/kg is necessary for successful weaning [4]. Safar and Kunkel [5] have reported that a VC of less than 1 liter would indicate that the weaning experience will be unsuccessful. Another valuable pressure measurement is that of the instantaneous peak negative pressure (PNP) during maximal inspiratory effort following a maximal expiratory effort. The measurement is made using an aneroid manometer connected to a T-piece. Values of –20 and preferably greater than –25 cm H_2O appear to be minimal requirements; if the PNP is more than –30, then one may predict with confidence that mechanical forces are adequate. It is important to begin weaning as soon as possible. Even minimal PNP, –10 cm, and very reduced VC, 4.5 ml/kg, allows one to initiate weaning. The whole process from the first few minutes off the respirator to successful extubation may take weeks, months, and in some cases, years.

Stetson [9] has reported that patients who are unable to maintain a resting minute ventilation of less than 10 liters are unlikely candidates for extubation. Others [6] have used the maximal voluntary ventilation (MVV), observing that in most cases, if the patient is unable to double his resting minute ventilation (MV), then discontinuation of mechanical ventilation is impossible. Because these measurements are so critical to proper patient care, all equipment employed in testing must be properly standardized and in good working order. This is of special import if electronic spirometers are employed.

All test results must be interpreted in light of the patient's baseline pulmonary status, remembering that the aforementioned tests, except the MV, require an alert, cooperative patient. Determinations of pulmonary mechanics in some patients may be misleading, for some patients are unable to perform the required maneuvers while intubated; also, the problem of increased airway resistance caused by the tube must be remembered.

A V_D/V_T of greater than 0.6 is generally felt to represent evidence that successful weaning will not be accomplished. However, a number of patients with V_D/V_T of greater than 0.6 have been successfully extubated [10]. This is especially true in young patients following pneumonia, when, for reasons that are unclear, the V_D/V_T remains abnormal even after the $AaPO_2$ has returned toward normal. Accurate assessment of V_D/V_T requires a thorough search for causes of increased carbon dioxide production such as fever, hypercatabolism, and added mechanical dead space, as well as taking into account the compressible gas in the ventilator tubing and system. Generally, the V_D/V_T remains a useful and accurate tool and a determination that can easily be calculated:

$$V_D = \frac{(Pa_{CO_2} - P_{E_{CO_2}})\, \dot{V}_E}{Pa_{CO_2}}$$

where V_D = dead space ventilation; Pa_{CO_2} = arterial carbon dioxide pressure; PE_{CO_2} = expired carbon dioxide pressure; $\dot{V}E$ = expired gas.

If the alveolar to arterial oxygen gradient is greater than 300 torr, or 350 torr while breathing 100% oxygen, then the discontinuation of controlled ventilation is unlikely. The same can be said of Pa_{CO_2} of greater than 50 torr, if the patient does not have chronic obstructive disease.

The achievement of a reasonably normal Pa_{CO_2} and arterial pH may be a necessary first step in weaning; frequently, patients ventilated for acute respiratory failure, especially those with normal lungs, have a marked hypocapnia and respiratory alkalosis. It should be recalled that renal compensation for respiratory acidosis is delayed and, in fact, imposes an added acid load just at a time when respiratory support is being discontinued. In general, alkalosis is detrimental to the organism not only for the above reason, but for the well-recognized problems of twitching, seizures, and cardiac arrhythmias that are associated with systemic alkalosis. Sawa and associates [7] have suggested a nomogram that may be useful as a guide to determine the amount of mechanical dead space needed to accomplish a given increase in arterial Pa_{CO_2}. This nomogram is based on the Bohr equation; its goal is to achieve as nearly as possible the patient's premorbid blood-gas status, thereby facilitating the entire weaning process.

It is clear that patients who meet all of the above criteria pose no major problem as far as discontinuance from the respirator. If such is the case, then a T-piece adapter from a source of humidified gas is connected to the endotracheal or tracheostomy tube, usually with a supplemental oxygen source somewhat above the FI_{O_2} employed while on mechanical support. This is to compensate for the expected drop in Pa_{O_2} during this transitional period. During initial respiratory discontinuance, not only should frequent blood gas determinations be done but careful clinical observation is mandatory, for this is a most critical period, and in many instances it is essentially a time of trial and error.

Adequate clinical observation should make special note of such events as changes in respiratory frequency, tidal volume (TV), MV, heart rate, Pa_{O_2}, Pa_{CO_2}, and the onset of respiratory distress. Gilbert et al. [2] have noted that generally TV is decreased and respiratory frequency increased during the initial phases of weaning. This should come as no surprise, for it stands to reason that patients who have received mechanical support with large tidal volumes at a slow respiratory rate will be unable to sustain such values after that mechanical support has been discontinued. Such a directional change in TV and respiratory frequency, if not extreme, should not interfere with weaning.

Interpretation and evaluation of arterial oxygen tension must be in light of the entire clinical setting; there is no magic number identifying a Pa_{O_2} which will guarantee rapid and successful weaning, nor is there any sure value that requires restarting mechanical ventilation. Some patients with chronic obstructive respiratory disease are able to tolerate extremely reduced levels of Pa_{O_2}, reflecting the amazing adaptive qualities of the human organism. Also, there are those patients who have dependence on their hypoxic respiratory drive, which in such instances necessitates that particular attention must be directed to the FI_{O_2}, in order to prevent a recurrence of respiratory failure from respiratory depression. On the other hand, if the drop in arterial oxygen is associated with restlessness, confusion, tachycardia, pallor, respiratory distress, sweating, or significant cardiac arrhythmias, then surely improved arterial oxygenation is required. Instances where alveolar collapse is responsible for the respiratory failure may be handled with a system of continuous positive airway pressure (CPAP). Those patients who hypoventilate, showing substantial increases in Pa_{CO_2} and a dangerous drop in pH (less than 7.25) require discontinuance of weaning and reinstitution of mechanical ventilatory support.

The timing of weaning should be correlated with the patient's general medical status; surely the unstable patient is not a prime weaning candidate. Particular attention should be paid to nutrition. These patients frequently are hypercatabolic and may require hyperalimentation. A particularly difficult type of patient to wean is the one who is unconscious, e.g., the stroke victim, where one cannot rely on standard criteria and where a system of trial and error must be employed.

Specified goals should be presented to the patient that are within his expected achievement, so the patient will not become discouraged.

The role of respiratory muscle retraining has received attention of late, especially in the patient who is difficult to wean. The retraining of respiratory muscles of patients on respiratory support may prove valuable.

After weaning is complete and the patient is stable, showing no changes in vital determinations after a few hours, then extubation can be accomplished.

Various approaches to the tracheostomized patient have been suggested. For example, Hedley-Whyte and Feeley [3] advocate the use of the fenestrated tracheostomy tube, a tube that allows the patient to talk, cough secretion up into the mouth, and if necessary that allows controlled ventilation to be reinstituted. Others prefer partial plugging of the standard tracheostomy tube. A major disadvantage of this system is its increased resistance to air flow.

The popularity and widespread use of positive end expiratory pressure (PEEP) may compound the problem of ventilator discontinuance. Weaning is usually begun when PEEP is reduced to a level of 10 cm H_2O or less. Frequently the patient may be weaned from controlled ventilation if a system of continuous positive pressure is available.

McPherson and his associates [4] have designed an ingenious circuitry (Figure 12-1) that allows for great flexibility during the weaning period. The patient may be weaned with a continuous flow of gas that is humidified, or the patient and the circuitry may be interfaced in a manner so as to receive CPAP. Intermittent mandatory ventilation (IMV), indeed, IMV with CPAP, may also be employed. This circuitry also allows for accurate TV measurements under all the circumstances described and a gas compressability factor in the ventilator circuit of only 0.5 cc per cm H_2O.

Construction notes as described by McPherson et al. [4] are simple, straightforward, and explicit. Mixed gas is supplied from a blender that is capable of providing flows from zero to 100 liters/min. Flow is set above the patient's peak in-

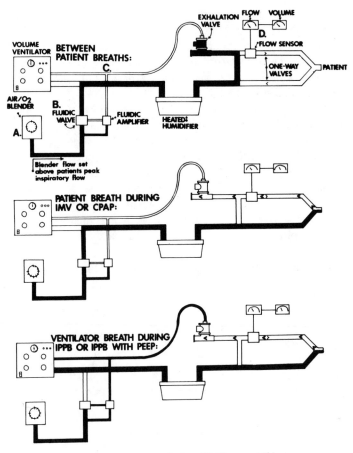

Figure 12-1. Continuous flow ventilation (McPherson [4]).

spiratory flow demand. A fluidic flow-interrupter switch (see Chapter 1), which works like an exhalation valve, interrupts flow from the blender if the ventilator cycles into inspiration. The signal pressure to the fluidic valve is supplied via a T in the exhalation valve line. Because the input pressure required to actuate the fluidic valve is 10 cm H_2O, the valve is not activated by CPAP up to 10 cm H_2O until the ventilator cycles into inspiration. When pressure exceeds 10 cm H_2O, the fluidic valve stops flow from the blender, so that tidal volumes are not significantly altered.

The ventilation monitor transducer is placed in line on the expiratory side of the one-way valved patient Y tubing, with a straight-through flow route from the blender and out the exhalation valve between patient inspirations. The continuous flow is accessible to the patient without being sensed by the transducer.

Intermittent mandatory ventilation was first advocated in the therapy of the infant respiratory distress syndrome; it is a system utilizing periodic machine-augmented breaths. Successful weaning of borderline patients, and, for that matter, routine use of IMV during weaning has been proposed by many authors, who point to the advantage of a smooth, slow transition from machine dependence to ventilatory discontinuance. Another area of usefulness for IMV is in those who have developed a psychic dependence on the ventilator and who are reluctant to begin weaning. Critics note the lack of hard data regarding the efficiency of IMV; there have to date been no controlled studies published.

This system can be adapted to existing constant volume respirators rather simply. A volume ventilator modified for IMV usually has its rate control altered to allow for an extended expiratory time; for example, on the Bennett MA-1 ventilator, an optimal expanded time circuit serves this purpose. Add-on devices, such as Healthdyne, consist mainly of a simple timing circuit which, when activated, triggers the ventilator. Typically, an accessory timer (Figure 12–2A) controls the rate of the ventilator. Between mandatory ventilator breaths the patient inhales aerosol produced by an aerosol generator (B) through a one-way valve in an H manifold (C) connected in line on the inspiratory side of the patient circuit, and exhales through the exhalation valve (D).

The technique of IMV employs the delivery of a volume of gas at preset intervals

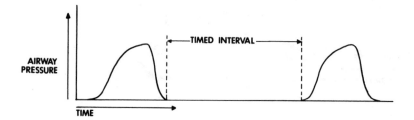

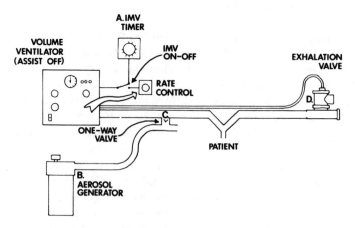

Figure 12–2. IMV: Intermittent mandatory ventilation.

without regard to the patient's respiratory pattern. The timing of the volume of gas to be delivered to the patient is therefore unpredictable, potentially minimizing the therapeutic value of the IMV.

Intermittent assisted ventilation (IAV), a system devised by the respiratory therapy department at St. Elizabeth's Hospital, allows the patient's inspiratory effort to cycle the ventilator, but only at preset intervals. The sensitivity mechanism of the Bennett MA-1 ventilator is adapted in a fashion that allows the machine to respond to the patient's inspiratory efforts. An aerosol generator is placed in line on the inspiratory side of the ventilator circuit, from which the patient breathes spontaneously. When the IAV module is activated, the MA-1 delivers a mechanically assisted breath. Should the patient be at the end of inspiration when the augmented breath is to be delivered, then expiration is completed and the next inspiration is the mechanically augmented breath. The assist mechanism can be isolated from the patient circuit either pneumatically with a solenoid valve (Figure 12-3A) and timer (B), or electrically with a relay (C) and timer (D). Between ventilator-assisted breaths the patient inhales aerosol produced by an aerosol generator (E) through a one-way valve in an H manifold (F) placed in line on the inspiratory side of the patient circuit. The patient exhales through the exhalation valve (G).

Intermittent assisted ventilation or IMV weaning makes TV determinations cumbersome, for the Bennett Spirometer does not function except during machine-assisted breaths. This problem can be avoided with the utilization of a Bennett MA-1 differential pressure sensitivity mechanism. During each inspiration, the bellows of the spirometer is emptied and allows for TV and apnea monitoring throughout the weaning process.

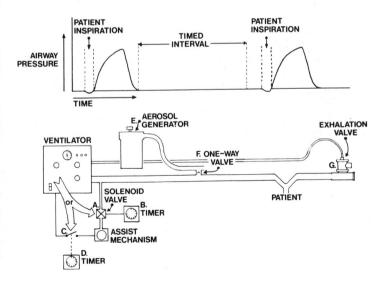

Figure 12–3. IAV: Intermittent assisted ventilation.

The physiologic benefit of IMV or IAV allows weaning time to be diminished. Intermittent mandatory ventilation may act to reinforce the proper coordination of diaphragmatic and accessory respiratory muscles [1].

The patient receiving PEEP requires a modified weaning program. When the time is appropriate to decrease the level of PEEP, as reflected in the arterial blood gases, we generally reduce it at increments of 1 to 2 cm per hour, carefully observing the patient's arterial oxygenation. Premature airway closure with intrapulmonary shunting may recur after PEEP has been discontinued for a number of hours; therefore, we usually continue controlled ventilation for at least 24 hours after discontinuation of PEEP. In the hard-to-wean patient, the routine use of CPAP has received support. If this system of weaning is to be adopted, the potential hazards of CPAP must be carefully considered.

Weaning is a complex and potentially dangerous procedure requiring great skill by those charged with this responsibility. Careful evaluation of the patient's premorbid pulmonary status, together with careful clinical observation, are invaluable guides during this critical period.

REFERENCES

1. Downs, J. B., et al. Intermittent mandatory ventilation: A new approach to weaning patients from mechanical ventilators. *Chest* 64, 1973, p. 331.
2. Gilbert, R., et al. The first few hours off a respirator. *Chest* 65, 1974, p. 152.
3. Hedley-White, J., and Feeley, T. W. Weaning from controlled ventilation and supplemental oxygen. *N. Engl. J. Med.* 292, 1975, p. 903.
4. McPherson, S. P., et al. A circuit that combines ventilator weaning methods using continuous flow ventilation. *Resp. Care* 20, 1975, p. 3.
5. Safar, P., and Kunkel, H. Prolonged artifical ventilation. *Respir. Ther.*, 1965, p. 126.
6. Sahn, S., and Lakshminarayan, S. Bedside criteria for discontinuation of mechanical ventilation. *Chest* 63, 1973, p. 1002.
7. Sawa, K., et al. A nomogram for deadspace requirement during prolonged artificial ventilation. *Anesthesiology* 29, 1968, p. 1206.
8. Stetson, J. Introductory essay in prolonged tracheal intubation. *Int. Anesthesiol. Clin.* 8, 1970, p. 774.
9. Teres, D., Roizen, M. F., and Bushnell, L. S. Successful weaning from controlled ventilation despite high deadspace-to-tidal volume ratio. *Anesthesiology* 39, 1973, p. 656.

Armand A. Lefemine

Tracheal Stenosis

13

Improved care of patients with respiratory failure has not been without problems. A particularly stubborn and nagging example is tracheal injury and stenosis. Knowledge of the anatomy of the trachea helps in understanding those circumstances that are liable to result in injury.

The trachea can be considered in three distinct sections: (1) the subglottic trachea, which basically comprises the cricoid cartilage; (2) the cervical trachea, which extends from the first tracheal ring to the sternal notch; and (3) the mediastinal trachea, which extends from the sternal notch to the carina and bifurcates into the bronchi at the junction of the first and second parts of the sternum (Figure 13-1). The trachea is kept distended by a series of C-shaped cartilagenous rings that are incomplete posteriorly in the so-called membranous portion of the trachea. These rings may also be attached to each other, lending some longitudinal stability as well as circumferential support. By extending the neck, approximately half of the trachea may be exposed by a cervical incision, and an additional length may be visualized by traction, because the carina is semimobile. Thus, about two-thirds of the trachea can be exposed by a cervical incision.

The cricoid cartilage is a critical part of the anatomy because of the attachment of the vocal cords through the cricothyroid and cricoarytenoid muscles. The recurrent or inferior laryngeal nerve, which lies in a groove between the trachea and esophagus, posterolaterally enters the larynx at the cricoid level and is closely related to the inferior thyroid artery. High tracheostomies involving the cricoid cartilage have a high incidence of subglottic stenosis and injury to the recurrent

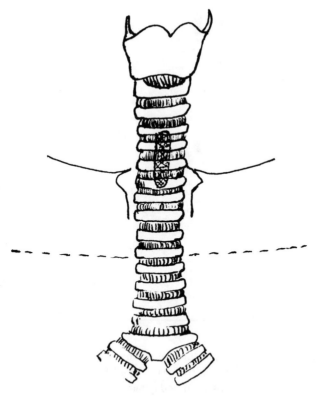

Figure 13–1. The relationship of the trachea to the clavicles. The hatched area at the sternal notch indicates the most common site for postintubation tracheal stenosis.

laryngeal nerve. The mediastinal trachea in the adult follows an inferoposterior course anterior to the esophagus to lie just behind the innominate artery and just medial and posterior to the ascending aorta.

The human trachea has a segmental blood supply. The upper trachea is supplied largely from branches of the inferior thyroid arteries. Other vessels supply the trachea and esophagus in common, arising from the thyrocervical trunk and upper intercostal vessels. The bronchial vessels supply the lower trachea and carina.

TRACHEOSTOMY AND TRACHEAL STENOSIS

Primary diseases of the trachea resulting in stenosis or malacia are rare. Carcinoma of the trachea unassociated with the larynx, goiter, and Hashimoto's disease are unusual entities. Tracheomalacia with local or general compression of the usual rigid breathing passage may result from an enlarged thyroid gland, from a general loss of cartilagenous rigidity, or from a localized absence of the cartilagenous support. These, too, are rare experiences in either the adult group or the pediatric group. Perhaps the most common cause of tracheomalacia is destruction of cartilage by pressure, infection, or both, following postintubation injury of the tracheal wall.

Unlike primary diseases of the trachea, stenosis and malacia of the trachea secondary to postintubation injuries are common and are seen with increasing frequency.
Cuffed tracheal tubes, long-term respiratory assistance, and tracheostomy can produce a variety of tracheal wall injuries that heal as cicatricial strictures (Figures 13-2,
13-3), as granulomas, or as membranes (Figures 13-4, 13-5). Tracheal malacia may
be associated with these lesions at some point in the process. Recognition of these
possibilities and the importance of cuffed tube design has brought about a progressive change in cuffed tubes, in the care and the technique of tracheostomy, and
finally in the development of resectional surgery for the trachea.

The incidence of postintubation stenosis and malacia are difficult to obtain. However, several studies such as those conducted by Grillo [17] and Pearson and
Andrews [36] give us reasonable estimates of the relative incidence of so-called
clinical and subclinical stenosis. There are many cases of tracheal injury that heal
with minor or moderate stricture and deformity and do not pose clinical problems
except, perhaps, under conditions of severe stress. The incidence of surgical obstruction requiring surgical correction is more evident. Grillo [17] reported that the
incidence of clinical upper airway obstruction in a vulnerable population of the
respiratory unit was 17 percent. Patients receiving respiratory support for a few days
are excluded from this group. Pearson and Andrews [36] reported a 20 percent
incidence. Another group at the Mount Sinai Hospital in New York reported a 12
percent incidence, and Gibson [16] in Australia indicated that the incidence of
stenosis was as high as 40 percent in the group in whom overdistention of the
trachea was visible on roentgenograms. Prospective studies indicate that the incidence of serious stenosis in patients undergoing prolonged respiratory assistance is
16 to 20 percent [16, 17, 36].

The true incidence of surgical and nonsurgical stricture is much more difficult to
define. Patients with an orifice of 5 mm or less have stridor at rest usually during
the inspiratory phase. Mild and moderate strictures are usually not detected at rest,
though severe exercise may elicit a wheeze or stridor. A brassy cough or difficulty
in raising sputum also are consistent with milder forms of stricture. A prospective
study (1971) by Pearson and Andrews [36] identified 32 (29 percent) functionally
significant strictures in a group of 153 survivors who required cuffed tube tracheostomy and assisted ventilation. Grillo [17] reported a 17 percent incidence (1967)
but excluded a large group of patients who received respiratory support for only 3
or 4 days. Gibson [16] (1967) at the Royal Perth Hospital in Australia found a high
incidence of tracheal ulceration and acute inflammation at the site of the tracheal
tube cuff (60 percent) at necropsies. However, in the 96 surviving patients, only 10
developed tracheal stenosis of varying severity, and 4 of these required operation.

Examination of the tracheas of patients after intubation with cuffed tubes during
life or at autopsy [9, 11] reveals a distinct pattern of injury, healing, and scarring.
Significant changes are found at the tube site in every patient, even with durations as
short as 1 day [11], though the degree of erosion and inflammation is related to
the duration of use of the tube. Damage is always at the site of the cuff [9] and is
characterized by mucosal erosion, dilation of the trachea, and exposure of the

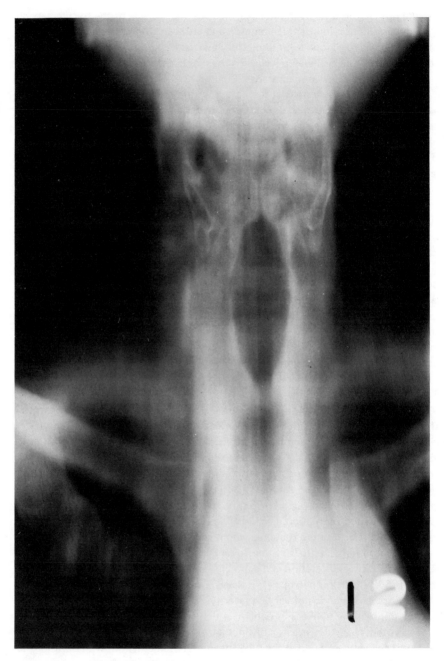

Figure 13-2. Typical hourglass deformity of a fibrous stricture resulting from a cuffed tube.

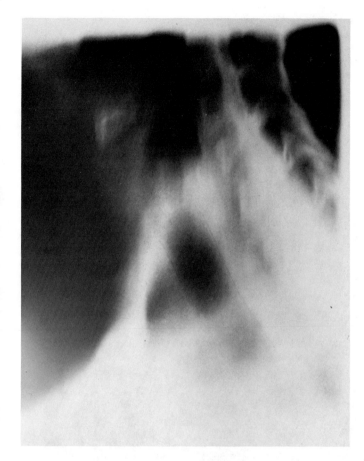

Figure 13-3. Postoperative laminagram following segmental resection of the stenosis in Figure 13-2.

cartilages. Superficial tracheitis with fibrin deposits is seen in the first 48 hours. Ulceration and baring of cartilages are seen in 3 to 7 days. Periods beyond this reveal softening and fragmentation of cartilage and bulging of the wall from continued pressure. Occasionally, erosion into the esophagus or an adjacent blood vessel may occur. Erosions at the tip of the tube are uncommon.

These gross pathologic findings are from an era of high-pressure cuffs. However, recent evidence [26] indicates that the tracheal wall is damaged even with the use of low-pressure cuffs. Significant surface alterations may be produced in man and dog by uncuffed and low-pressure cuffs in 2 hours. Surface morphology following uncuffed tubes revealed ciliary disorientation or ciliary denudation. The addition of low-pressure cuffs inflated to the seal point results in extensive damage to the cilia, particularly over the tracheal rings. Diffuse ciliary denudation is found under the

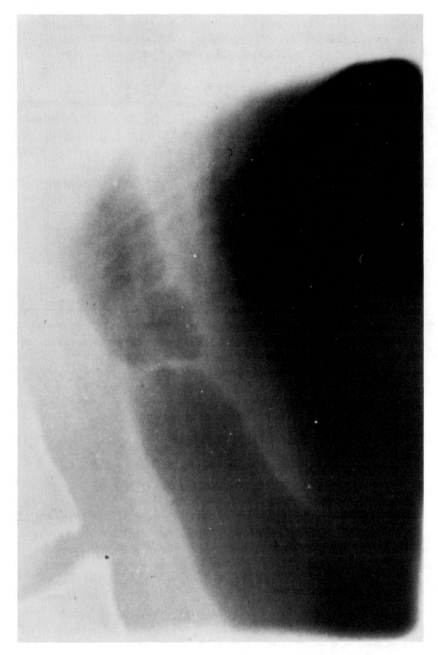

Figure 13-4. A thin membraneous stenosis producing severe obstruction following insertion of an endotracheal tube for 18 hours.

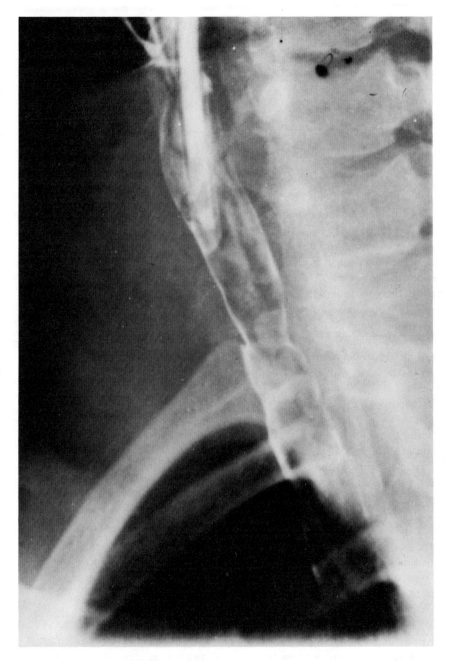

Figure 13–5. Tracheogram following transbronchoscopic resection of the lesion in Figure 13–4. This patient has remained asymptomatic for three years.

area of the cuff, with red blood cells and inflammatory cells attached to the surface. Regeneration of cilia may occur at 48 hours, but this is usually not of normal character. By 7 days, ciliation may be complete except for a few isolated areas. In man, squamous metaplasia may result. The loss of architectural support and healing by scar results in various degrees of stenosis, usually an hourglass deformity 1 to 2 cm in length.

Infection appears in a high percentage of patients with tracheostomy. Pathogenic organisms may be found in as many as 88 percent of those cultured [19], though this should vary with the routines employed. These organisms include coliform bacteria, *Pseudomonas pyocyanea, Staphylococcus aureus, Klebsiella pneumoniae, Hemophilus* species, and *Candida albicans.* Mixed infections are common. Most infections are superficial, though small abscesses have been noted in the wall of the trachea. Infection undoubtedly plays a significant role in addition to the previous phenomena.

A common observation during the care of a patient on prolonged cuff tube support is the gradual increase in the volume of air needed for cuff occlusion. This volume is associated with erosion, destruction of cartilage, and overdistention of the trachea. This overdistention may be noted by x-ray picture and is an ominous sign. Gibson [16], in a review of 125 x-ray studies of patients maintained on cuffed tubes, found that in 23 the cuffs had been distended beyond the limits of the trachea. In the patients in whom there was no visible overdistention of the trachea, only 4 of 62 survivors (6 percent) developed tracheal stenosis, whereas 6 of 15 survivors (40 percent) with visible overdistention of the trachea developed significant stenoses.

Tracheoesophageal fistula and tracheoinnominate artery fistula are seen in rare instances. These conditions usually relate to more prolonged support and more extensive damage to the tracheal support rings, though they can occur in as short a period as 2 weeks [10]. Various reports of tracheoesophageal fistulas attribute the tracheal injury to the cuff or balloon and not the tube tip [14, 20, 41]. Uncuffed tracheal tubes may erode into the innominate artery from tip injury in children [32, 40].

ETIOLOGY OF POSTINTUBATION STENOSIS

A tracheostomy and the use of a cuffed tube may damage the trachea at three distinct points: at the sites of (1) the tracheostomy, (2) the cuff, and (3) the tip of the tracheostomy tube. The mechanism for each site is unique. Stomal site problems do not apply to prolonged use of nasotracheal or orotracheal tubes, though they share in other pressure-induced complications involving the nose and vocal cords. Stomal site problems involve obstruction or stenosis caused by granuloma formation and tracheal ring destruction secondary to infection and/or extensive tracheal injury at the time of tracheostomy. Extensive resection of the tracheal wall to form the stoma, or dilatation of the stoma with resulting stellate tears, may be the source of anterior stenosis and granuloma. Infection with local destruction of mucosa and cartilage will lead to tracheal malacia that will result in stenosis as its final outcome. Although superficial infection is common and almost inevitable, invasive pathologic infection may produce enough local destruction of the wall or its supporting cartilage to result in early or late stricture. Strictures related to the tracheostomy site are usually anterior and may comprise a significant percentage of the total incidence of strictures.

Experimental and Clinical Background

Tracheal stenosis was regarded as a rare complication of tracheostomy until the production of cuffed tracheostomy tubes and their prolonged use for controlled and assisted ventilation. Early cases of tracheal stenoses occurred because of high tracheostomies involving the larynx, the cricoid cartilage, and the first ring of the trachea. In 1921, Jackson [21] condemned the high tracheostomy because of a high incidence of laryngeal stenosis. There were few experiences with the problem until 1960, when the occurrence of tracheal stenosis after tracheostomy for respiratory assistance began to appear in the Belgian, French, and American literatures, coinciding with the extensive use of cuffed tracheostomy tubes and ventilators. Large series of tracheostomies without prolonged ventilatory support or use of cuffed tubes indicate that the incidence of tracheal stenosis is very low [13, 19]. Atkins [3] subsequently reported pressure necrosis from cuffed tubes, and Aboulker et al. [1] reported significant tracheal stenosis in 22 out of 600 patients undergoing tracheostomy with assisted ventilation; 150 others had subclinical tracheal narrowing.

Almost simultaneously there appeared reports of several isolated cases of tracheal resection and end-to-end anastomosis, such as those of Witz et al. [46], Van Wein et al. [43], and Binet and Aboulker [5]. In 1965, Murphy, MacLean, and Dobell [30] reported 4 cases resulting from cuffed metal tubes for assisted ventilation, and could not reproduce tracheal stenosis on animals except by a tracheostomy and a cuffed cannula such that the cuff traversed the stoma. Gibson [16] in 1967 stressed that pressure necrosis may result from overinflation of a tracheostomy tube, particularly in patients with impaired circulation. Fraser and Bell [15] in 1967 reported a case of stricture 1 month following a prolonged tracheostomy with cuffed tube treated successfully by resection and end-to-end anastomosis. The stricture was the usual 2-cm long stricture 5 cm distal to the stoma. The excised stricture consisted of mature fibrous tissue without cartilagenous rings.

Evidence that confirms the hazard of prolonged cuffed tubes was developed by Cooper and Grillo [9] and Shelly, Dawson, and May [41]. In dogs, pressures in the cuff inflated to occlude at a ventilatory pressure of 40 cm H_2O were about 200 torr. Ching [7] found that cuff pressures ranged from 35 to 214 torr. Cuff pressures and lateral wall pressures against the trachea differ because lateral pressure does not develop until contact is made with the tracheal wall. Cuff pressures and lateral wall pressures do not coincide until a large-volume, soft cuff is used. Thus, in a distended, modified Portex tube, the occlusive cuff pressure is the same as the lateral wall pressure, and generally this can be maintained in the 10 to 30 torr range, instead of the 100 to 200 torr found in standard latex cuffs. Excessive pressures can be produced in high volume cuffs if more than the occlusive volume is introduced.

The overwhelming evidence in favor of pressure necrosis resulting from the cuff of tracheostomy tubes has led to the search for less traumatic or low-pressure cuffs. Cooper and Grillo [9] presented experimental data in which large-volume, very compliant, low-pressure cuffs produced minimal damage when compared with the high-pressure, low-volume cuffs. The extension of this principle to clinical practice has been evident in the last four years with the addition of a number of design variations to control lateral wall pressure within the 10 to 30 torr range. Clinical evaluation of these newer cuffs is not complete, but the information at hand indicates that even though trauma is reduced, it is not eliminated, and pressure necrosis can occur though at an ameliorated rate [18].

Comparisons of similar groups with high-volume and low-volume cuffs revealed that 68 percent of the patients with the high-volume cuff showed no areas of exposed cartilage, whereas none of the patients with the high-pressure, low-volume cuffs were in this category [18]. For the low-pressure, high-volume cuff the average cuff pressure was 33 torr, whereas with the older standard cuffs, the average cuff pressure was 270 torr at a peak respiratory pressure of 28 torr.

Variations of this principle have been successfully applied by other groups. An ingenious cuff was described by Magovern [26] in which the cuff pressure is controlled by an external balloon that would eliminate the hazards of overinflation. Intermittent inflation of the cuff to produce occlusion only during the inspiratory phase of the ventilator is another approach that has been successfully applied [40]. Ochsner [35] states that ischemia was not seen even after one month of continuous assisted ventilation. Cuffless endotracheal and tracheostomy tubes have been described by Miller [27]. These are "flange tubes" that employ multiple thin collapsible Silastic flanges instead of an air-filled balloon.

These new designs, although an improvement over the old, do not prevent mucosal or even tracheal wall damage. It is apparent that any foreign material in contact with tracheal mucosa, even without pressure, will produce deleterious changes [23]. Low-pressure cuffs and even cuffless tubes in contact with the mucosa produce definite inflammatory or denuding changes, though the incidence of ulceration is much less [18, 43]. High-volume cuffs, however, may present other problems related to the size and position of the cuff on the tube. An overdistended, floppy cuff may protrude over the tip of the tube, causing obstruction to ventilation. High-volume cuffs also may not collapse spontaneously when positive pressure ventilation is not needed, thereby restricting air passage around the tube, unless suction is applied.

CLINICAL COURSE

The appearance of obstructive symptoms after removal of the tracheostomy tube may be quite variable, from days to months. Murphy et al. [30] reported the occurrence of tracheal stenosis 12 to 29 days after removal of the tracheostomy tube, which had been in place 6 to 24 days. The patient reported by Fraser and Bell [15] developed stenosis one month after a tracheostomy tube had been in place for 2 weeks. Grillo [17] found that the majority of patients developed symptoms from 10 to 42 days after extubation, though time intervals may be as small as a few days or as long as 18 months. Rarely, a granuloma at the tip of this tube may cause obstruction while the tube is still in place.

Tracheal stenosis usually manifests itself by stridor and difficult breathing. In milder cases, this is manifest only with severe exercise, though the patient will complain of difficulty in clearing the throat or coughing up secretions. Any patient who develops stridor or wheeze or difficulty clearing secretions should be suspect if he has had a tracheostomy or a prolonged intubation.

Definitive diagnosis may be made by laminagrams of the trachea in the anteroposterior and lateral views (see Figure 13-2). Most of the stenoses are just below or at the sternal notch and will not be seen well on routine anteroposterior or lateral films of the neck. A high tracheal or subglottic lesion may be seen clearly on routine lateral films of the neck. Bronchoscopy is an important means of evaluating the presence and degree of stenosis. This procedure is usually tolerated well so long as dilatation or forceful passage of a bronchoscope are not attempted. The fiberoptic bronchoscope facilitates the safe observation of these lesions. There is a definite hazard of precipitating obstruction in the very tight stenoses, and of needing a small endotracheal tube or bronchoscope through the stenosis as an emergency airway.

Any techniques that require the installation of fluid or dyes in the trachea for contrast studies or even anesthesia are best avoided, for these substances may precipitate an acute respiratory insufficiency if the functional margin has reached the critical stage. A tracheostomy tube, if present, should be removed prior to x-ray studies, and the possibility of immediate replacement should be provided for. It is well to mark the tracheostomy when the films are taken. At times, tracheal resection must be carried out immediately after a bronchoscopy because the patient cannot be without a rigid tube to stent the stenosis. Tracheostomies, although providing a good temporary solution, add the undesirable elements of infection and possible destruction of some tracheal length needed for a tension-free anastomosis.

Pulmonary functions are helpful indicators for diagnosis. A slow inspiratory time is suggestive of a critical lesion. Vital capacity (VC) and forced expiratory volume of 1 second may be severely impaired in the patients with critical stenosis. Perhaps the most helpful is the flow-volume loop formed by taking full inspiration (100 percent VC), exhaling maximally to residual volume, and then forcing inspiration. Narrowing of a major airway by a rigid lesion creates a plateau on both the inspiratory and expiratory loops (see Chapter 4). The diameter of the stenosis can be estimated. In nonrigid stenosis only one limb of the loop may be deformed. Stridor at rest is usually associated with a lumen of less than 5 mm.

The mild or moderate stricture without symptoms at rest are more difficult to identify. Pearson and Andrews [36] found that these strictures constitute about half of all strictures in a prospective study. These patients are often tagged and treated as having chronic bronchitis or lung diseases because of a brassy cough, limited exercise tolerance, or difficulty clearing secretions. Occasionally, a wheeze arises during exercise. There is always a question of therapy in this group, and this must be determined by the degree of disability and stenosis. Here, bronchoscopy and tracheograms are definitely helpful, as are tomograms.

SURGICAL THERAPY

Surgical treatment of these stenotic lesions should be defined by the specific type of deformity or obstruction. The hourglass deformity of the cervical trachea below the cricoid cartilage, the most common type of lesion, is resected with end-to-end anastomosis. Dilatation of these hard fibrotic lesions is generally unsuccessful, even on a short-term basis, and often causes acute obstruction. Dilatation may improve these lesions temporarily by removal of granulation tissue that adds to the narrowing. However, this tissue is rapidly replaced and accounts for the rather brief effects of dilatation in this kind of lesion. Subglottic or cricoid stenosis is a more complicated lesion that requires specialized techniques of partial cricoid resection.

The less common granuloma at the ostium or the thin membranous obstruction are generally treated by segmental resection, though occasionally these conditions lend themselves to partial though effective resection through a bronchoscope. Dilatation and stents should have a minimal role in the management of any of the lesions. Experience indicates that conservative treatment of stenosis results in a high percentage of failures and complications. Occasionally patients are managed by a permanent tracheostomy and tube through the stenotic area.

Surgical technique and approaches must be tailored to the location and extent of the lesion. Most operations are elective, preferably without a tracheostomy in place because of additional technical difficulties and possibility of infection. At times, the operation is performed as an emergency because of obstruction resulting from bronchoscopy and dilatation. Preparation should include adequate bacterial culture and antibiotic therapy for any evident infection, or should include antibiotics prophylactically for 24 to 48 hours before the operation. If a tracheostomy is not present, anesthesia may be difficult. Introduction and intubation may be a very tense and dangerous period. We have witnessed cardiac standstill on two occasions during this period because of inadequate ventilation. Generally, the endotracheal tube is placed above the stenosis, though on one occasion a small tube was forced through the stenosis as a solution to the emergency. A rigid bronchoscope, in several sizes, should be available for passage across the stenosis if this is needed for emergency reasons. There should also be a variety of cuffed endotracheal tubes and sterile connecting tubing on the operating table for cannulation of the trachea distally when the stenosis is resected.

Cervical Stenosis

The trachea is exposed by a long transverse cervical incision with division of the sternocleidomastoid muscles if needed. This procedure allows good exposure of the trachea for lesions involving the proximal two-thirds of the trachea and allows resection of the trachea up to 4 cm in length (Figure 13–6). The trachea is exposed from the cricoid cartilage to the sternum anteriorly and is dissected circumferentially only in the area of the stenosis. Fibrosis and scarring at the site of a current or old tracheostomy makes the dissection difficult, and the recurrent laryngeal nerves

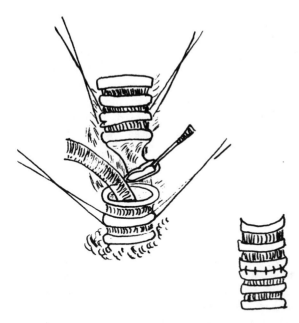

Figure 13-6. Resection of the stenosis and end-to-end anastomosis. Ventilation is provided by the cuffed tube into the distal segment until the posterior wall is closed.

are avoided by dissecting only the tracheal wall. At this stage, extension of the neck and even traction sutures are required to expose a cuff stenosis in the neck, because this stenosis is usually at the level of the sternum. Stomal strictures are easily accessible in the cervical exposure but may involve the cricoid cartilage by scar or malacia; they often present as subglottic strictures.

The principles of successful tracheal resection and reanastomosis involve preservation of the blood supply, avoidance of excessive tension, and bacteriologic control. Circumferential dissection is avoided except at the site of the stricture and one or two cartilages needed for placing sutures for the anastomosis. A plexus of fine vessels exists on the surface of the trachea communicating to a submucosal plexus that should bleed freely at the time of anastomosis. The trachea is freed from the surrounding tissue anteriorly to the carina. The blood supply reaches the trachea principally from the lateral aspect, with some approaching posteriorly from the esophagus. Branches from the inferior thyroid and superior intercostal arteries reach the upper trachea, and branches from the bronchial arteries reach the lower trachea.

Pearson and Andrews [36] do not free the lateral or posterior trachea except for the segment adjacent to the anastomosis. Grillo [17] frees the posterior aspect for additional mobilization; however, extensive mobilization is usually not required for the excision of 2 to 4 cm of trachea that is required for the usual cuff stricture. The trachea is transected distal to the stenosis and a cuffed endotracheal tube is inserted for ventilation while the strictured segment is removed and posterior portion of the anastomosis completed. Traction sutures are placed laterally on both ends of the trachea. Interrupted sutures of 3–0 Tevdek with generous bites around a tracheal cartilage are placed so that the knots are on the outside and spaced about 4 mm apart. The neck is flexed and posterior sutures are tied while the traction sutures approximate the ends without tension. The peroral endotracheal tube is then pulled down and placed in the distal tracheal segment, and the other tube is removed before the anterior sutures are placed. The neck is flexed maximally for the anastomosis. There should be no air leak. The tissues are lavaged with an antibiotic solution, and the tissue spaces are drained by closed sterile suction. The sterno-cleidomastoid muscles are reapproximated. The platysma is closed as a separate layer. Infected tissue around a tracheostomy is generally removed during the skin incision. The tracheal stoma is removed as part of the resection so that there remains only a single clean suture line without tension.

Subglottic Stenosis

Stomal stenoses often involve the cricoid cartilage, even the thyroid cartilage, if there has been extensive infection, a high tracheostomy, removal of a large piece of tracheal wall, or rough dilatation of the original tracheal stoma. The subglottic lesion is particularly difficult because of the limitations placed upon resection by the involvement of the cricoid cartilage, to which the arytenoid muscles of the vocal cords are attached. Total resection of the cricoid cartilage would destroy the voice and may produce obstruction at the cords, neither being a good solution to the problem. In the past, these patients often represented the failures in high tracheal lesions because stenosis remained above the anastomosis, usually requiring permanent tracheostomy.

The general technique of exposure is the same as in the lower cuff lesions, though additional exposure of the larynx is needed. Internal stents of Silastic with an anterior tracheostomy tube have been used to splint this area and provide a means of suctioning and auxiliary ventilation. Our experience with the Montgomery tube has not encouraged us to continue its use because of progressive buildup of inspissated secretions on the inside, eventuating in complete obstruction and sudden death. More recent techniques for this defect offer a way of partially resecting the deformed cricoid cartilage, which is usually the site of obstruction, without destruction of vocal cord function. A portion of the cricoid cartilage may be removed anteriorly with impunity. Pearson et al. [39] have devised a technique for resection of the cricoid cartilage that may solve the problem of high subglottic stenosis. The distal tracheal resection line is fashioned to form a complete ring for mucosa-to-mucosa anastomosis within 1 cm or less of the vocal cords.

Low Tracheal Stenosis

An uncommon type of lesion, a low tracheal stenosis may result from a peroral endotracheal tube or from tip injury of a tracheostomy tube. In this type, a more extensive mediastinal exposure of the trachea is required. Partial sternotomy involving two or three interspaces allows good exposure of the trachea down to the carina, though it does not provide well for extensive mobilization of the carina or bronchi.

All patients undergoing resection for tracheal stenosis should be positioned and prepared for a possible sternal-splitting incision. The principles of mobilization and blood supply are the same for this lesion as for the higher cervical types. End-to-end anastomosis is accomplished without tension if no more than 4 cm of trachea is excised. In the event that a longer resection is required, mobilization of the upper trachea by hyoid-releasing techniques and mobilization of the carina by freeing the mainstem bronchi is used. These maneuvers are rarely needed for the localized stricture and are more apropos for the tracheal tumor, whose extension can be difficult to determine preoperatively. The technique of resection and anastomosis remains the same except for the added mediastinal exposure. Drainage of this potentially infected closed space is important, for a serious infection or hematoma may easily destroy the operation.

Extended Resections

The long tracheal resection, another recent major contribution to this field, is the ability to extend resections of the trachea beyond the usual 3 to 4 cm without the need for a prosthesis or a mediastinal tracheostomy. Until recently, 5-cm segments represented the limit for end-to-end anastomosis. A combination of releasing techniques at the carina and at the larynx allows resection of lengths up to 8.5 cm with primary anastomosis [36, 38].

Division of the inferior pulmonary ligament and mobilization of the right hilum offer additional length, but these procedures are troublesome because they require a formal thoracotomy with the morbidity that can result. Almost the entire trachea lies in the mediastinum when the neck is fully flexed.

Laryngeal release techniques [11, 29] facilitate the sleeve resection of the trachea when additional length is needed, because of suture line tensions of greater than 1,000 gm (Figure 13-7). The suprahyoid technique is preferred because it interferes with deglutition the least and provides an amount of additional length equal to the laryngeal release. The usual horizontal skin incision is made. This is extended superiorly to the hyoid bone for development of a subplatysmal skin flap. The sternohyoid muscles and the thyroid isthmus are divided for complete exposure of the cervical trachea. The stenosis is opened and the distal trachea cannulated in the usual fashion. The stenotic segment is removed and the body of the hyoid bone is exposed. The muscle attachments to the superior surface of the hyoid bone are transected, as are the lesser and greater cornua of the hyoid bone, allowing the body of the hyoid bone, the larynx, the cricoid cartilage, and the proximal tracheal segment to drop inferiorly. An end-to-end anastomosis is then performed in the usual manner. This procedure may give an additional 1 to 2 cm for tension-free anastomosis. A similar releasing technique can be applied anteriorly between the thyroid and hyoid cartilages.

The place for complete circumferential replacement of a segment of trachea is not established as yet. Though there have been extensive experimental trials of prosthetic as well as natural tissue replacement of the trachea, there does not appear to be an ideal artificial replacement for the trachea.

Success with circumferential or partial wall replacement has been achieved in a

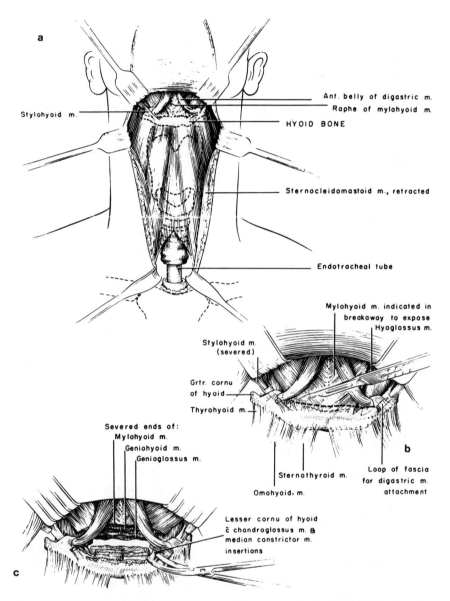

a

Ant. belly of digastric m.

Raphe of mylohyoid m.

HYOID BONE

Stylohyoid m.

Sternocleidomastoid m., retracted

Endotracheal tube

Mylohyoid m. indicated in
breakaway to expose
Hyoglossus m.

Stylohyoid m.
(severed)

Grtr. cornu
of hyoid

Thyrohyoid m.

Severed ends of:
Mylohyoid m.
Geniohyoid m.
Genioglossus m.

Sternothyroid m.

b

Loop of fascia
for digastric m.
attachment

Omohyoid. m.

Lesser cornu of hyoid
c̄ chondroglossus m. &
median constrictor m.
insertions

c

Figure 13–7. (a) Endotracheal tube bridging gap between proximal and distal tracheal ends after tracheal stenosis has been resected. Anterior cervical skin flap has been elevated to suprahyoid region. (b) Muscle attachments to superior surface of hyoid bone transected, exposing preepiglottic space. (c) Lesser cornu of hyoid bone is palpated and transected with heavy scissors. Mylohyoid, geniohyoid, and genioglossus muscles are separated from hyoid bone, exposing preepiglottic space. (d) Dotted lines indicate point where hyoid bone is sectioned, separating its body from the greater horn on each side. (e) Site for hyoid bone incision imme-

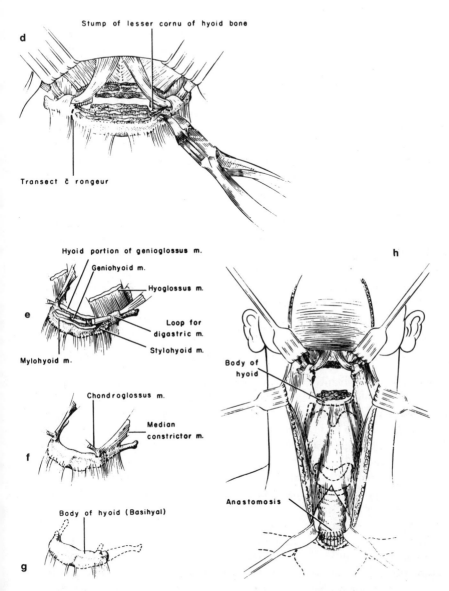

Stump of lesser cornu of hyoid bone

d

Transect č rongeur

Hyoid portion of genioglossus m.

Geniohyoid m.

Hyoglossus m.

e

Loop for digastric m.

Stylohyoid m.

Mylohyoid m.

Chondroglossus m.

Median constrictor m.

f

Body of hyoid (Basihyal)

g

h

Body of hyoid

Anastomosis

diately anterior to tendinous attachment of digastric muscle to hyoid bone. (f) Relationship of chondroglossus and medial constrictor muscles to bone incisions that separate greater and lesser cornua of hyoid bone from its body. (g) Greater and lesser cornua of hyoid bone have now been separated from the body of the hyoid bone and its inferior muscle attachments. (h) Termination of operation, anastomosis of distal to proximal trachea has been done. (Reproduced with permission from W. W. Montgomery, Suprahyoid release for tracheal anastomosis. *Archives of Otolaryngology* 99, 1974, p. 1255.)   Copyright 1974, American Medical Association.

few patients and at times offers the only solution to an impossible situation. Extensive involvement by primary or secondary tumor is the usual indication, though it is an uncommon entity. Moghissi [28] has recently presented a series of 13 patients in whom he accomplished this form of reconstruction using a combination of Marlex mesh and pericardium. Two of these represented circumferential replacement, and one is alive and well 4 years later. The others represented one-half to three-fourths circumference excision and replacement with good results. Nine of the remaining 11 patients are alive and well. The Marlex tube or patch is fashioned at the time of surgery. The outer surface of the Marlex is covered by a free or pedicled graft of pericardium. Most of these patients represented carcinoma of the lung with extension to the trachea, and the procedure was combined with a lobectomy or pneumonectomy. Only 3 patients had primary mucoepidermoid carcinoma of the trachea.

The use of Marlex substitutes in the past has been attended by problems of air leak, infection, and recurrent stenosis [4, 37]. Being firm and rough, it may also cause erosion of nearby vessels. It is not clear whether circumferential replacement is attended by restitution of a ciliated mucosa, though this is apparently restored with good functional results if a portion of the wall remains. Borrie and Redshow [6] and Neville et al. [33] have used a Silastic tracheal prosthesis. The combination of a rigid porous prosthetic device and a graft of natural tissue appears to have merit.

Results

The results of conservative treatment such as dilatation have been poor when applied to the fully developed circumferential hourglass type of deformity. There is almost always a rapid recurrence of obstruction, usually in days, and the repeated procedures carry the disadvantage of discomfort, bleeding, and acute obstruction. Dilatation has been used successfully, however, for the stricture that occurs after a primary resection [2].

Segmental resection and primary anastomosis remains the basic technique. Grillo [17] reported the results in 30 patients operated upon between 1965 and 1969. There was one death in this group. The cervical route only was used in 16 patients; 8 required cervicomediastinal exposure, and 5 a transthoracic approach. One required a tracheal reconstruction using staged skin flaps. There were 24 good to excellent results (80%). The poor results were related, for the most part, to anastomotic separation, residual malacia above the anastomosis, and wound infection, though several of these were improved by additional surgery or by bronchoscopy [17]. Pearson and Andrews [36] reported good results in 33 of 37 strictures managed by resection of 1 to 5-cm segments. Two were operative deaths (6%) and 1 required reconstruction by staged plastic reconstruction. Of interest is the fact that about half of the lesions were stomal in location. Webb et al. [45] reported 20 patients with one death and one recurrence. Three of this group required subsequent bronchoscopic removal of granulation tissue from the suture.

Restenosis

A significant number of patients who undergo segmental resection of the trachea for stenosis will develop restenosis. In Pearson's series, this was approximately 17%. These are usually due to excessive tension, infection, and other reasons producing a disruption of the suture line. Reoperation appears to be the most effective approach, though it has been possible in our experience to avoid this by judicious dilatation in 2 patients.

PREVENTION OF STENOSIS

Prevention of cuff or posttracheostomy stenosis involves all steps of the process of instituting ventilatory assist—the technique of tracheostomy, the selection of tube and cuff, and finally but not least, the care of the patient while the tube is in place. Though tracheal stenosis can occur at any tracheostomy site irrespective of duration, it is unusual if the tube or tracheostomy are in place for only a few days. However, any cuff, low-pressure or high-pressure, may institute changes in the mucosa and even in the submucosal tissue within hours of placement, and any respiratory difficulty in the first few months after ventilatory assistance should raise the possibility of tracheal stenosis. The technique of performing a tracheostomy should be reviewed. There is a large variation in technique and details among house and senior staff. The philosophy is often that it is a simple, uncomplicated procedure and that any technique works well. Many tracheostomy sets include two-blade and three-blade dilators that fracture the trachea in several directions, producing an extensive irregular tear that probably heals with some contracture. Excision of circles, squares, and the like produce defects that heal by contracture. Stellate incisions with inversion of corners of the tracheal wall into the lumen may provide the nidus for granulation tissue obstruction.

The size of the tracheostomy tube also plays a role in the size of the defect that must heal and also in the production of adjacent malacia that may add to narrowing by destruction of supporting cartilaginous rings and local indentations of the wall. The care of the tube and tracheostomy during the ventilatory assist become most critical when the process is prolonged for more than a few days. Prevention or control of lateral wall pressure and of infection become primary requirements.

There is some evidence that intermittent inflation of the cuff cycled by the ventilator is effective in preventing cuff complications. Intermittent deflation of the cuff once an hour is probably a good principle if the patient's condition allows it. Inflation of the cuff by measuring pressure and volumes just to the point of occlusion is the safest way of monitoring and controlling lateral wall pressure. This should be done intermittently because the volume of a cuff may change under the influence of the gas mixture [42]. A large-volume low-pressure cuff should be used routinely during surgery as well as for tracheostomy tubes. Cuffed tubes should be removed as early as possible and replaced by noncuffed tubes. Tracheostomy tubes larger than a 6 mm size are best avoided. Tracheostomy tubes should be changed at least every 48 hours and possibly every 24 hours, if secretions are difficult to aspirate or if purulent infection is present.

A prospective study by Webb et al. [45] in 92 patients is pertinent to the subject of prevention. Each had a tracheostomy performed with a vertical incision in the trachea, and each had a tracheostomy tube with a self-inflating foam cuff that could not exceed atmospheric pressure. Of these patients, 23 died of their primary diseases, and postmortem examinations in 17 did not show evidence of significant tracheal damage. The remainder of the patients followed clinically and by bronchoscopy for 5 to 18 months also have shown no evidence of stenosis.

TECHNIQUE OF TRACHEOSTOMY

The simplest approach to the trachea in adult or child is a longitudinal incision in the cervical midline extending from the cricoid cartilage to the sternal notch. Many prefer a transverse incision because of its superior cosmetic result, though this may prolong exposure and may be less safe in children. The platysma is divided and the strap muscles are separated at the midline. Occasionally, veins must be ligated or sutured. The thyroid gland, which presents below the strap muscles, is usually retracted inferiorly by releasing its fascial attachment above to expose the pretracheal fascia. Occasionally, in a long neck with a low incision, the thyroid is retracted superiorly or the isthmus may even be divided between sutures for exposure of the pretracheal fascia. The fascia is opened longitudinally for exposure of approximately three rings. The first tracheal and cricoid cartilages are avoided because of the dangers of tracheomalacia and tracheal stenosis in the subglottic region. The trachea is grasped with hooks on either side of the midline and a longitudinal incision through two or three tracheal rings is made with a no. 11 blade. Segments of tracheal rings are not excised. The edges of the incision are retracted by the hooks and a no. 6 tracheal tube is inserted in the adult. In the child, the technique is the same, though the tracheal tube used may be a smooth soft tube without cuff in order to obtain maximum lumen and to avoid the dangers of pressure erosion potentially produced by the cuff.

TRACHEAL STENOSIS IN INFANTS AND CHILDREN

There are special problems connected with infants and children because of their size and because of variations in tension, permissible length of resection, and growth potential. The cause and prevention of problems in the young are the same as in the adult. Cuffed tubes are best avoided, and nontraumatic tracheostomy tubes without cuffs can be used for positive pressure ventilation by virtue of the fit. Maeda and Grillo [25] have developed experimental evidence in puppies and adult dogs that indicate that the level of permissible tension in puppies is roughly half that of the adult. In addition, tracheal growth was more restricted at the anastomotic site when resection rather than transection was done, though all puppies with resection in the permissible range grew without stenotic signs. Muscall and his associates [31] resected a 3.5-cm long circumferential stenosis in a 6-year-old patient equivalent to 65% of the whole tracheal length. Of interest is the recent experience with a conservative approach to certain tracheal stenoses in children that prevent extubation after tracheostomy. Ofherson [34] has used a combination of dilatation, intraluminal stenting, and steroid administration in high doses over a period of 4 weeks to treat 4 children with severe tracheal strictures followed by successful removal of the tracheal cannula.

REFERENCES

1. Aboulker, P., Lissac, J., and Saint-Paul, O. Respiratory accidents due to laryngo-tracheal stricture post tracheostomy. *Acta Chir. Belg.* 59, 1960, p. 533.
2. Andrews, M. J., and Pearson, F. G. An analysis of 59 cases of tracheal stenosis following tracheostomy with cuffed tube and assisted ventilation with special reference to diagnosis and treatment. *Br. J. Surg.* 60, 1973, p. 208.
3. Atkins, J. P. Tracheal resection following the use of cuffed tracheostomy tubes. *Ann. Otol. Rhinol. Laryngol.* 73, 1964, p. 1124.
4. Beall, A. C., Jr., et al. Tracheal reconstruction with heavy Marlex mesh. *Arch. Surg.* 86, 1963, p. 112.
5. Binet, J. P., and Aboulker, P. Un cas de sténose trachéale après trachéotomie: Resection—suture de la trachée querison. *Mem. Acad. Chir.* (Paris) 87, 1961, p. 39.
6. Borrie, J., and Redshow, N. R. Prosthetic tracheal replacement: Silastic tracheal prosthesis with subterminal Dacron suture cuff. *J. Thorac. Cardiovasc. Surg.* 60, 1970, p. 829.
7. Ching, N. P., et al. The contribution of cuff volume and pressure in tracheostomy tube damage. *J. Thorac. Cardiovasc. Surg.* 62, 1971, p. 402.
8. Cooper, J. D., and Grillo, H. C. The evaluation of tracheal injury due to ventilatory assistance through cuffed tubes. A pathologic study. *Ann. Surg.* 169, 1969, p. 334.
9. Cooper, J. D., and Grillo, H. C. Experimental production and prevention of injury due to cuffed tracheal tubes. *Surg. Gynecol. Obstet.* 129, 1969, p. 1235.
10. Cooper, J. D., and Grillo, H. C. Analysis of problems related to cuffs on intratracheal tubes. *Chest* 62, 1972, p. 21S.
11. Dedo, H. H., and Fishman, N. H. Laryngeal release and sleeve resection for tracheal stenosis. *Ann. Otol. Rhinol. Laryngol.* 78, 1969, p. 285.
12. Donnelly, W. H. Histopathology of endotracheal intubation, an autopsy study of 99 cases. *Arch. Pathol.* 8, 1969, p. 511.
13. Dugan, D. J., and Samson, P. C. Tracheostomy: Present day indications and technics. *Am. J. Surg.* 106, 1963, p. 290.
14. Flege, J. B., Jr. Tracheoesophageal fistula caused by cuffed tracheostomy. *Br. J. Surg.* 54, 1967, p. 302.
15. Fraser, L., and Bell, P. R. Distal tracheal stenosis following tracheostomy. *Br. J. Surg.* 54, 1967, p. 302.
16. Gibson, P. Aetiology and repair of tracheal stenosis following tracheostomy and intermittent positive pressure respiration. *Thorax* 22, 1967, p. 1.
17. Grillo, H. Surgery of the trachea. *Curr. Prob. Surgery* July, 1970, p. 3.
18. Grillo, H. C., et al. A low pressure cuff for tracheostomy tubes to minimize tracheal injury. *J. Thorac. Cardiovasc. Surg.* 62, 1971, p. 898

19. Head, J. M. Tracheostomy in the management of respiratory problems. *N. Engl. J. Med.* 264, 1961, p. 587.

20. Hedden, M., Ersoz, C. J., and Safar, P. Tracheoesophageal fistulas following prolonged artificial ventilation via cuffed tracheostomy tubes. *Anesthesiology* 31, 1969, p. 281.

21. Jackson, C. High tracheostomy and other errors, the chief cause of chronic laryngeal stenosis. *Surg. Gynecol. Obstet.* 32, 1921, p. 329.

22. Johnston, J. B., Wright, J. S., and Hercus, V. Tracheal stenosis following tracheostomy. *J. Thorac. Cardiovasc. Surg.* 53, 1967, p. 206.

23. Klainer, A. S., et al. Surface alterations due to endotracheal intubation. *Am. J. Med.* 58, 1975, p. 674.

24. Lindholm, C. E. Prolonged endotracheal intubation. *Acta Anaesthesiol. Scand.* (Suppl.) 33, 1970, p. 1.

25. Maeda, M., and Grillo, H. C. Effect of tension on tracheal growth after resection and anastomosis in puppies. *J. Thorac. Cardiovasc. Surg.* 65, 1973, p. 658.

26. Magovern, G. J. Discussion of paper by Ching, N. P., et al. *J. Thorac. Cardiovasc. Surg.* 62, 1971, p. 410.

27. Miller, D. R. Discussion of paper by Grillo, H. C., et al. *J. Thorac. Cardiovasc. Surg.* 62, 1971, p. 906.

28. Moghissi, K. Tracheal reconstruction with a prosthesis of Marlex mesh and pericardium. *J. Thorac. Cardiovasc. Surg.* 69, 1975, p. 499.

29. Montgomery, W. W. Suprahyoid release for tracheal anastomosis. *Arch. Otolaryngol.* 99, 1974, p. 255.

30. Murphy, D. A. MacLean, L. D., and Dobell, A. R. C. Tracheal stenosis as a complication of tracheostomy. *Ann. Thorac. Surg.* 2, 1966, p. 44.

31. Muscall, I., et al. Stenosis of the trachea—resection and end-to-end anastomosis. Report of two cases. *Arch. Surg.* 87, 1963, p. 726.

32. Myers, R. S., and Pilch, Y. H. Temporary control of tracheoinnominate artery fistula. *Ann. Surg.* 170, 1969, p. 149.

33. Neville, W. E., et al. Replacement of the intrathoracic trachea and both stem bronchi with a molded Silastic prosthesis. *J. Thorac. Cardiovasc. Surg.* 63, 1972, p. 569.

34. Ofhersen, H. B., Jr. Steroid therapy for tracheal stenosis in children. *Ann. Thorac. Surg.* 17, 1974, p. 254.

35. Oschner, J. L. Discussion of paper by Ching, N. P., et al. *J. Thorac. Cardiovasc. Surg.* 62, 1971, p. 410.

36. Pearson, F. G., and Andrews, M. J. Detection and management of tracheal stenosis following cuffed tube tracheostomy. *Ann. Thorac. Surg.* 12, 1971, p. 359.

37. Pearson, F. G., et al. Reconstruction of circumferential tracheal defects with a porous prosthesis: An experimental and clinical study using heavy Marlex mesh. *J. Thorac. Cardiovasc. Surg.* 55, 1968, p. 605.

38. Pearson, F. G., et al. Adenoid cystic carcinoma of the trachea. *Ann. Thorac. Surg.* 18, 1974, p. 16.

39. Pearson, F. G., et al. Primary tracheal anastomosis following resection of the cricoid cartilage with preservation of recurrent laryngeal nerves. Presented at

the 55th Annual Meeting of the Association for Thoracic Surgery, April 14–16, 1975.

40. Reich, M. P., and Rosenkrantz, J. G. Fistula between innominate artery and trachea. *Arch. Surg.* 96, 1968, p. 401.

41. Shelly, W., Dawson, R. C., and May, I. A. Cuffed tubes as a cause of tracheal stenosis. *J. Thorac. Cardiovasc. Surg.* 57, 1969, p. 623.

42. Stanley, T. H., and Liu, W. S. Tracheostomy and endotracheal tube cuff volume and pressure changes during thoracic surgery. Presented at the 11th Annual Meeting of the Society of Thoracic Surgeons, January 20–22, 1975, Montreal, Canada.

43. Van Wein, A., et al. Tracheal stenosis after tracheostomy. *Acta Chir. Belg.* 60, 1961, p. 85.

44. Webb, W. R. Discussion of paper by Ching, N. P., et al. *J. Thorac. Cardiovasc. Surg.* 62, 1971, p. 409.

45. Webb, W. R., et al. Surgical management of tracheal stenosis. *Ann. Surg.* 179, 1974, p. 819.

46. Witz, J. P., et al. Low stenosis of the thoracic trachea post-tracheotomy. *Mem. Acad. Chir.* (Paris) 86, 1960, p. 123.

Robert E. Flynn

Controlled Ventilation: Neuromuscular Blocking Agents

14

The treatment of patients with acute and chronic respiratory failure often requires total or partial control of the neuromuscular components of breathing. This control is most effectively achieved by the use of a variety of pharmacologic agents whose site of action is the neuromuscular junction. An understanding of the anatomic, physiologic, and pharmacologic characteristics of the neuromuscular control of breathing provides the basis for the proper utilization of drugs that may be used clinically to achieve controlled ventilation. This chapter focuses on neuromuscular function as it relates to the mechanics of breathing, and on the drugs that are used to control neuromuscular activity. It is not concerned with the many complex and interrelated neuropulmonary reflexes of the central nervous system that are involved in the physiology and pharmacology of respiration.

NEUROMUSCULAR ANATOMY

The muscles involved in breathing are the skeletal muscles that are attached to the rib cage. Skeletal muscles are voluntary muscles that are innervated by both motor and sensory nerves. The physical act of breathing, that is, the movement of the diaphragm, rib cage, and abdomen, is accomplished by the contraction of these skeletal muscles.

Although the act of breathing is under some voluntary control, the basic pattern of the act is at a reflex level (Figure 14-1). The mechanisms involved in both the voluntary and reflex activities are directly related to the nervous system by structural components that interact at several levels of the central nervous system.

277

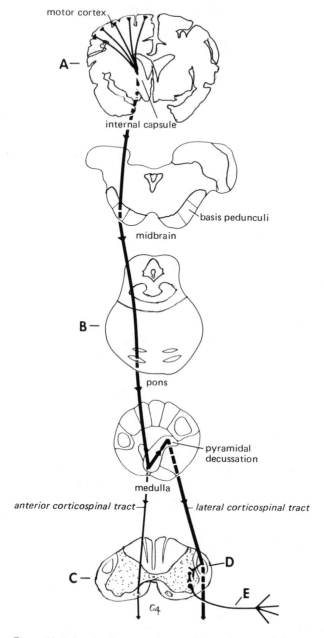

Figure 14–1. Levels of motor system and sites of sensory influence on breathing. (A) Cerebral hemisphere—voluntary, emotional; (B) pons and medulla—central homeostatic reflexes; (C) spinal cord—basic motor and sensory reflexes; (D) anterior horn—motor neuron; (E) motor axon. (Adapted from Curtis, Jacobson, and Marcus. *Introduction to Neurosciences*. Philadelphia: Saunders, 1972.)

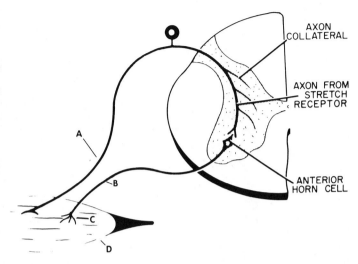

Figure 14-2. Pathway for monosynaptic stretch reflex, basic reflex involved in muscle contraction. (A) Sensory nerve; (B) motor nerve; (C) motor end-plate; (D) muscle. (Adapted from Curtis, Jacobson, and Marcus. *Introduction to Neurosciences.* Philadelphia: Saunders, 1972.)

The levels of control extend from the cerebral hemisphere where the basic pattern of voluntary (total body) motor and sensory function is represented, to the central homeostatic centers located in the pons and medulla. Nerve impulses interact at various levels of the brain and exert their influence on the act of breathing by way of neural connections that descend through the brain to the spinal cord. At that level the motor axons synapse with the anterior horn cells in the cervical and thoracic spinal cord. The reflexes involved in the mechanics of breathing are dependent on the complex integration of sensory input from the muscles, tendons, and joints of the muscles of respiration with the central and peripheral motor system involved in respiration (Figure 14-2). For the purpose of this chapter, attention is focused on the voluntary and involuntary motor aspects of the act of breathing.

Control of respiration can be pharmacologically achieved at both the central and peripheral sites. However, central control is nonspecific, for the drugs that effect central structures, for example, benzodiazephine compounds (Librium and Valium), narcotics (morphine), and barbiturates, also effect consciousness, behavior, and the central homeostatic reflexes. Therefore, control of the motor system is most effectively and specifically obtained by pharmacologic manipulation in the peripheral neuromuscular system of the functional unit of the peripheral motor system, the motor unit.

The motor unit is composed of a motor neuron, an axon, and the group of muscle fibers innervated by a single axon. Each motor nerve is composed of several axons, and each skeletal muscle is composed of many muscle fibers. At the neuromuscular

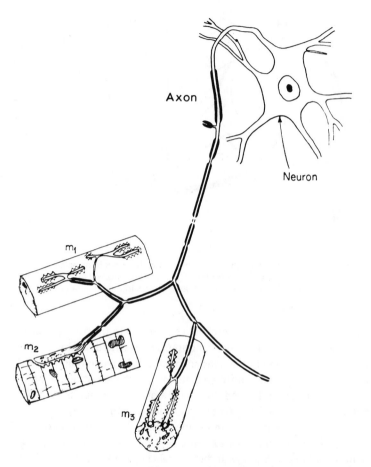

Figure 14-3. The axon branches of a motor neuron are shown terminating on several muscle fibers (M_1, M_2, M_3). (From Ochs, S. *Elements of Neurophysiology.* New York: Wiley, 1965.)

junction, which is the site of the innervation of the individual muscle fiber, a specialized anatomic structure, the motor end-plate, is located (Figure 14-3).

The nerve impulses are conducted from the lower motor neurons (anterior horn cells) by way of myelinated nerve fibers to the motor end-plate, which is located within the muscle fiber. At the motor end-plate, the axon loses its myelin sheath and forms an invagination with the sarcoplasm of the muscle fiber. This invagination, which is continuous with the axon, is composed of the terminal membrane, which encloses a group of synaptic vesicles within the motor nerve. The vesicles contain the neurotransmitter acetylcholine.

Within the sarcoplasm of the muscle, adjacent to the neural elements, is the postjunctional membrane. The space between the terminal membrane (neural) and the postjunctional membrane (muscular) is called the *subneural space*. The terminal

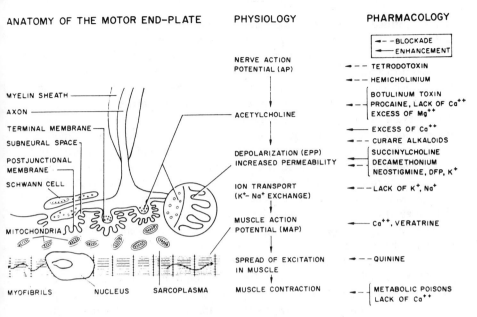

ANATOMY OF THE MOTOR END-PLATE   PHYSIOLOGY   PHARMACOLOGY

Figure 14-4. Sites of action and interrelationship of miscellaneous agents at the neuro-muscular junction and adjacent structures. (From Goodman, L. S., and Gilman, A. *The Pharmacological Basis of Therapeutics* (5th ed.). New York: Macmillan, 1975. Fig. 28-1, p. 581.)

membrane, the subneural space, and the postjunctional membrane constitute the structural motor end-plate. Here the nerve impulse is transmitted to the skeletal muscle by the liberation at the motor end-plate of the chemical substance acetyl-choline. At this point the transmission of the conducted nerve impulse changes from a conducted circuit flow to one of chemical transmission. This latter process is defined as the neurohumoral transmission of nerve impulses. Except in the postganglionic sympathetic fibers, acetylcholine is the neurohumoral transmitter. In postganglionic sympathetic fibers this function is effected by the neural transmitter norepinephrine (Figure 14-4).

NEUROHUMORAL TRANSMISSION

The transmission of the nerve impulse by the axon to the motor end-plate is an electrical phenomenon associated with a change in the membrane potential of the axon. The nerve, like other cells of the body, maintains a resting potential. The size of this resting potential is determined by the relative permeability of the cell membrane to the sodium (Na^+) and potassium (K^+) ions (the greater the ratio of permeability to potassium to the permeability to sodium, the greater the membrane potential).

When, by mechanical or chemical means, the membrane potential undergoes changes unique to excitable cells, the resultant sequence is termed an *action potential*. The nerve cell membrane in the resting state is permeable only to potassium and is identified as a *potassium membrane.* The active membrane, that is, one in which permeability to sodium is present, is termed the *sodium membrane.* The development of an action potential is characterized by a sudden change from a potassium to a sodium membrane plus a rapid change back to a potassium membrane. Such a change produces a local circuit of current that is reproduced along the nerve membrane. This propagating change produces an action potential at a constant rate along the nerve and as such constitutes the nerve impulse. The depolarization of the axon, that is, the conducted action potential or nerve impulse, causes a release of acetylcholine at the terminal membrane of the axon. When released, acetylcholine passes through the subneural space to the receptors on the negatively charged postjunctional membrane and contiguous subneural space. This neurotransmitter acetylcholine is probably synthesized from choline and acetic acid in the area of the axon terminal by the enzyme choline acetylase. Acetylcholine is stored in the synaptic vesicles within the portion of the axon enclosed by the terminal membrane of the axon.

With partial depolarization there is an increased permeability of the postjunctional membrane to sodium and potassium. The alteration of the end-plate potential eventually produces an impulse similar to that which had been propagated along the axon. This impulse eventually causes a contractile process in the muscle fiber. Therefore, as the postjunctional membrane is depolarized above its threshold, the effect of the nerve impulse is transmitted to the muscle fiber. This process ultimately results in shortening of the muscle fiber. This change in the length of the muscle fiber is associated with complex reversible biochemical, electrical, and structural changes within the muscle that result in contraction and relaxation of muscle.

At the postjunctional membrane there are probably two types of acetylcholine receptors. One of these receptors is concerned with end-plate depolarization, the other with the enzymatic destruction of acetylcholine by the enzyme acetylcholinesterase (AChE).

The exact chemical nature of the receptors is not known. They are probably negatively charged lipoproteins of the subneural or postjunctional membrane. The neutralization of these receptors by acetylcholine allows for the exchange of sodium and potassium and the subsequent membrane depolarization. Acetylcholine is converted to choline and acetic acid by the enzyme acetylcholinesterase. Choline and acetic acid appear to pass back across the subneural space to be resynthesized in the nerve and stored as acetylcholine in the synaptic vesicles.

NEUROMUSCULAR BLOCKING AGENTS
The neuromuscular blocking agents are classified according to the manner by which the nerve impulse is blocked at the myoneural junction of skeletal muscle. This classification identifies substances as competitive agents and depolarizing agents. Tubocurarine chloride is the classic competitive blocking agent. Succinylcholine chloride (Anectine) is representative of a depolarizing or noncompetitive

agent. This classification is physiologically important and particularly useful in the clinical application of the pharmacologic properties of the drug. However, the neuromuscular blocking agents, under particular circumstances that relate to the dose of an agent, to the patient's idiosyncratic responses to that agent, and to the enhancing or inhibiting effect of other agents, may exert both competitive and depolarizing effects in the same individual patient.

The competitive agents tubocurarine chloride, gallamine triethiodide (Flaxedel), and pancuronium bromide (Pavulon) combine with the cholinergic receptor sites on the postjunctional membrane and block the reception of acetylcholine at the receptor site. The nerve impulse whose transmission is dependent on neurohumoral transmission is effectively blocked at the level of the motor end-plate. Acetylcholine is destroyed locally by the enzyme acetylcholinesterase, which hydrolizes acetylcholine into choline and acetic acid.

The neuromuscular block that is produced by the competitive blocking agents can be overcome by the use of anticholinesterase compounds such as neostigmine methylsulfate (Prostigmin) and edrophonium chloride (Tensilon).

The depolarizing drugs such as succinylcholine chloride probably produce their effect by persistent depolarization of the end-plate and the sarcoplasmic membrane. Although the mechanism of action of the depolarizing drugs is not as clear as with the nondepolarizing or competitive agents, it is clear that the clinically useful anticholinesterase compounds such as neostigmine and edrophonium increase the depolarizing block produced by succinylcholine but antagonize the competitive neuromuscular block produced by curare-like or competitive agents. The depolarizing drugs (succinylcholine), therefore, resemble acetylcholine in their initial reaction. However, with depolarizing agents, the postjunctional membrane remains depolarized and thus less sensitive to the spread of electrical impulses from nerve to muscle. The end-plate undergoes gradual repolarization after continued exposure to depolarizing drugs. However, even though repolarized to a degree, the end-plate is much less sensitive to the effect of acetylcholine. This phenomenon is frequently termed a *dual block*. The desensitization appears to be related to the dose and manner of administration of the depolarizing agents.

Competitive Nondepolarizing Agents

Tubocurarine chloride is available in 1.5 ml ampules, each containing 15 mg; 5 ml bottles containing 50 mg (10 mg/ml); and vials providing 3 mg/ml.

The routine dose for single intravenous injections is 0.5 mg per kilogram of body weight. The onset of action is between 2 to 4 minutes and lasts for approximately 30 minutes, with some residual effect often noted for up to 4 hours [5]. Levels of tubocurarine in the plasma decrease rapidly during the first 10 to 12 minutes as equilibrium is established among the drug bound to plasma protein, the drug in solution, and the drug at the motor end-plate. In facilitating the management of patients undergoing mechanical ventilation, 1.0 mg for a 70 kg patient should be employed as the initial dose and the dose monitored and adjusted based on the patient's response. The drug is excreted by the kidney and appears to be stored in muscle and liver. Within 24 hours approximately 80 percent of the total dose is excreted as tubocurarine in the urine or eliminated in the bile. The kidneys are the primary source of elimination, and about one-third of the dose is eliminated within several hours independent of the manner of administration.

Gallamine triethiodide USP (Flaxedel) is a synthetic compound with pharmacologic activity similar to tubocurarine. It is available as a sterile solution containing 20 mg/ml or 100 mg/ml, 2 and 3 ml ampules containing 80 and 120 mg, and 100 ml rubber-capped bottles containing 400 mg (40 mg/ml). Neuromuscular blockade occurs within 1.5 to 2 minutes and lasts approximately 20 minutes [5]. The suggested dose tends to be about 1 mg per kilogram of body weight. No more than 100 mg should be injected at any one time regardless of the weight of the patient. For prolonged block this compound may be reinjected after an interval of 30 to 40 minutes using 0.5 to 1.0 mg/kg. The frequency of injection and the dose must be determined by the patient's response.

Pancuronium bromide (Pavulon) is a nondepolarizing neuromuscular blocking agent that possesses the characteristic pharmacologic actions of the curariform class of drug on the myoneural junction. Pavulon is considered to be approximately five times as potent as tubocurarine chloride. It is available in 2 ml ampules, 2 mg/ml; 5 ml ampules, 2 mg/ml; and 10 ml vials, 1 mg/ml. When 0.08 mg/kg is administered, pancuronium bromide has an onset of action of about 30 seconds and a peak effect within 3 minutes [5]. In adults the initial intravenous dose range is 0.04 to 0.l mg/kg. For continued use incremental doses starting at 0.01 mg/kg may be used. At all times the dose is ultimately determined by the patient's response to the medication.

Depolarizing Agents

Succinylcholine chloride USP (Anectine) is available as a sterile solution containing 20, 50, or 100 mg/ml. It is available in 2 ml ampules containing 100 mg, and 10 ml rubber-capped bottles containing 1 gm (50 mg/ml). The optimal intravenous dose for an adult is approximately 20 mg, although amounts in excess of 30 mg may be required. For continuous intravenous infusion, doses from 0.5 to 5.0 mg per minute may be given. The average rate of continuous intravenous administration is 2.5 mg per minute. Anectine Flo-Pack, 500 mg sterile powder, and Flo-Pack, 1,000 mg sterile powder, are available for preparation of dilute solutions for intravenous drip only.

Approximately 90 percent of succinylcholine is hydrolyzed within 1 minute by the enzyme pseudocholinesterase. This reaction is directly related to the serum concentration of succinylcholine, for the enzyme is active only while succinylcholine is present in the serum. The degradation takes place in two steps. Succinylmonocholine, which is itself a weak neuromuscular blocker, and choline are produced during the first stage of degradation. In the second stage, which takes place slowly, succinylmonocholine is hydrolyzed to succinic acid and choline. Excretion is primarily through the kidney. Approximately 70 percent of a dose of succinylcholine, in the form of succinylmonocholine, is found in the urine within 7 to 8 hours after the drug has been administered.

The enzyme pseudocholinesterase is produced in the liver. Approximately 95 percent of the population are homozygous for the normal enzyme. The remainder are either homozygous for one of the abnormal enzymes or heterozygous for two abnormal enzymes. The abnormal pseudocholinesterases have decreased affinity for succinylcholine, and patients who carry the abnormal enzyme may experience prolonged neuromuscular block. The duration of the abnormal block is greater in patients who carry predominantly abnormal enzymes [6].

Patients with liver disease, malnutrition, or significant anemia; patients who have had cytotoxic drugs; and patients with renal insufficiency may also experience prolonged block.

After a dose of 30 mg of succinylcholine chloride muscle relaxation begins in a minute and peaks at 2 to 3 minutes, usually preceded by muscular fasciculations. During constant infusion of succinylcholine the degree of muscular relaxation can usually be modified within 60 seconds by adjustment of the rate of infusion.

Muscle pain has been described following the use of succinylcholine. The pain seems most prominent in the neck, shoulders, and chest muscles.

CLINICAL CONSIDERATIONS

It should be recalled that whatever agent is used to control a patient's breathing, the primary purpose is to establish controlled ventilation. This is true whether it be a patient with acute or chronic respiratory failure, a patient in status epilepticus or tetanus, or an agitated patient with drug overdose. In most circumstances the period of controlled ventilation is prolonged and the patient is frequently conscious during the entire period. Indeed the ideal state of block is one in which the patient is awake and capable of some movement. In order to achieve this state the clinician should be aware of all those factors that influence the degree of neuromuscular block; he should also be aware of the associated side effects of the drugs. There is a great degree of individual patient response to medication, and therefore continued careful clinical observation provides the best method for preventing untoward reaction and for determining effective dose schedules.

The psychological phenomena associated with total body paralysis must not be overlooked in the care of patients on controlled ventilation. The patient should be informed, whenever possible, of the effects of the neuromuscular blocking agents.

The effects of curare-like drugs on the awake patient are unpleasant and frightening. The patient experiences a feeling of lightheadedness and notes difficulty in focusing. The jaw muscles become weak, and ptosis, diplopia, dysarthria, and dysphagia are noted. The extremities become weak and heavy. Diaphragmatic breathing develops as intercostal muscles are paralyzed. The patient may experience a sensation of shortness of breath, and frequently the sensation of choking occurs as saliva accumulates in the pharynx. Recovery from paralysis usually begins with the facial muscles and diaphragm, followed by the extremities, trunk, hands, feet, and pharynx. There is no central nervous system effect of clinical significance.

The paralysis produced by succinylcholine usually involves the neck, arm, and leg muscles, with only slight weakness of the facial and pharyngeal muscles.

Independent of the type of neuromuscular blocking agent that is used, in the awake patient the feeling of total helplessness and dependency produces fear and anxiety. Those in attendance must always keep in mind that the totally paralyzed patient may be awake and alert to all that is going on in the unit. Discussions about the patient's care, dose of medication, and effect of medication should take place away from the patient's bedside. A pleasant but serious manner provides the patient with the confidence needed to withstand the routine of intensive pulmonary care and controlled ventilation. The use of Librium 10 to 25 mg or Valium 5 to 10 mg every 6 to 8 hours is frequently helpful in controlling the patient's anxiety. Dosage should depend on the patient's response; in most instances an awake and cooperative patient is the goal of the combined therapy of neuromuscular blockade and sedation.

Succinylcholine may produce bradycardia and hypotension. The bradycardia is most marked with successive intravenous doses or prolonged intravenous infusion. Atropine will inhibit the bradycardia. With constant intravenous infusion succinylcholine may produce tachycardia and hypertension. Ventricular arrhythmias and asystole have been reported following intravenous infusion of succinylcholine. Ventricular arrhythmias are also said to occur in digitalized patients.

The hypotension associated with tubocurarine is dose related. The rapid intravenous injection of tubocurarine may cause a rapid fall in blood pressure. The hypotension is probably due to a fall in peripheral resistance secondary to blockade of sympathetic ganglia. Histamine release and direct myocardial depression may also contribute to the hypotension. Patients who are hypovolemic and patients with excessive positive airway pressure are particularly likely to develop hypotension.

Tubocurarine, which may cause histamine release, has been reported to cause bronchospasm and increased bronchial secretions. However, this effect is most likely to occur with a single intravenous injection of tubocurarine. Continued intravenous infusion of tubocurarine is not usually associated with bronchospasm. The clinician must be aware of this eventuality and must be prepared to institute appropriate therapy if it is encountered.

Pancuronium is described as having little effect upon the circulatory system other than a slight rise in pulse rate. However, transient rise in blood pressure has been reported in some patients [2]. Pancuronium has no known effects on consciousness, pain threshold, or cerebration. An occasional transient rash is noted accompanying the use of this drug. Histamine release rarely occurs with pancuronium, which is metabolized in the liver and excreted by the kidney. All patients in renal failure require titration of the drug [3].

Prolonged apnea after the use of succinylcholine usually represents overdosage of the drug. Patients with abnormal pseudocholinesterase may also experience prolonged paralysis and apnea. There is no specific antidote for prolonged block associated with depolarizing agents. However, the clinical setting in which controlled ventilation is utilized provides immediate treatment of apnea, which is the most serious complication of prolonged block. Prolonged block after the use of nondepolarizing agents may be antagonized by the intravenous use of neostigmine at a dose of approximately 0.06 mg per kilogram of body weight, not to exceed a maximum dose of 2.5 mg. The side effects associated with the anticholinesterase compounds such as abdominal cramps, increased salivation, and bronchial secretions, plus the variety of hemodynamic effects on the heart, usually bradycardia and hypotension, should be treated by combining atropine sulfate 0.6 to 1.2 mg with neostigmine.

Persistent apnea following discontinuance of neuromuscular blocking agents requires careful search for other causes of apnea such as the effect of narcotics, a reduction in arterial carbon dioxide pressure, hypoxia, hypercapnia, metabolic acidosis, and hypokalemia.

Patients with myasthenia gravis may have an increased sensitivity to nondepolarizing blocking agents (tubocurarine chloride, gallamine triethiodide, pancuronium bromide). Individuals with the Eaton-Lambert syndrome, which is a myasthenia-like syndrome associated with small cell carcinoma of the lung, as well as patients with neuromyopathic syndromes associated with malignancy, also frequently demonstrate increased sensitivity to neuromuscular blocking agents.

DRUG INTERACTION

Bacitracin, colistimethate, gentamicin, kanamycin, neomycin, and polymyxin B, when used with nondepolarizing (curare-like) neuromuscular blockers, may result in prolonged block [4]. It is assumed that the antibiotic agents reduce the amount of acetylcholine released at the motor end-plate. Clinically the phenomenon has been observed more often after intrapleural or intraperitoneal instillation of the antibiotic or is associated with overdosage of the antibiotic in children.

Antiarrhythmic drugs such as diphenylhydantoin, propranolol, and quinidine may act at pre- and postneuromuscular junctional sites; in some cases prolonged block has been associated with the use of nondepolarizing blockers.

The effects of body temperature on neuromuscular block are variable. Increase in body temperature may potentiate the curare-like drugs, and a decrease in body temperature has a similar potentiating effect on the action of depolarizing agents.

Alteration in serum concentrations of sodium (Na^+) and potassium (K^+), the calcium (Ca^{++})-magnesium (Mg^{++}) ratio, and the hydrogen (H^+) ion concentration affect the action of the neuromuscular blocking agents. The ratio of intracellular potassium to extracellular potassium is a major factor that influences neuromuscular transmission. A rise in extracellular potassium causes an increased sensitivity to depolarizing drugs and a decreased sensitivity to nondepolarizing drugs. If the ratio of intracellular potassium to extracellular potassium remains constant, the resting membrane potential does not change. However, with a reduction of total body potassium, a relatively small shift in the ratio may effect the sensitivity to neuromuscular block.

Hyperkalemia associated with succinylcholine has been described in burned patients, patients with muscle trauma, and a variety of neuromuscular disorders.

Gronert and Theye [1] indicate that succinylcholine should not be used in patients who have thermal trauma, muscle trauma, or any neurologic disorder with motor deficit. The hyperkalemic phenomenon begins 5 to 15 days after injury and can persist for 2 to 3 months in patients who have been burned or who have suffered muscle trauma.

It appears that alkalosis antagonizes the block produced by tubocurarine and enhances the block produced by gallamine and succinylcholine. Acidosis produces the opposite effect.

The maintenance of the calcium-magnesium ratio is essential for normal neuromuscular function. An increase in concentration of magnesium and a decrease of calcium produces a degree of neuromuscular block by inhibiting the release of acetylcholine. There are rare clinical reports that suggest that magnesium sulfate administration potentiates neuromuscular blockade.

Patients who require controlled ventilation frequently experience changes in their acid-base balance along with other changes in their metabolic states. The constant monitoring of blood gases and electrolytes and the institution of the therapeutic programs needed to maintain homeostasis usually provides adequate protection from the adverse effects that pH changes could produce on the sensitivity of neuromuscular blocking agents.

Effect in Pregnancy
In the conventional dose range neither tubocurarine nor succinylcholine crosses the placental barrier. As much as 500 mg of succinylcholine has been administered during pregnancy before any drug was detected in the infant's circulation. However, the safe use of tubocurarine chloride, pancuronium bromide, gallamine triethiodide, and succinylcholine chloride has not been established with respect to the possible adverse effects upon the fetus. Therefore, the drugs should not be used in women of child-bearing potential unless the physician judges the potential benefits to outweigh the unknown hazards.

Pediatric Patients
Neonates may demonstrate some resistance to depolarizing drugs and hypersensitivity to the nondepolarizing drugs. The recommended dose in children is based on body weight, and dosage schedules are provided in package inserts.

Glaucoma
Succinylcholine causes a slight increase in intraocular pressure during the period when muscle fasciculations are noted. The effect is brief and appears to be due to contraction of the extraocular muscles. The effect is probably not sufficient to contraindicate the use of the drug in patients with glaucoma who may require succinylcholine for controlled ventilation.

Opiates

The selective control of neuromuscular function obtained with neuromuscular blocking agents seems to be the most effective method of maintaining an awake patient who is capable of cooperating through a prolonged period of controlled ventilation. However, some physicians prefer the more general and nonspecific method of control that is provided by the use of morphine. Indeed, the euphoria and sense of well-being often produced by morphine may be helpful in the patient in whom the relief of constant pain is a part of the therapeutic program. Morphine is a narcotic analgesic that produces analgesia, drowsiness, and mood change. Although some patients experience euphoria, a significant number often experience anxiety and apprehension. The intensity of the effect is dose related. Morphine depresses all phases of respiration—rate, minute volume, and tidal exchange—by direct effect on the brain-stem respiratory centers. In addition, patients given morphine can demonstrate an indifference to breathing and remain apneic unless urged to breathe. Such a characteristic of morphine-induced apnea can be useful in patients in whom controlled ventilation is required. Maximal respiratory depression occurs within 7 to 10 minutes after intravenous administration of morphine.

Nausea and vomiting occur as a result of direct stimulation of the central chemoreceptor trigger zone for vomiting. Hypotension, gastric and intestinal immobility, constipation, urine retention, and biliary tract spasm may occur in patients who are taking larger and regular doses of morphine. A dose of 10 mg of morphine given subcutaneously has a duration of action of 4 to 5 hours. Ninety percent of morphine and conjugated morphine will be excreted within 24 hours after injection.

The effects of morphine may be antagonized by the use of narcotic antagonists. Naloxene hydrochloride (Narcan), which is available in 2 ml ampules and 10 ml multiple dose vials with a concentration of 0.4 mg/ml, does not possess the morphine-like properties of the other narcotic antagonists. The onset of action is within 2 minutes. The initial dose is 0.4 mg intravenously (1 ml). The dose may be repeated at 2- to 3-minute intervals. Failure to respond after 2 to 3 ml should alert the clinician to look for additional causes of prolonged apnea.

A SUMMARY OF CLINICAL ATTITUDES

Controlled ventilation can be a life-saving procedure in patients with acute and chronic respiratory failure or status epilepticus and tetanus. Ideal control is obtained when the patient is awake and capable of some limited motor activity. Such control is best obtained when the patient's fears and anxiety are considered along with the careful selection of the appropriate pharmacologic agent. A pleasant, optimistic professional attitude is essential to achieve these goals. The choice of appropriate sedatives, tranquilizers, and neuromuscular blocking agents should be based on one's experience and skill in the use of specific drugs. It is important to become familiar with the action, side effects, and unusual reactions of all the drugs that are used. Although suggested initial dose schedules for drugs have been provided, it is imperative that adjustment to patient response be the cornerstone of therapy.

A cookbook or standing order approach should be avoided. Rather, a constant, orderly monitoring of the patient's level of consciousness, appropriateness of behavior, motor activity, vital signs, and metabolic status is necessary for good patient care. Changes in any of the above parameters require an immediate differential review of the patient's status.

REFERENCES

I. Gronert, G. A., and Theye, R. A. Pathophysiology of hyperkalemia induced by succinylcholine. *Anesthesiology* 43, 1975, p. 89.
2. Loh, L. The cardiovascular effects of pancuronium bromide. *Anesthesia* 25, 1970, p. 356.
3. Miller, R. D., Stevens, W. C., and Way, W. L. The effect of renal failure and hyperkalemia on the duration of pancuronium neuromuscular blockade in man. *Anesth. Analg.* (Cleve.) 52, 1973, p. 661.
4. Pittinger, C., and Adamson, R. Antibiotic blockade of neuromuscular function. *Annu. Rev. Pharmacol.* 12, 1972, p. 169.
5. Pryor, W. J., and Bush, D. C. *A Manual of Anesthetic Techniques*. Chicago: John Wright (distributed by Year Book), 1973.
6. Whittaker, M. Genetic aspects of succinylcholine sensitivity. *Anesthesiology* 32, 1970, p. 143.

SELECTED BIBLIOGRAPHY

Campbell, E. J. M., Agostoni, E., and Davis, J. N. *The Respiratory Muscles: Mechanics and Neural Control.* Philadelphia: Saunders, 1970.

Dripps, R. D., Eckenhoff, J. E., and Vandam, L. D. *Introduction to Anesthesia: The Principles of Safe Practice* (4th ed.). Philadelphia: Saunders, 1973.

Foldes, F. F. *Muscle Relaxants.* Clinical Anesthesia Series. Philadelphia: Davis, 1966.

Goodman, L. S., and Gilman, A. *The Pharmacological Basis of Therapeutics* (5th ed.). New York: Macmillan, 1975.

Mark, L. C., and Papper, E. M. *Advances in Anesthesiology: Muscle Relaxants.* New York: Hoeber Division, Harper & Row, 1967.

Kenneth F. MacDonnell

Chronic Obstructive Pulmonary Disease

15

Chronic obstructive pulmonary disease (COPD) encompasses a group of diseases that are joined by a common pathophysiologic abnormality. It is the most common form of chronic lung disease, estimated to be present in 5 to 20 percent of adult American males, and found to be present in 6.5 percent of all autopsies. Its economic impact is enormous. For example, emphysema, which is one of the COPD categories, ranks second only to arteriosclerotic heart disease as a cause of disability in the United States.

However, there has been a good deal of confusion regarding terminology and definition among the various illnesses recognized as COPD. In an effort to clarify the situation, an international symposium was convened in 1959 [2] with the specified goals of categorizing and defining COPD, considered at that time to include emphysema, bronchitis, bronchiectasis, and asthma. More recent work suggests the inclusion of an additional category, that of small airways disease.

In order to establish a clearer understanding of obstructive lung disease, it is best to recall the normal structure and function of the lung. During expiration, there are clear limits to the rate at which one can blow air out. Once maximal flow is attained, then further patient effort does not increase expiratory flow (Figure 15-1).

The factors that influence an individual's ability to generate gas flow are multiple and complex. Often overlooked in this equation are the simple and obvious, for example, airway caliber. Airway caliber is dependent upon anatomic and physiologic influences such as (1) intrinsic size, which is genetically determined, and (2) the state of distention of the walls.

A.

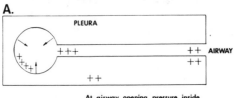

At airway opening pressure inside
airway equals pressure in the pleura

B.

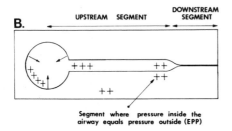

Segment where pressure inside the
airway equals pressure outside (EPP)

C. IN COPD:

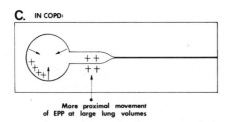

More proximal movement
of EPP at large lung volumes

Figure 15–1. Normal structure and function of the lung: Equal pressure point.

It should be recalled that the airways are formed early in fetal life as a centrifugal outgrowth from the floor of the pharynx, and this growth is genetically determined. On the other hand, alveolar development occurs during the seventh intrauterine month and occurs first at the periphery. At birth, there are approximately 20 million alveoli, and the development of alveoli continues until approximately the age of 8 years. When fully grown, the normal lung contains about 300 million alveoli. Alveoli will continue to grow until maturity, but they will not increase in number. Such a developmental scheme allows for dysanaptic growth, that is, disproportionate growth within an organ. The scene is set for fetal injury to result in altered growth and development that may result in a decreased flow rate and perhaps a predisposition for COPD.

Resistance to air flow at high lung volume is located centrally within the first 7 to 10 generations of the tracheobronchial tree. Resistance per unit length drops at bifurcations of the tracheobronchial tree when the total cross-sectional area of the daughter branches is greater than 1.4 times the cross-section of the parent bifurcation. This is accomplished in the normal lung by the sixth generation. However, at low lung volume, this cross-sectional increase is not attained and resistance is more peripherally located. Thus, alterations in the complex geometric relations of the lung architecture can have profound physiologic consequences.

The major supporting structure of the lung consists of elastic and collagen fibers that are helical in shape with multiple crosslinks. It is this construction which allows for normal expansion. The analogy to the mechanics of an old-fashioned door spring may help in the understanding of lung expansion. The spring elongates, but the length of the spring remains constant, and torsional strain throughout the helix closes the door. The helical arrangement of fibers in the alveolar ducts provide reactive forces, providing that the collagen and elastin are normal.

The alveoli represent curved surfaces with an air-liquid interface, and as such they are subject to the effects of surface tension, as described by La Place's relationship of a sphere. Under these conditions, the pressure necessary to inflate is related directly to two times the surface tension, and inversely to the radius. It is readily apparent that if two spheres of unequal size are connected in series, that inflation will preferentially occur in the larger sphere with resultant collapse of the second sphere. If this were the case in the lung, there would result large-scale atelectasis. Fortunately, the type II pneumocyte secretes a phospholipid that lowers surface tension and allows for filling of all alveoli.

The normal lung, as previously noted, has a fixed maximal flow capacity that is effort independent. In order for flow to occur, there must be a pressure drop, and the driving pressure will depend on elastic recoil. When the pressure outside the airway is equal to the pressure inside, flow is fixed; this is at the equal pressure point. Maneuvers of testing that employ forced expiration reflect these events. Thus, a common pathophysiologic thread to explain obstruction to flow during expiration emerges, e.g., emphysema decreases elastic recoil and therefore there is less driving pressure; with bronchiectasis, a diseased wall, mucous plugs, and edema result in premature airway closure.

The National Tuberculosis Association [8] classifies emphysema and related conditions in the following manner: (1) pulmonary emphysema: (a) centrilobular, (b) panlobular, (c) paracicatricial lobular, (d) unclassified; (2) pulmonary overinflation: (a) obstructive (formerly localized obstructive emphysema), (b) nonobstructive (formerly compensatory emphysema); (3) asthma; (4) chronic bronchitis.

PULMONARY EMPHYSEMA

The word *emphysema* is derived from the Greek, meaning to "puff up." At the Ciba Guest Symposium in 1959 [2], emphysema was defined pathologically as a condition of the lung characterized by an increase beyond the normal size of air spaces distal to the terminal bronchiole from dilatation or destruction. The American Thoracic Society [1] states that emphysema must include both destruction of alveolar walls and overinflation. Reid [9] defined emphysema as "a condition of the lung characterized by increase beyond the normal in the size of the air spaces distal to the terminal bronchioles, i.e., the acinus." Laennec [5], in 1826, said, "Elle consiste dans la simple dilatation des vesicules ou cellules dont elle compose," which Forbes [6], in 1827, translated: "it consists simply in the dilatation of the air cells."

The acinus is the functional unit of the lung and includes all the lung distal to the terminal bronchiolus; it is roughly 0.5 to 1 cm in diameter. The secondary lobule is the smallest segment of the lung that can be consistently identified by a connective tissue septum; each lobule contains 3 to 5 acini. The two major classifications of emphysema refer either to the lobule or the acinus.

Panacinar or panlobular emphysema (Figure 15-2) is a destructive disease that unselectively affects all the lung distal to the terminal bronchiole. There may be no preceding symptoms of chronic bronchitis. It occurs both as a hereditary and as a nonhereditary disease. Laurel and Eriksson [7] first identified the hereditary form of emphysema. In 1963, they described four patients with chronic obstructive pulmonary disease who also had low serum concentrations of alpha I antitrypsin.

Subsequent investigations have revealed a complex inheritance pattern, and family studies have shown this defect to be transmitted as an autosomal dominant trait [3]. This serum glycoprotein alpha I antitrypsin is one of many protease inhibitors and is a major endogenous inhibitor of human leukocyte collagenases and elastases. That proteases are capable of producing emphysema has been well established in animal models. Papain, leukocyte proteases, and, interestingly, cadmium, which is found in cigarettes, are capable of producing experimental emphysema. It has been suggested that patients lacking this protease inhibitor in their serum suffer

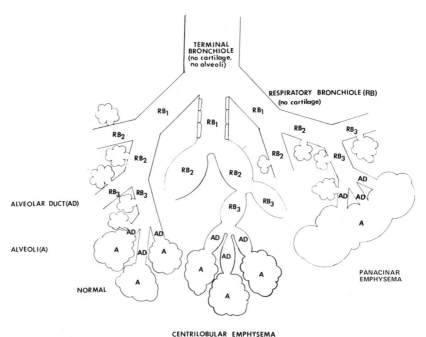

Figure 15-2. Panacinar and centrilobular emphysema.

from a sort of "self-digestion" of their lungs because of the unchecked action of such agents as leukocyte proteases.

Some instances of alpha I antitrypsin deficiency have been associated with childhood cirrhosis. This circulating enzyme inhibitor is produced by the liver under the control of 13 fully penetrant dominant allelels with at least 20 phenotypes identified. Children with associated cirrhosis have had the ZZ phenotype. The SZ and FZ phenotypes, along with the ZZ phenotype, have been identified in adults with cirrhosis. In patients with PiZZ, there may be a number of defects in the protease inhibitors ranging from steric hindrance to deficient sialyltransferase activity. There is a resultant defective transport of the antitrypsin out of the hepatocytes, where it is synthesized in the rough endoplasmic reticulum. The subsequent storage of this material within dilated cisternae of the rough endoplasmic reticulum somehow injures the cell, and cirrhosis may result.

Antitrypsin levels identifying homozygous and heterozygous individuals can be determined. Such information may be of value in job counseling and as a deterrent to smoking.

The clinical picture of the patient with hereditary alpha antitrypsin deficiency differs from the usual patient with COPD and serves to alert the clinician to the diagnosis. These patients may be quite young; there is a relatively even male to female ratio; there may be little or no cough. No history of cigarette smoking may be noted. These patients are rather typical of the type A or "pink puffer" patient.

As a result of the destructive process there is loss of ventilation-perfusion ratio ($\dot{V}/\dot{Q}$). Thus hypoxia and cor pulmonale are late manifestations, and if either is present, the prognosis is less favorable [4]. Pulmonary function studies depict overinflation, a low diffusing capacity, and normal blood gases (see Chapter 4).

The nonhereditary panlobular type of emphysema is found more commonly in males, usually in the older age group (greater than 50 years old), and can be found uniformly throughout the secondary lobule. Frequently, the areas most severely involved are the lower lobes. There may or may not be a prior history of cough and sputum production; cor pulmonale and abnormal blood gases are very late manifestations of the illness. Physical examination of the chest may disclose a generalized absence of breath sounds and no wheezing, rales, or rhonchi. It is a most distressing illness for the clinician to deal with, for there is very little hope for cure, and mainly one directs therapy toward preventing a superinfection while attempting to make the patient more comfortable and asymptomatic.

Much effort has been directed to exercise programs, the results of which are still unclear. Steroids and bronchodilators have not been shown to be useful in the majority of these patients, although occasionally an individual trial of therapy has been successful, probably indicating a complicating bronchospastic type of illness. Centrilobular emphysema (see Figure 15-2), on the other hand, starts in the center of the secondary lobule with parenchymal destruction and dilatation occurring initially at the level of the respiratory bronchioles; there are up to eight orders of respiratory bronchioles; evidence of bronchiolar wall thickening with associated inflammation, both acute and chronic, is frequent. Commonly, it is upper lobe in its distribution and is frequently associated with a history of chronic bronchitis. The male-female ratio has been estimated to be as great as 20:1. Frequently, it will occur in younger patients in the age group of the 40s and 50s. Relatively early ventilation-perfusion imbalance leads to abnormal blood gas levels and cor pulmonale. The lungs are not as hyperinflated as they are with the panlobular type, and on physical examination there may be signs of coarse rhonchi with wheezing. These patients may respond favorably to the treatment of their cor pulmonale and also to bronchodilator therapy. Associated infection should be treated with appropriate antibiotic therapy.

Chest x-ray studies in both the hereditary and nonhereditary forms of emphysema may be diagnostic , albeit a late finding. The major criteria are a low, flat, and poorly moving diaphragm with a large retrosternal area; a narrow vertical heart with a large pulmonary trunk and small peripheral vessels; and localized avascular areas suggesting bullae. Fraser [4] has correlated arterial deficiency emphysema with a primary emphysematous form contrasted with a chest x-ray with increased markings representative of emphysema with bronchitis. Listed below are specific roentgen signs of emphysema.

Hyperlucency	Small vertical heart
Presence of bullae	Cor pulmonale
Increased anteroposterior diameter	Low, flat diaphragm
of the chest	Visible phrenocostal detachments
Kyphosis	Diminished diaphragmatic excursions
Anterior bowing of the sternum	Prominent pulmonary arteries at the hili
Increased retrosternal space	with abrupt attentuation

Fluoroscopy may show diminished diaphragmatic excursions in a more reliable fashion. Along with localized air trapping and bullae, these findings are late manifestations of pulmonary emphysema.

Patients with emphysema of either type frequently accommodate to the illness and, in fact, will deny any respiratory symptoms, claiming virtual "perfect health prior to a precipitous onset" of symptoms. It is hard to imagine in such a circumstance that normal pulmonary functions did, in fact, precede; rather, it seems more likely that the patient has made life-style accommodations sometimes so subtle and insidious that he is unaware of them.

Scar emphysema refers to the distention of air spaces and alveolar wall destruction adjacent to a fibrotic area of the lung, either gross or microscopic. In the unclassified lobular emphysema, the original location, because of the extent of the destruction, can no longer be defined and may be manifested by bullae. Bullous emphysema, of course, refers to the large, thin-walled cystic air spaces formed by the destruction of many alveoli and also of the intralobular septum.

Senile emphysema is in fact a misnomer. The term refers merely to the changes accompanying intrathoracic cage alteration with age. Obstructive overinflation is seen with check valve obstruction of an airway, such as with a foreign body or with a tumor. Nonobstructive overinflation was formerly called compensatory emphysema and is seen frequently after pneumonectomy, or perhaps with large areas of persistent atelectasis.

CHRONIC BRONCHITIS

Chronic bronchitis is defined on clinical grounds as chronic or recurrent excessive mucous secretion in the bronchial tree, marked by chronic productive cough occurring for at least three consecutive months for at least two successive years, occurring in patients without any other explanation such as the presence of another disease. The pathologic basis for hypersecretion of mucus is due to hypertrophy of the mucus-secreting structures, that is, the bronchial submucosal glands and the bronchial epithelial goblet cells (Figures 15-3, 15-4). In chronic bronchitis, in patients over 3 years, the bronchial submucosal glands are located in airways with cartilage in their walls, with a gland-to-wall ratio greater than one-third in 10 to 12 fields. The bronchial epithelial goblet cells, which normally are found in large airways, may appear in large numbers in small airways.

A very important consideration in hypersecretion of the lower airway is the common accompaniment of hypersecretion in the upper airway. Thus, in the patient with bronchitis, a thorough examination of the nose and sinuses and surrounding areas is required, as well as a thorough history searching for information suggestive of a chronic postnasal drip. If such a condition is discovered, then appropriate treatment should be instituted. A predisposing condition should also be searched for, such as a family incidence suggestive of a heterozygote alpha I antitrypsin deficiency, or perhaps a history of cigarette smoking that clearly is associated with the development of chronic bronchitis.

Patients with lowered host resistance are susceptible to developing chronic bronchitis. Illnesses such as agammaglobulinemia, and specifically IgA deficiency associated with the triad of sinusitis, situs inversus, and bronchiectasis (Kartagener's syndrome), should be carefully considered in the differential diagnosis of chronic bronchitis.

Cystic fibrosis, especially in the older individual, may be quite subtle and easily mistaken for a routine case of chronic bronchitis. The pathognomonic sweat test loses much of its diagnostic value when the patient is older than 19 years. The number of forme fruste instances of cystic fibrosis is undetermined; to establish the diagnosis, a high index of suspicion must be maintained. Recent insight into cystic fibrosis has disclosed a serum factor that is capable of suppressing ciliary activity and of disrupting sodium transport. Abnormal staining properties of the skin fibroblast in a number of patients with cystic fibrosis and in some members of their families has been demonstrated. These observations serve to substantiate the suspicion that cystic fibrosis is indeed a systemic disease.

The advanced chronic bronchitic patient or "blue bloater" typically displays cough, sputum, cyanosis, and cor pulmonale. Pulmonary function tests may show a

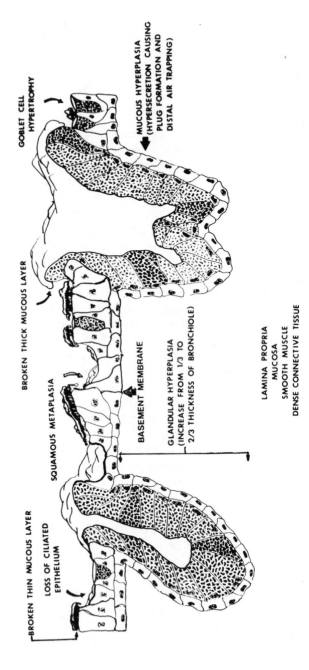

Figure 15-3. Chronic bronchitis: Hypertrophy of the mucus-secreting structures.

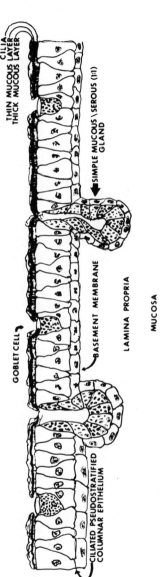

Figure 15–4. Normal mucus-secreting structures.

THIN MUCOUS LAYER
THICK MUCOUS LAYER
CILIA

SIMPLE MUCOUS \ SEROUS (1:1) GLAND

GOBLET CELL

BASEMENT MEMBRANE

LAMINA PROPRIA

MUCOSA

SMOOTH MUSCLES

DENSE CONNECTIVE TISSUE

CILIATED PSEUDOSTRATIFIED COLUMNAR EPITHELIUM

minimally elevated functional residual capacity (FRC) and a diffusing capacity that is usually normal (see Chapter 2). However, the arterial blood gases may be distinctly abnormal. The x-ray picture is of little value in establishing the diagnosis.

Treatment is first directed at removing inciting agents such as smoking and infection. Any associated bronchospasm may be treated with bronchodilator agents. Cardiac decompensation is appropriately treated with diuretic agents and digitalis. Expectorants may also be of some value.

BRONCHIECTASIS

Bronchiectasis is characterized by irreversible dilatation of the bronchial tree (Figure 15-5). This disease has been classified by a variety of methods. A particularly useful method has been suggested by Reid and Simon [10] that is based on the number of subdivisions of the tracheobronchial tree that can be counted macroscopically or microscopically. Normally, 17 to 20 divisions of the tracheobronchial tree can be discerned. With cylindrical bronchiectasis, only 16 subdivisions can be identified; also, there can be mucous plugging with dilatation along with inflammatory infiltrates in the bronchial wall.

Varicose bronchiectasis allows for the identification of only 6.5 divisions macroscopically and 8 divisions microscopically, mucous plugging with purulent secretions, and local constriction giving an appearance similar to varicose veins, hence the name. Saccular (cystic) bronchiectasis is the most serious and destructive form of the illness, a maximum of 5 divisions of the tracheobronchial tree being identifiable.

The diagnosis of bronchiectasis is established with a bronchogram. The most commonly incriminated etiologies are pneumonia, congenital defects, and central mucoid impaction.

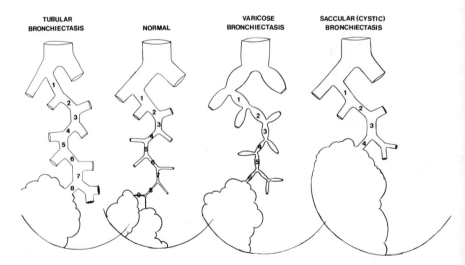

Figure 15-5. Bronchiectasis.

SMALL AIRWAYS DISEASE

The lung is divided into three sections: large airways, small airways, and parenchyma. In the past, the small airways have been the silent zone of the lung, literally and figuratively. Air flow in airways smaller than 2 mm are not capable of generating noise and until recently were not reflected in standard function studies. If the major area of disease is located in the bronchioles, there results premature airway closure, air trapping, higher residual volume, and an elevated alveolar-arterial oxygen gradient. If lung parenchyma is also involved, it is reflected by lower flow rates and lower elastic recoil pressure.

The resistance of the smaller airways — those less than 2 mm in diameter — contributes about 10 percent of the total airway resistance, making it possible to have a substantial amount of small airway disease and obstruction with little effect on total airway resistance.

In children, the cross-sectional area of the bronchiolar bed is not much greater than that of the bronchial bed, and the diagnosis of small airways disease is more commonly recognized — for example, acute bronchiolitis as contrasted with adults, where there may be considerable obstructive disease in the small airways without any significant effect on airways resistance, but with a marked effect on alveolar ventilation and gas exchange. This results from obstructed units being ventilated with dead space gas by means of collateral ventilation, thus setting the stage for severe ventilation-perfusion mismatches. As a consequence, some areas of lung will have high ventilation-perfusion ratios (that is, perfusion in excess of ventilation). This ventilation-perfusion ratio abnormality is one of the earliest manifestations of small airways disease and can result in an increase in the alveolar-arterial blood oxygen gradient. This may be reflected in a decrease in the tension of oxygen in the systemic arterial blood. Figure 15-6 shows the regional variation in ventilation and perfusion from top to the base in the upright position. Regional ventilation increases from the apex to the base. Perfusion of blood also shows an increase from the apex to the base, the relative increase in perfusion being more than that of ventilation. At the extreme base of the lung there is some decrease in perfusion.

It has been suggested that small airways disease may represent the earliest phase of COPD. Morphologic studies have shown goblet cell hyperplasia and hyper-

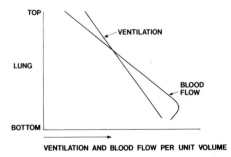

Figure 15-6. Regional gradient of ventilation and perfusion in the upright lung.

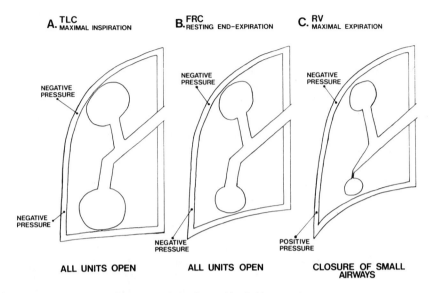

Figure 15-7. The principle of closing volume: Normal lung.

secretion with obstruction of bronchioles, peribronchiolar fibrosis, and general distortion of the normal small-airway architecture. As mentioned before, the physiologic consequence of this condition is basically maldistribution of inspired air
rather than significantly increased airway resistance. The inspired air initially will go
to areas where there is little or no small airways disease.

Pulmonary function tests (see Chap. 4) useful in establishing the diagnosis of small
airways disease include the determination of closing volume and flow-volume loops.
Figures 15-7 to 15-9 illustrate the principle of closing volume. At maximal inspiration (Figure 15-7A) all the lung units are open. As the patient exhales the negative
pressure in the pleura decreases. The pressure at the base is less negative compared
to that of the apex (B). Below FRC (C) the pleural pressure at the base becomes
gradually positive, causing closure of lung units in this region. Figure 15-10 depicts
flow-volume loops under various sets of circumstances. (A) is a normal flow-volume
loop. The flow is fairly constant and maximal during the major part of inspiration.
During expiration after breathing maximum (peak flow), the flow decreases uniformly. (B) In COPD there is a uniform decrease in flow throughout expiration.
(C) In restrictive diseases flow is maintained without any decrease. (D) In bronchial
asthma flow decreases uniformly throughout expiration with improvement following
the use of bronchodilator agents.

Patients with small airways disease may experience such traditional symptoms as
cough, increased sputum production, and dyspnea; in fact, they may suffer respiratory failure. Chest x-ray pictures may show a coarse reticulation pattern without
emphysematous changes. Hypoxemia occurs early in the course of the disease. As
stated previously, standard pulmonary function tests and diffusion studies may be

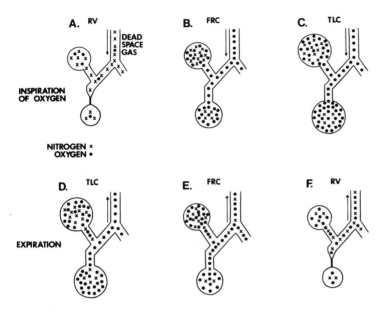

Figure 15-8. Resident gas technique of determining closing volume.

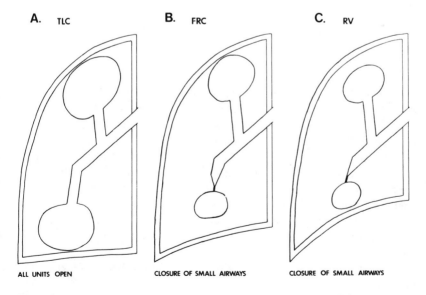

Figure 15-9. Closing volume in chronic obstructive pulmonary disease. (B) Rest expiration.

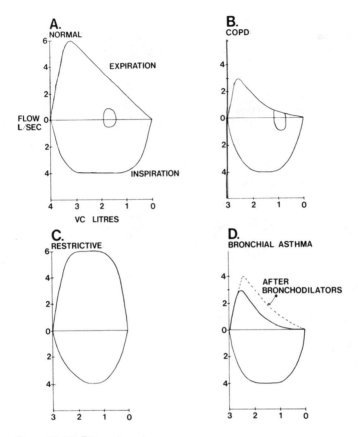

Figure 15–10. Flow-volume loops.

entirely normal. The maximum midexpiratory flow rate (determined from the forced vital capacity maneuver) may be abnormal early in the disease. As the disease progresses, the residual volume increases, but the total lung capacity may remain normal, as does the functional residual capacity.

Some patients' clinical course is that of small airways disease and they may die a cardiopulmonary death related to this condition. Others, perhaps the majority, progress to larger airways disease and have any of the numerous complications associated with COPD. There is no reason to believe that small airways disease is a distinct entity. Rather it may take several forms; that is, it may occur in a patient with chronic bronchitis, in a patient with bronchiectasis, and as an early stage of emphysema.

Asthma, the last of the categories included under COPD, will be considered in the following chapter.

REFERENCES

1. American Thoracic Society. Statements of definitions and classifications of chronic bronchitis, asthma, pulmonary emphysema. *Am. Rev. Respir. Dis.* 85, 1962, p. 762.

2. Ciba Foundation Symposium. Terminologies, definitions and classification of chronic pulmonary emphysema and related conditions. New York: American Elsevier, 1959.

3. Fagerhol, M. K., and Gedde-Dahl, T., Jr. Genetics of the Pi Serum type; family studies of the inherited variants of serum alpha I antitrypsin. *Hum. Hered.* 19, 1969, p. 354.

4. Fraser, R. G. Alpha I-antitrypsin and obstructive disease, a community study. *N. Engl. J. Med.* 292, 1975, p. 278.

5. Laennec, R. T. H. *Traité de L'Auscultation Médiate et des Maladies de Poumons et du Coeur* (2nd ed.). Paris: Chaude, 1826.

6. Laennec, R. T. H. *On the Diseases of the Chest and on Mediate Auscultation.* Translated from the French by John Forbes, 2nd ed. London: Underwood, 1827.

7. Laurell, C. B., and Eriksson, S. The electrophoretic alpha I globulin pattern of serum in alpha I antitrypsin deficiency. *Scand. J. Clin. Lab. Invest.* 15, 1963, p. 132.

8. National Tuberculosis Association. *Chronic Obstructive Emphysema, A Manual for Physicians.* New York: The National Tuberculosis Association, 1963.

9. Reid, L. The Pathology of Emphysema. In *Lynne Reid Year Book.* Chicago: Medical Publishers, 1976.

10. Reid, L., and Simon, G. Unilateral lung transradiancy. *Thorax* 17, 1962, p. 230.

Maurice S. Segal
Kenneth F. MacDonnell

Bronchial Asthma: Nature and Management

16

NATURE OF THE DISEASE

Bronchial asthma is a distressing, frightening type of dyspnea characterized by acute, recurrent, chronic, or protracted bronchial hyperactivity occurring through several pathogenic mechanisms. There may be specific immunologic mechanisms involved. Extrinsic atopic asthma, immediate hypersensitivity type I reaction (see Chapter 8) occurs more commonly in the younger patient and is mediated by reaginic antibodies (IgE) now readily determined by the radioallergosorbent test (RAST) technique. A more delayed type III asthma reaction (Pepys), more common in adults, has been referred to as extrinsic nonatopic asthma, and is usually mediated by circulating antibodies (IgG, IgA, and IgM) [11]. Intrinsic asthma occurs principally in adults, is not associated with any clear-cut immunologic mechanisms, and is usually more severe and progressive than is extrinsic atopic asthma.

It was once the belief that bronchial asthma provided a likely assurance of long life. This is far from reality. The acute attack is episodic, erratic, labile, and usually reversible; however, the chronic form is debilitating and recurrent over the years or even a lifetime. The protracted form, status asthmaticus, is potentially lethal.

In fatal instances, pathologic examinations may show little more than a hyperinflated lung; on the other hand, there may be thick, tenacious mucus impacted in airways throughout. It is these mucous casts that account for the well-known Curschmann's spirals seen with asthma (see Chapter 5). Degenerating eosinophils account for the Charcot-Leyden crystals also seen with this condition. Typically, there is subepithelial edema with a diffuse eosinophilic infiltrate along with hypertrophy of the smooth muscle surrounding the airway.

   The pharmacologic mediators incriminated in the asthmatic reaction are slow-reactive substance of anaphylaxis (SRS-A), histamine, eosinophilic chemotactic factor of anaphylaxis (ECF-A), bradykinin, serotonin, acetylcholine, and prostaglandin F. Altering the release or thwarting the adverse target effect of these substances has been the main thrust of therapy. Definition of the patient relative to the type of asthma, with identification of perhaps a predominance of one or another mediator, holds therapeutic promise, thus aiding the clinician to tailor each patient's treatment regimen (Figure 16–1). The reader is referred to the sections on therapeutics (Chapters 19, 20, 24) for examples of pharmacotherapeutics directed at a specific mediator or type of asthma. During the acute stages of the severe asthmatic reaction, a careful study of the blood gas profile is mandatory. Staging by blood gas

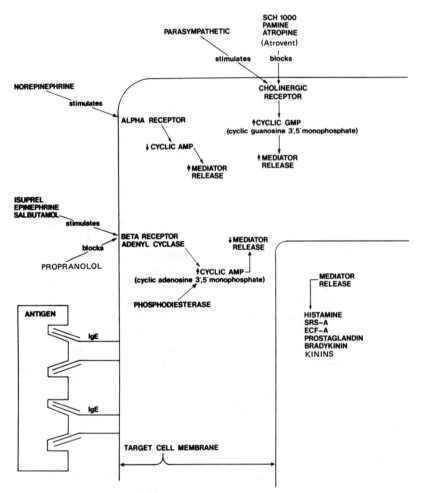

Figure 16–1. Mediators and the cause of asthma.

Table 16-1. Blood gas profile during asthma attack

Stage	PO_2	PCO_2	pH	Airways Obstruction
I	normal	decrease	increase	mild
II	mild decrease	decrease	increase	mild to moderate
III*	moderate to severe decrease	normal	normal	moderate to severe
IV	severe decrease	increase	decrease	severe

*Crossover point at stage III, at which stage patient is unable to hyperventilate, indicating severe obstruction.

levels guides the therapy, alerts the clinician to a potentially explosive situation (Table 16-1), and reflects the patient's therapeutic response. For example, particular attention must be paid to patients with stage III and stage IV asthma, potentially lethal situations requiring close clinical observation and a maximal therapeutic climate, i.e., respiratory intensive care unit. Death in stage III or IV might result from cardiac arrest or arrhythmias, a sudden drop in oxygen tensions, or inappropriate management.

Included in the diagnosis of bronchial asthma are the following categories: (1) extrinsic asthma; (2) intrinsic asthma; (3) asthmatic bronchitis; (4) aspirin sensitivity, nasal polyps, and asthma, the ASA triad; (5) exercise-induced asthma; and (6) variant asthma.

Extrinsic Asthma
Extrinsic asthma is characterized by acute, labile, reversible paroxysms of wheezing and dyspnea in a patient who may display many or all of the following features: a family history of atopy, a modest degree of blood eosinophilia, an elevation of immunoglobulin E, a predominance of sputum eosinophils, the demonstration of positive skin tests to various antigens, the identification of an extrinsic antigen responsible for the onset of clinical symptoms, and finally, the onset of symptoms, usually before the age of 40 years. Extrinsic asthma is usually caused by inhaled, ingested, or injected allergens. The clinical course of extrinsic asthma is generally typical and usually is easily identified.

Intrinsic Asthma
The designation intrinsic asthma implies a disruption of normal bronchial tone originating from within the organism, in contrast to extrinsic asthma, where the initiation of the illness presumably originates outside the organism, as in the form of an external antigen, such as ragweed. Intrinsic asthma has been defined as resulting from toxic materials or from neurotic, reflex, or infective causes. Infection of the respiratory tract, with a postulated nonimmunologic release of asthmatic mediators, is frequently incriminated in intrinsic asthma. However, the distinction between intrinsic and extrinsic asthma, on the basis of the presence of infection, may be quite difficult, for infection is a common precipitant in the extrinsic group as well. To confuse matters more, the findings on physical examination may be identical in both groups. Typical signs of allergic phenomena are generally absent with intrinsic

asthma, in spite of the fact that intrinsic asthma may represent altered host response such as negative skin test, normal or indeed low levels of immunoglobulin E, and usually a negative family history of atopy. The clinical presentation and course with intrinsic asthma may differ greatly from extrinsic asthma. Intrinsic asthma is generally a disease affecting older individuals, having its onset after the age of 30 to 40 years, and is usually more resistant to therapy; spontaneous remissions are unlikely.

Asthmatic Bronchitis

Asthmatic bronchitis is considered by many to be a subgroup of intrinsic asthma where the predominant clinical manifestation is the bronchitis. This illness generally occurs in patients with the typical clinical history and physical findings of chronic bronchitis, but further complicated by either continuous or paroxysmal episodes of wheezing. The history is the key in distinguishing asthmatic bronchitis from intrinsic and extrinsic asthma.

It is not at all unusual for the initial episode of wheezing to follow a particularly severe bout of bronchitis or pneumonia. Commonly, these patients complain of recurrent sinusitis or a chronic postnasal drip (frequent clearing of the throat, which the patient may easily overlook). Wheezing episodes may be terminated with clearing of sputum. On physical examination, even during periods of quiescence, diffuse rhonchi, coarse breath sounds, and wheezing may be elicited. Occasionally, the inspiratory component of the wheeze is striking.

Chest x-ray studies, aside from the usual asthmatic hyperinflation, may demonstrate peribronchial thickening, and unlike typical extrinsic asthma the roentgenogram may remain abnormal during periods of relative clinical quiescence.

Frequently the query is encountered, How does bronchitis result in paroxysms of bronchial constriction and wheezing? The usual explanation employs the experimental observation that denuding the tracheal mucosa in animals results in reflex bronchoconstriction, presumably a result of exposure of the tracheal sensory receptors. There is no requirement for allergic phenomena in asthmatic bronchitis.

ASA Triad

Aspirin sensitivity, nasal polyps, and asthma (the ASA triad) describes a group of patients with either intrinsic or extrinsic asthma who display a sensitivity to acetylsalicylic acid, as manifested by severe exacerbations of their asthma. The exact incidence of this association is rather elusive, but has been estimated to occur in 2 to 10 percent of patients with asthma. The salient features of the ASA triad are (1) temporal relation of symptoms, usually less than 2 hours after the ingestion of the aspirin; (2) a diagnosis of asthma, the majority being intrinsic; however, the syndrome can also occur in the extrinsic group; (3) nasal polyps reported in about half the cases; (4) middle age, although the age span ranges from 27 to 70 years; (5) females affected more often than males; (6) possibly a positive skin test to aspirin; (7) demonstrated sensitivity to other drugs such as codeine, morphine, aminopyrine; (8) provocative testing with aspirin ingestion; (9) does not occur with other salicylate compounds, underlining the importance of the acetyl group.

Most patients with this syndrome have intrinsic asthma, although an occasional patient may suffer from extrinsic asthma. Generally, there is a strong history of perennial rhinitis. Other nonspecific agents, such as environmental irritants, may also precipitate episodes of asthma. These patients are generally "nonallergic" with normal IgE levels. The observed nasal polyps are nonallergic. These polyps result primarily from local alteration in capillary permeability with an accumulation of edema both intracellularly and extracellularly; as the edema progresses, there is a forward protrusion of the mucous membrane with mucosal herniation.

Exercise-Induced Asthma

Following exercise, a marked decrease in air flow and increase in airway resistance has been observed in certain asthmatic patients. Recent observations suggested that catecholamines may be the mediators of exercise-induced wheezing in the asthmatic patient, having noted a greater increase in norepinephrine in the exercised asthmatic subject than in the control group [2]. Supporting these observations has been the demonstration of alpha receptors in the human lung. In order for this increased secretion of catecholamines to induce an asthmatic attack, it is suggested that a predisposition must exist. Nonasthmatic subjects with elevated levels of norepinephrine or epinephrine do not respond with bronchospasm. One such patient with a history of bronchial asthma was shown to have elevated plasma histamine levels after exercise and exercise-induced wheezing. After exercise, the patient suffered episodes of wheezing and pruritis. Elevation of plasma histamines has not been demonstrated in other cases.

Lefcoe [6] found postexercise decreases in forced expiratory volumes in both normal subjects and asthmatic patients, citing hyperventilation as the postulated mechanism. Prevention of the predicted decrease in forced expiratory volume in the postexercise state in 10 asthmatic subjects was accomplished with the inhalation of 7% carbon dioxide. The role of any metabolic acidosis generated by the exercise remains speculative. Acidosis renders the beta receptors less responsive to both exogenous and endogenous stimulators.

Variant Asthma

A variant of asthma has been described where the presenting symptoms are not paroxysmal wheezing or dyspnea but protracted paroxysms of cough. This cough is resistant to the usual antitussive medications and is particularly severe in the early morning. The hallmarks for this variant of asthma are (1) no history of wheezing or dyspnea; (2) a vague or no history in the past of allergic diathesis; (3) an essentially normal examination; (4) a mild decrease in one-second forced expiratory volume that may respond to bronchodilation; (5) an increase in total peripheral eosinophil count; (6) marked response to short-term steroids.

CORRELATION OF CLINICAL AND PHYSIOLOGIC STATUS OF THE ASTHMATIC PATIENT WITH THERAPY

Clinical signs and symptoms (subjective evaluation) at best should serve only to assist and not be the sole guide for regulating therapy. Appropriate therapy requires the accurate diagnosis of bronchial asthma from the very outset.

Delay in diagnosis, or misdiagnosis, will lead to inappropriate management, a feature that can be lethal. Bronchospasm is frequently associated with various types of (functional) hyperventilation syndromes, and particularly in many types of heart disease, e.g., mitral stenosis in rheumatic heart disease, acute coronary occlusion, paroxysmal dyspnea of left ventricular failure origin (cardiac asthma), and congenital heart diseases, and also in many types of lung diseases, e.g., mucoviscidosis (pancreatic cystic fibrosis), bronchiolitis, allergic alveolitis, pulmonary fungal diseases, congenital airway anomalies, lung tumors, pulmonary embolism, and the obstructive-airway lung diseases (croup, bronchitis, bronchiectasis, and emphysema). The associated bronchospasm in these entities often responds partially to bronchodilating drugs. On the other hand, the patient with bronchial asthma who is misdiagnosed and treated for one of the above diseases will be inappropriately managed and may shortly reach a critical stage. Thus, a careful analysis of the clinical and laboratory data is helpful in establishing the correct diagnosis (see Table 16-2).

There is a serious need for correlating simple clinical observations and physiologic data to determine appropriate therapy and its effects in preventing progressive development of lethal states. Auscultatory wheezing, prolonged expirations, and dyspnea alone are not adequate guides for therapy in critical patients. The retraction of the sternocleidomastoid and intercostal muscles may be equated with a severe obstructive state. More recently, it was demonstrated that the presence of such retractions was indicative of a forced expiratory volume of less than 1 liter [4]. The presence of pulsus paradoxus [5] with a drop of the peak systolic pressures of greater than 10 torr should be looked for in severe acute bronchial asthma [3]. Further correlations were noted in the amplitude of the pulsus paradoxus and pulmonary function changes in the one-second forced expiratory volume and the peak expiratory flow rate, indicative of the severity of the bronchial asthma [4]. The evolving critical state is additionally surmised from these and other simple clinical-physiologic correlations [12]. The critical significance of oxygen and carbon dioxide pressure relationships in the evolution of the lethal state must be understood [7].

THE PROFILE OF THE RISK ASTHMA PATIENT
It is essential to recognize this profile in order to avoid increased morbidity and mortality in their management. The risk asthma patient can be determined by the following criteria.

1. The excessive use of adrenergic bronchodilator aerosols, and xanthines, indicating increased bronchial reactivity or progressive airways obstruction from mucous plugs, detached bronchial epithelium, thickened basal membranes, and bronchial walls infiltrated with eosinophils.

2. Therapeutic failures, including (a) the failure to respond to aminophylline therapy in the face of adequate theophylline plasma levels of 10 to 20 μg/ml or even elevated levels above 20 μg/ml, and (b) the clinical evidence of steroidism with failure of eosinopenic response to increasing steroid dosages.

3. Clinical observations of cyanosis (hypoxemia), inspiratory neck and intercostal retractions, pulsus paradoxus, and cardiac irregularities.

4. Personality disturbances with or without actual central nervous system changes.

5. Progressive fatigue and exhaustion with the slightest physical effort.

6. Overinflated lungs, by both clinical and radiologic examinations, fixed or minimal movements of the diaphragm under fluoroscopy with careful, slow, deep breathing maneuvers.

7. Persistent airways obstruction confirmed by pulmonary function testing. Failure of significant improvement in the 1-second forced expiratory volume and forced vital capacity, and particularly in the maximal midexpiratory flow rates or similar selected timed intervals of the forced vital capacity curves, after the administration of bronchodilator aerosols would indicate severe airways obstruction.

8. Reduction in the arterial oxygen pressure below 80 torr and increase in the arterial carbon dioxide pressure above 45 torr, provided that the pH is lowered below 7.3.

LABORATORY PROCEDURES FOR OPTIMAL AND SAFE THERAPY

1. The periodic determination of blood, sputum, and nasal smears for eosinophils (although this procedure can be used as a guide for steroid needs, the absence of eosinophils does not contravene the use of steroids); for blood electrolytes (sodium, potassium, and chlorides); for blood sugar; for hemoglobin and hematocrit; and testing for blood in stool in patients on steroids.

2. The periodic determination of pulmonary function with emphasis on procedures to determine the degree of reversibility of airways obstruction, e.g., failure of significant improvement in 1-second forced expiratory volume and forced vital capacity after administration of bronchodilator aerosols. The possible presence of small airway disease in patients who are doing well may be determined by maximal midexpiratory flow rates (25 to 75 percent) and more sophisticated laboratory procedures, e.g., flow-volume curves, plethysmography, and pulmonary compliance.

3. The determination of the hypothalamic-pituitary-adrenal function by testing for insulin and metypyrone stimulation and measuring the plasma compound S (11-deoxycortisol) before the start of continuous steroid therapy and periodically thereafter. In general, the latter rises in patients who do not have adrenal suppression to about 10 to 15 mg percent after the administration of metypyrone. This provides (a) a means for detecting a primary form of adrenocortical insufficiency; (b) insight in the patient's future steroid needs; (c) particular precautions to be followed during stress situations; (d) indication as to whether any adrenocortical insufficiency can be attributed (iatrogenically) to the subsequent use of steroids [8].

4. Finally, it is essential to monitor biochemical, arterial blood gas, ventilatory, and other hemodynamic functions in the critically ill patient in order to provide optimal care, reduce morbidity, and prevent fatality.

Contemporary treatment remains largely symptomatic. Measures to prevent or

Table 16–2. Differential Diagnosis of Bronchial Asthma

Diagnosis	History	Physical Examination	Laboratory	Differential Diagnosis
Asthma				
Extrinsic asthma	Paroxysms of wheezing and dyspnea; Family history of atopy; Generally under 40 years of age	Polyphonic wheezing, mainly expiratory; Rhonchi scattered throughout, variable	Modest blood eosinophilia; Sputum: eosinophils, Charcot-Leyden crystals, Curschmann's spirals; Chest x-ray: hyperinflation	Positive skin tests to various antigens; Increased IgE levels
Intrinsic asthma	Paroxysms of wheezing and dyspnea; Negative family history of atopy; Older age group, usually over 30 years of age	Polyphonic wheezing, mainly expiratory; Rhonchi; Nasal polyps in some cases	May or may not have blood eosinophilia; Sputum: few eosinophils	Generally negative skin tests; Normal or low levels of IgE; Frequently sensitive to aspirin
Asthmatic bronchitis	Chronic productive cough; Older age group, usually over 30 years; Smoking history is frequent	Polyphonic wheezing, both inspiratory and expiratory, with coarse rhonchi throughout	Chest x-ray may show signs of chronic infection with peribronchial thickening and increased markings; Sinusitis may be present; Sputum: polymorphonuclear leukocytes; possibly bacteria	Typical history of bronchitis with negative allergy workup; Sputum shows few eosinophils
Exercise asthma	May be the only symptom of asthma; Type of exercise that induces attack may be quite variable	May be negative at time of examination	Decrease in $FEV_{1.0}$ after exercise	Induction of episode with exercise
Aspirin sensitivity, nasal polyps, and asthma	Asthma, usually intrinsic; Temporal relation; More common in females than in males	Polyphonic wheezing and rhonchi; Rhinitis; Nasal polyps	X-ray sinusitis in some cases; IgE generally normal	May have a positive skin test to aspirin and demonstrate a positive challenge to aspirin ingestion
Variant asthma (similar to allergic cough)	Paroxysmal coughing; Vague or nonexistent history of allergy	May be normal	Reversible decrease in $FEV_{1.0}$; Blood: mild to moderate eosinophilia	Marked response to steroids

Nonasthmatic Diseases

Disease	History	Physical Examination	Laboratory	Comments
Pulmonary embolism	Predisposition: pregnancy, postoperative state, stasis, oral contraceptives, etc. Sudden shortness of breath; Pleuritic chest pain; Hemoptysis; Apprehension; Cough	Polyphonic wheezing; Signs of right heart strain and failure with large embolus; Increased S_2P; Shock; Tachypnea; Tachycardia; Rales (focal); Cyanosis; Pleural friction rub	Hypoxemia; Pulmonary scan: ^{131}I albumin scan; ventilation-perfusion scan is quite helpful; Impedance phlebography; Pulmonary arteriogram; Abnormal electrocardiogram; Chest x-ray: oligemia, local and general; atelectasis; increased size of pulmonary artery; focal pleural effusion; increased alveolar-arterial O_2 gradient	Pulmonary arteriogram is definitive procedure for most cases
Cardiac asthma	History of heart disease; Paroxysmal nocturnal dyspnea; Orthopnea; Pedal edema	Polyphonic wheezing may be prominent during inspiration; Fine moist inspiratory rales S_3S_4 gallop; cardiomegaly; hoarseness; Jugular venous distention; Hepatojugular reflux	Increased venous pressure; Increased pulmonary wedge pressure; Electrocardiographic evidence of heart disease; Chest x-ray: increased heart size; vascular congestion; effusions	History of prior cardiac disease; absence of previous episodes of asthma; if both illnesses are present, differential diagnosis is most difficult; Response to diuretics and cardiac support
Central airways obstruction	Wheezing episodes, frequently terrifying; May have syncope; Negative family history	Extrathoracic inspiratory stridor, intrathoracic expiratory wheezing; Monophonic or polyphonic wheezing; May have position change factor in physical findings	Chest x-ray may disclose lesion; Blood: no eosinophilia; Sputum: no eosinophilia	Laminagrams of large airways may reveal obstruction; Bronchoscopy to reveal obstruction; Xerography to reveal obstruction
Angioedema	Occurs spontaneously or following trauma; Gastrointestinal colic; Episodic shortness of breath; May have family history of sudden death	Inspiratory stridor, crowing respirations	In hereditary form, C1 esterase inhibitor deficiency; Laminagram of larynx; Xerography: narrowed air column	In hereditary form, diagnosis rests on demonstration of a decrease of or ineffective C1 esterase inhibitor; In nonhereditary form, no specific laboratory test is available

Table 16–2 *(continued)*

Diagnosis	History	Physical Examination	Laboratory	Differential Diagnosis
Pulmonary aspiration	Predisposing causes: Neurological disease, e.g., cerebrovascular accident Hiatal hernia with reflux Sudden onset of symptoms in young child; foreign body Seizures Alcoholism Carious teeth	Monophonic wheeze Reflex bronchoconstriction with diffuse wheezing Occasional click over foreign body	X-ray Xerography Bronchoscopy, bronchography	Always consider aspiration as cause of cough and and wheeze in predisposed individuals
Carcinoid syndrome	Gastrointestinal symptoms, e.g., diarrhea or episodes of wheezing and hemoptysis Dermatologic findings: violescent rash	Red-violescent rash spreading from face to trunk Hypotensive spells Tricuspid-pulmonic murmurs	Increased 5-HIAA in urine; increased serotonin in blood; increased bradykinin X-ray: GI series, tumor; lung, coin lesion	Unusual to present as asthma Provocative testing: alcohol ingestion and injection; catecholamines; norepinephrine; dopamine; histamine and calcium infusion Biopsy of tumor
Bronchiolitis	Usually infant under 2 years of age 1 to 2 days of upper respiratory infection, then sudden respiratory distress	Diffuse polyphonic wheezing Fine inspiratory and expiratory rales Severe retractions, nasal flaring Cyanosis (severe cases) Mild fever	Immunofluorescent identification of respiratory syncytial virus Chest x-ray; hyperinflated, focal atelectasis	Asthma generally rare in infancy Lymphocytosis greater than 15,000 cells/ml; whooping cough
Cystic fibrosis	Meconium ileus Prolapsed rectum Pancreatic insufficiency Recurrent infections	Diffuse inspiratory and expiratory rhonchi and wheezing Barrel chest (advanced cases)	Thick viscid sputum Sweat test positive Chest x-ray variable from hyperinflation to	When disease has its onset in adult life, the sweat test loses much of its reliability

	Failure to thrive Cough	Cachexia (advanced cases) Digital clubbing; cyanosis	bronchiectasis "Serum factor" inhibits ciliary function Metachromatic staining of skin fibroblast	Diagnostic test is the sweat test
Environmental and industrial toxins (e.g., toluene diisocyanate, Yokahama asthma)	Exposure history, which may be quite subtle	Diffuse polyphonic wheezing	May have blood eosinophilia May have positive skin or inhalation challenge	Detailed geographic and work history is needed May have both type I and type III hypersensitivity
Psychogenic illness	Hysteric personality Recent stress	Normal	Normal	Frequent deep sighing respirations Voluntary hyperventilation PaO$_2$ normal (or high)

Pulmonary Infiltration with Eosinophilia (PIE)

Löffler's syndrome	Frequent drug ingestion, e.g., penicillin Shortness of breath Prior infectious illness Parasitic infestation	Wheezing may be present Areas of decreased breath sounds	Chest x-ray Blood: mild to moderate eosinophilia Pulmonary functions combined: obstructive and restrictive	Combination of fluffy infiltrates (lasting up to 6 weeks) associated with peripheral eosinophilia Response to corticosteroids
Chronic PIE	Frequently with history of asthma May last for weeks or years	Normal Percussion dullness; moist rales	Modest to spectacular eosinophilia Dense pneumonic infiltrates in peripheral pattern	Lung biopsy: alveoli filled with large mononuclear cells and eosinophils May have normal eosinophil count
Tropical eosinophilia	Recent residence in tropics Predominantly pulmonary symptoms	Wheezing diffuse, polyphonic	Eosinophilia 2,000/ml Positive filarial complement fixation test	Clinical response to diethylcarbamazine within 2 weeks Other worms, such as Ascaris, may be involved
PIE with aspergillosis	Allergy history Cough	Wheezing diffuse, polyphonic	Sputum: brown, with eosinophils IgE markedly increased Identification of fungus in sputum	Wheeze upon inhalation challenge with Aspergillus Marked increase in IgE Therapeutic response to steroids

Table 16-2 *(continued)*

Diagnosis	History	Physical Examination	Laboratory	Differential Diagnosis
PIE with vasculitis	Older person More common in males than in females Evidence of systemic vasculitis	Diffuse wheezing	Eosinophilia Hematuria	Tissue biopsy, granulomatous vascular reactions

Source: MacDonnell, K. F. Differential Diagnosis of Asthma. In Weiss, E. B., and Segal, M. S. (Eds.), *Bronchial Asthma: Mechanisms and Therapeutics.* Boston: Little, Brown, 1976. Chapter 52.

minimize the severity of attacks are available; immunologic diagnosis and therapy have advanced significantly; but nevertheless, cure is not at hand.

SUMMARY

Most patients who complain of paroxysmal episodes of wheezing and dyspnea, and who seek a physician, suffer from bronchial asthma. Any atypicality, however, should serve to alert the clinician and to cast doubt on this presumptive diagnosis. Even in routine cases, a high index of suspicion of the differential diagnosis is in order.

The specificity of the therapeutic program, and the prognostic implication of the many illnesses capable of masquerading as asthma, compels as precise a diagnostic definition as is possible, e.g., bronchial asthma versus congestive heart failure. This can be achieved in many instances by a careful analysis of the entire clinical situation, together with a logical and orderly analysis of the laboratory data. During the acute episode, however, diagnostic distinction may be impossible and a therapeutic trial directed at all factors is justified.

It is first by an awareness of those disorders that may be confused with bronchial asthma that the clinician is able to properly direct what may, in many instances, be life-saving therapy.

REFERENCES

1. Godfrey, S. Exercise induced asthma. Clinical, physiological and therapeutic implications. *J. Clin. Immunol.* 56, 1975, p. 1.
2. Griffith, J., et al. Sequential estimation of plasma catecholamines in exercise-induced asthma. *Chest* 69, 1972, p. 527.
3. Katz, L. H., and Gauchat, H. W. Observations on pulsus paradoxus: With special reference to pericardial effusion. *Arch. Intern. Med.* 33, 1924, p. 350.
4. Knowles, G. K., and Clark, T. J. H. Pulsus paradoxus as a value sign indicating severity of asthma. *Lancet* 2, 1973, p. 1356.
5. Kussmaul, A. Ueber schwielige mediastino-pericarditia und den paradoxen puls. *Klin. Wochenschr.* 1873, p. 445.
6. Lefcoe, N. M. Postexercise bronchoconstriction in normal subjects and asthmatics. *Am. Rev. Respir. Dis.* 104, 1971, p. 562.
7. MacDonnell, K. F. Differential Diagnosis of Asthma. In Weiss, E. B., and Segal, M. S. (eds.), *Bronchial Asthma: Mechanisms and Therapeutics.* Boston: Little, Brown, 1976, Chapter 46.
8. Melby, J. A. Pharmacology and Endocrinologic Considerations in the Use of Corticosteroid Therapy in Bronchial Asthma. In Weiss, E. B., and Segal, M. S. (eds.), *Bronchial Asthma: Mechanisms and Therapeutics.* Boston: Little, Brown, 1976, Chapter 52.
9. Patel, K. R. Atropine, sodium chromoglycate, and thymoxamine in PGF-induced bronchoconstriction in extrinsic asthma. *Br. Med. J.* 2, 1975, p. 360.
10. Pepys, J., et al. Inhibitory effects of disodium cromoglycate on allergen-inhalation tests. *Lancet* 2, 1968, p. 134.
11. Pepys, J. Nonimmediate Asthma Reactions. In Weiss, E. B., and Segal, M. S. (eds.), *Bronchial Asthma: Mechanisms and Therapeutics.* Boston: Little, Brown, 1976, Chapter 15.

12. Rebuck, A. S., and Read, J. Assessment and management of severe asthma. *Am. J. Med.* 51, 1971, p. 788.
13. Segal, M. S. Aminophylline: A clinical overview. *Adv. Asthma Allergy* 2, 1975, p. 17.
14. Thorn, G. W., and Lauler, D. P. Treatment Schedules with Steroids. In Weiss, E. B., and Segal, M. S. (eds), *Bronchial Asthma: Mechanisms and Therapeutics.* Boston: Little, Brown, 1976, Chapter 53.

Kenneth F. MacDonnell

Adult Respiratory Distress Syndrome

17

The appellation adult respiratory distress syndrome (ARDS) was first used by Petty and Ashbaugh [5] to describe a group of 12 patients with severe respiratory distress, an identical roentgenographic picture, and, in fatal instances, similar pathologic findings. The usefulness of this classification has been questioned. However, if the traditional interpretation of a clinical syndrome is maintained, then there is value in retaining this terminology. A syndrome is a "running together," "the sum of signs associated with any pathological process" [6].

Thus, the diagnostic umbrella of the adult respiratory distress syndrome serves to focus our attention on the many noncardiac forms of alveolar edema. The illnesses responsible share a common pathophysiologic mechanism and in many instances require similar respiratory support.

A review of the structural and functional interrelationship of the human alveolus will help in a better understanding of the role of the air-blood barrier in the adult respiratory distress syndrome. The human lung is an enormously sophisticated organ having a surface area of 70 to 80 square meters; its functional unit is the acinus, which includes all of the lung distal to the terminal bronchiolus and which is roughly 0.5 to 1 cm in diameter.

With the aid of the electron microscope, we have been able to unveil the fine architecture and cytologic features of the alveolus. Thus, a number of long-standing controversies have been resolved. For example, the cells lining the alveolar walls are indeed epithelial and possess a basement membrane. In fact, the ultrafine structure consists of a continuous layer of two types of epithelial cells and a basement mem-

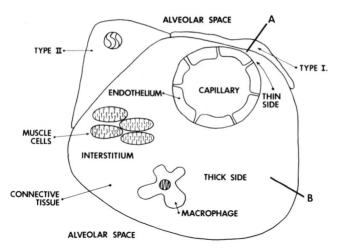

Figure 17-1. The alveolar membrane.

brane. The type A (type I) cell is a markedly attenuated supporting cell (Figure 17-1) that stretches throughout the alveolus. This type I cell does not possess microvilli and is quite thin (about 0.2 μ in thickness). The other cell is the type II (type B) alveolar lining cell, which is almost cuboidal, with microvilli and osmophilic lamellar bodies, and which is thought to be the main source of alveolar surfactant. Nagaishi [4] has suggested the terms squamous gas exchange cell for type I, and cuboidal secretory cell for type II, as reflecting more accurately their structure and function.

Electron and scanning microscopic examination of the alveolar capillaries demonstrate that the endothelial cells with their basement membrane are back to back with the basement membranes of the epithelium (A in Figure 17-1). Therefore, the air-blood barrier is composed of a type I or type II cell with its basement membrane, endothelial basement membrane, and an endothelial cell. The thinnest portion of the alveolar-capillary membrane is approximately 0.15 μ thick.

The other constituent of the alveolus is connective tissue that serves as support along with regulating alveolar volume. The alveolar connective tissue cells are of three types: fixed, granular, and wandering.

The structural characteristics of the various components of the alveolus are critical to the maintenance of an effective surface capable of gas delivery and exchange. The alveolar epithelial cells are quite impermeable to particles; on the other hand, the alveolar endothelial cells have spaces at their interdigitations, allowing for the flux of some small particles, a point of some importance in the pathophysiology of the adult respiratory distress syndrome. If these spaces become greater than 60 angstroms in width, then there is a movement of particles of size sufficient to result in an oncotic draw into the alveolus, and pulmonary edema may ensue. Figure 17-2 depicts (1) the alveolar capillary membrane, which normally is relatively imperme-

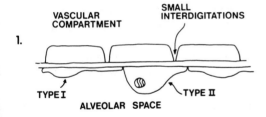

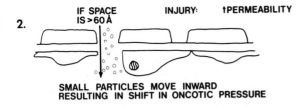

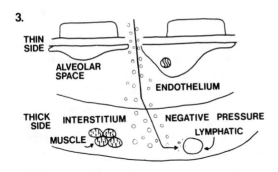

Figure 17-2. Permeability of the alveolar membrane.

able. (2) With injury this permeability is altered, with influx of fluid and particles. (3) The fluid first accumulates in the interstitium. When the capacity of the interstitium is exceeded, then the alveoli are filled, causing congestive atelectasis.

There is a thick and a thin side to the alveolar membrane (see Figure 17-1). The thin side (A in Figure 17-1) is the area of primary gas exchange and is last to be involved in interstitial edema. Animal experimentation, utilizing rapid freezing techniques, has verified these observations, demonstrating that edema preferentially occurs on the thick side (B in Figure 17-1) of the alveolar membrane, the site where the connective tissue and the interstitial lymphatic vessels are located. The movement of fluid is determined by the negative pressure relationships in the interstitium.

When the capacitance of the interstitium is exceeded, backup then occurs and alveolar edema accumulates. The spatial characteristics are such that once a critical amount of alveolar edema accumulates, then total obliteration of the alveolus results, and atelectasis with intrapulmonary shunting is observed.

Thus, the formation of pulmonary edema depends upon the disruption of the normal relationship between tissue pressure, oncotic pressure, and hydrostatic pressure (the Starling equation).

In the case of the adult respiratory distress syndrome, which is characterized by alveolar edema, the common denominator seems to be injury to the alveolar capillary membrane, and in particular to the pulmonary capillaries. It has been estimated that approximately 150,000 patients annually suffer from the adult respiratory distress syndrome. Early diagnosis and treatment have resulted in a marked improvement in survival figures upward of about 50 percent; however, this is still an unacceptably high mortality level. The major illnesses responsible are trauma, hemorrhaghic shock, aspiration pneumonia, viral pneumonia, narcotic overdose, hemorrhagic pancreatitis, pulmonary fat embolism, sepsis, DIC (disseminated intravascular coagulation), neurologic injuries, post pump lung, toxins (phosgene), transfusion with unfiltered blood, and oxygen toxicity. A specific etiology must, of course, be carefully searched for in each instance.

The establishment of the correct diagnosis depends in large measure on obtaining an accurate clinical history, a thorough physical examination, and selective use of laboratory information.

The clinical manifestations of the adult respiratory distress syndrome are those of acute respiratory distress, although dyspnea, restlessness, and apprehension may be late findings. The earliest laboratory finding is arterial hypoxemia, so in the appropriate clinical setting, careful monitoring of arterial blood gases is mandatory. The observed hypoxemia results from multiple microscopic areas of congestive atelectasis, which may not be detected initially by chest roentgenogram. The finding, then, of arterial hypoxemia should serve as a warning beacon to the clinician, a harbinger of impending disaster. Early recognition, with the institution of appropriate therapy with supplemental oxygen, along with careful clinical observation may save the patient.

Progression of illness results in increasing shortness of breath and cyanosis in spite of supplemental oxygen therapy. In severe instances, there may be carbon dioxide retention and a combined respiratory and metabolic acidosis indicative of massive lung involvement. This correlates with the clinical picture of profound respiratory failure and the roentgenologic picture of a "whiteout" of the lung. Vigorous therapy must be instituted immediately, or there is little hope of patient survival.

Pathologic examination of the lungs at this point discloses them to be soggy, wet, heavy, airless, and hemorrhagic (Figure 17-3). Microscopic examination is characterized by interstitial and alveolar protein-rich edema and congestive atelectasis (Figure 17-3 A, C, D); there is cellular debris filling alveolar spaces (B, C, D), along with intervascular congestion (A) and leukocyte infiltration (B, C, D). Hyaline membranes (D) also may be present. Progression of this process results in a universally consolidated lung. If this inflammatory process is countered successfully, then it is completely resolved; if the products of inflammation are incompletely removed, then all levels of residua may remain.

The patient who is left with varying amounts of pulmonary fibrosis may suffer significant respiratory embarrassment, or there may be only a slight physiologic disruption without any clinical symptoms. Whether the patient will be more susceptible to future injury (infectious or other) has not been established.

Therapy during the early stages is supportive unless the clinical condition warrants a more aggressive, invasive form of respiratory therapy. Because of requirements for supplemental oxygen, there is the potential of oxygen toxicity. Reduction in lung compliance causes an increase in the work of breathing and tachypnea, and is a reflection of lung stiffness as alveolar and interstitial fluid accumulates and congestive atelectasis spreads. At this stage, the x-ray picture shows a diffuse alveolar pattern without signs of cardiac failure.

The pulmonary wedge pressure may be normal or low, a helpful finding in sorting this clinical and x-ray picture from typical cardiac failure. It should be recalled that the adult respiratory distress syndrome and congestive heart failure are not mutually exclusive; they can and do coexist. Indeed, the patient with acute respiratory failure is particularly vulnerable to fluid overload, a tendency that is exaggerated if mechanical ventilation or positive end expiratory pressure (PEEP) is employed.

Of special importance is the presence of infection, either primary or secondary, in the clinical setting of the patient suffering with shock, for it is a far more serious prognosticator than simple hypovolemia. Clowes et al. [2] have attempted to define a specific circulating agent responsible for the pulmonary injury seen with sepsis. Others have suggested that mediators such as histamine, serotonin, prostaglandin, and endotoxin themselves may cause pulmonary venoconstriction and a subsequent increase in pulmonary capillary pressure. Albumin normally accounts for about 60 percent of serum oncotic pressure, and sepsis is commonly associated with hypoalbuminemia. Thus, in the case of sepsis, the combination of a capillary leak, increased pulmonary capillary pressure, and decreased oncotic pressure can result in a net flux of fluid out of the vascular compartment, resulting in noncardiac alveolar edema. Salt poor albumin, in this instance, will help to reestablish normal oncotic pressure; corticosteroid therapy has been advocated because of its antiinflammatory action, which serves to reduce the amount of capillary leak, a view that is disputed.

If the process worsens, then the adult respiratory distress syndrome becomes clear. Intrapulmonary shunts of greater than 20 percent of the cardiac output are not unusual; alterations in pulmonary mechanics are reflected in reductions in functional residual capacity and compliance, a result of progressive congestive atelectasis and the previously described pathologic findings. Epithelial cell damage results in a decrease in surfactant synthesis. It should be recalled that surfactant, along with stabilizing alveolar volume, plays a vital role in bacteriostasis of the lower respiratory tract; thus secondary bacterial infection is not unexpected. Common to all

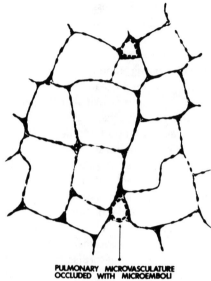

PULMONARY MICROVASCULATURE
OCCLUDED WITH MICROEMBOLI

A

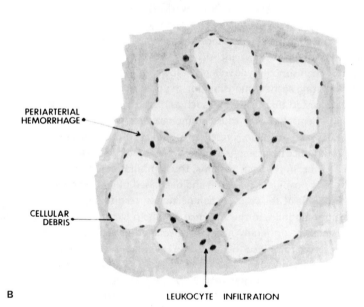

PERIARTERIAL
HEMORRHAGE

CELLULAR
DEBRIS

B

LEUKOCYTE INFILTRATION

Figure 17–3. Four examples (A–D) of pathologic states of the lung.

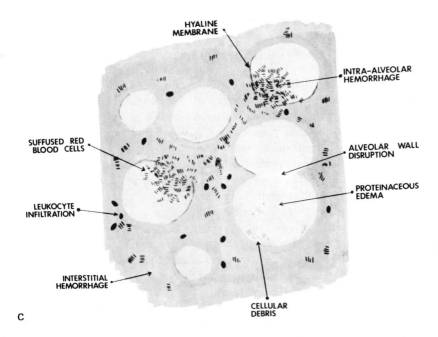

C

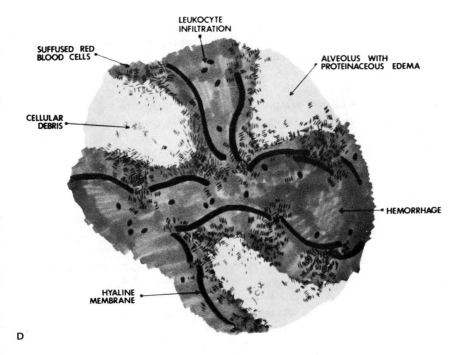

D

patients with the adult respiratory distress syndrome is the necessity for scrupulous attention to fluid balance, and the maintenance of adequate tissue oxygen.

It is impossible to define what level of arterial oxygen tension will supply cells with enough oxygen to maintain vital function. Arbitrarily, an arterial oxygen tension of 60 torr (see Chapter 10) is strived for; however, individual requirements and circumstances must always be taken into account. For example, a patient with long-standing lung disease may have a baseline arterial blood gas of less than 60 torr. Situations where great increases in inspired oxygen concentration result in negligible alterations in arterial oxygen pressure require careful adjustment and monitoring of oxygen therapy. Progressive respiratory failure frequently demands positive pressure ventilation, continuous positive airway pressure (CPAP), or positive end expiratory pressure, the mainstays in the therapy of the adult respiratory distress syndrome. Recruitment of collapsed alveoli by positive end expiratory pressure results in a marked decrease in intrapulmonic shunting (Figure 17-4). This effect is demonstrated by an increase in functional residual capacity. Indeed, patients with illnesses characterized by an increase in functional residual capacity, such as emphysema, are not benefited and may even be harmed with positive end expiratory pressure. Starting at a level of approximately 5 cm H_2O, PEEP has proved satisfactory in our hands for adult respiratory distress syndrome, with increases or decreases being dictated by the patient's physiologic and laboratory response. Levels up to 10 cm H_2O PEEP are well tolerated. Various methods have been proposed to select the "best" or optimal positive end expiratory pressure.

Illustrative of the variety of illnesses responsible for the adult respiratory distress syndrome are the following cases, again noting that proper treatment requires accurate diagnosis of the underlying etiology.

FAT EMBOLISM SYNDROME

Mrs. D. was a 77-year-old, widowed, white female brought to the hospital because of right hip pain after falling down at home. The patient was alert and cooperative, complaining of pain in her right hip. The remainder of her physical examination and past medical history was unremarkable. X-ray examination disclosed a subcapital fracture of the femur. While the patient was being interviewed in the accident ward, she became comatose. Her breathing became labored, and intubation was required. Examination of tracheal secretions disclosed fat globules; a chest x-ray picture (Figure 17-5) showed bilateral lower lobe infiltrates. Positive end expiratory pressure at 10 cm H_2O was instituted, along with the administration of heparin and steroids; measurement of central venous and pulmonary wedge pressures was normal. The fracture was stabilized. However, the patient did not respond; she remained comatose and expired suddenly 5 hours after admission. Autopsy demonstrated diffuse pulmonary and systemic fat emboli.

The unusual aspect of this case was the rapidity of progression from the onset of symptoms to death. Usually patients who suffer from the fat embolism syndrome have a period of about 24 to 72 hours from the time of injury to the appearance of

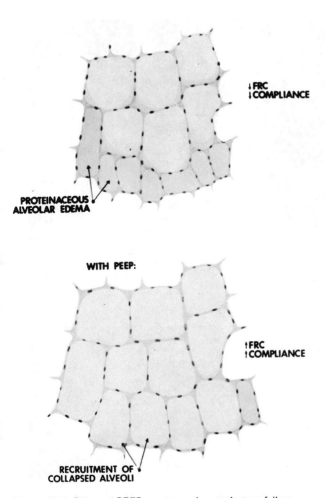

↓FRC
↓COMPLIANCE

PROTEINACEOUS
ALVEOLAR EDEMA

WITH PEEP:

↑FRC
↑COMPLIANCE

RECRUITMENT OF
COLLAPSED ALVEOLI

Figure 17–4. Effect of PEEP on progressive respiratory failure.

this syndrome. It is possible, in this instance, that the fracture was sustained at an earlier date, with completion of the fracture occurring just prior to admission. There have been a number of postulated mechanisms put forth to explain the pathophysiology of the fat embolism syndrome, ranging from a purely mechanical disruption of marrow fat, with the fat globules being intravasated into the low pressure veins and then circulating as emboli, to an ill-defined biochemical disruption of fat stability in plasma. However they are formed, they may be trapped in the pulmonary capillary network; those that escape may traverse the lung and appear as systemic emboli. In fact, cerebral emboli at one time were postulated as being responsible for the ARDS seen with the fat embolism syndrome, a form of neurogenic pulmonary

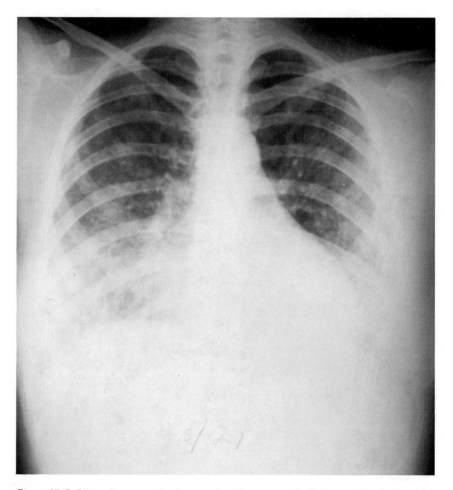

Figure 17-5. Bilateral asymmetric air space densities, greatest in the lower lobes, in fat embolism syndrome.

edema. This hypothesis has generally been discarded, for many patients without cerebral involvement display flagrant pulmonary abnormalities.

The mechanisms of injury caused by the trapped fat in the pulmonary microcirculation appears to be twofold: (1) mechanical vascular obstruction, and (2) the release of free fatty acids as a result of hydrolysis of the emboli. The mechanical aspects are similar to other types of embolic events (blood clots, etc.); it is immediate and may be catastrophic, undoubtedly the terminal event in the above-described patient. On the other hand, the second stage of fat emboli may be subtle and delayed, requiring a high index of suspicion if the correct diagnosis is to be made; hypoxemia is the earliest physiologic derangement and one that calls for prompt treatment.

The pulmonary response to the trapped fat and released fatty acids may be analogous to the dermal changes that have been observed in the skin as a result of fat emboli to dermal vessels. Abnormal gaps between endothelial junctions and the dermal postcapillary venules have been found by electron microscopy, presumably in response to the release of mediators such as serotonin and bradykinin. The end result is significantly altered permeability characteristics. If a similar sequence is operative in the lung, then the combined effect of released fatty acids and mediators could result in an increased alveolar-capillary permeability, and in its full-blown clinical manifestation, the adult respiratory distress syndrome.

Therapy requires stabilization of the fracture to prevent further embolic showers, along with vigorous fluid replacement. If blood is given, then Millipore filters should be used. Scrupulous attention to the patient's respiratory status is mandatory; frequent blood-gas determinations, with prompt oxygen therapy if any hypoxemia is noted, must be carried out. If further respiratory failure ensues, then the system of continuous positive airway pressure or intubation and respiratory support with positive end expiratory pressure may be indicated. Various adjuncts to therapy have been recommended, such as heparin, intravenous alcohol, low molecular weight dextran, and steroids.

Heparin increases lipase activity, and, if used early, it may disrupt the large fat globules, allowing them passage through the microcirculation. Also, disseminated intravascular coagulation may be precipitated by fat emboli; if heparin therapy is properly timed, it might be useful. Those who dispute the efficacy of heparin indicate that if the fatty acids released are damaging the lung, heparin would serve only to enhance their release and aggravate the situation. The use of heparin with major trauma also carries a risk of untoward bleeding complications. Along the same line, alcohol and low molecular-weight dextran infusion have been suggested, although their efficacy have not been established. Steroids, because of their antiinflammatory properties, remain as part of the standard therapeutic program used in the fat embolism syndrome.

SHOCK LUNG

This 63-year-old white male was admitted to the hospital with the chief complaint of back pain, predominantly in the lumbar area. The pain had worsened in the lumbar area for the past two years prior to admission, with accelerated worsening during the past few weeks. The patient's past history was significant in that he had suffered a myocardial infarction 16 years prior to admission and had had several episodes of angina for which he was taking nitroglycerin. A long-standing cigarette smoker of a pack or more a day, he had a chronic cough productive of small amounts of white and green sputum. The only significant physical finding was that he had an increase in the anteroposterior diameter of his chest and had coarse breath sounds. He was admitted to the hospital and an aortogram was carried out that showed a calcified abdominal aortic aneurysm extending into the bifurcation of the aorta.

The patient was operated on with resection of the aneurysm and an insertion of a

Dacron Y graft. He had substantial bleeding during the operation, required multiple transfusions, and had a period of 15 minutes of hypotension. Postoperatively, hypoxia developed that was resistant to oxygen delivered by means of face mask. The patient's pulmonary status progressively worsened over the next 12 hours, as reflected by progressive hypoxemia, dyspnea, tachypnea, and the x-ray picture shown in Figure 17-6. Intubation and respirator support with positive end expiratory pressure was instituted. A striking improvement in the blood gas levels was noted, and treatment was continued with 10 cm H_2O of PEEP for the next 4 days. Weaning off the positive end expiratory pressure and subsequent extubation was uneventful. The x-ray picture cleared; the arterial blood gas levels returned to normal, and the patient was discharged in good health.

Patients with cardiopulmonary bypass and those with major aortic surgery formerly constituted a high percentage of the adult respiratory distress syndrome victims seen in the hospital. These patients share the hazard of having substantial periods of low blood volume, along with receiving large volumes of fluids, colloids, blood, and blood products. Frequently, the transfused blood is administered using standard blood filters, allowing debris in the stored blood to be delivered into the vein to be trapped in the filtering system of the lung microvasculature. With the use of the Millipore filter, there is effective removal of this debris. To ensure continued effectiveness, these filters should be changed frequently.

Since we have used this system, we have not observed any instance of ARDS in a nonseptic graft or bypass patient, further supporting the observation of many investigators that the presence of a state of shock requires some other accompanying event to wreak the havoc that is recognized as the adult respiratory distress syndrome. Blaisdell [1] dramatically demonstrated this by developing a shock model by cross-clamping the infrarenal aorta; in so doing, the lung was not deprived of blood flow. Reestablishment of flow from the injured tissue allowed for the migration of platelet masses. These microemboli then became lodged in the pulmonary microcirculation. If flow is modified so that blood from the injured area is directed to the liver, the lung is spared from injury, or if only one lung is perfused with "injured" blood, then only that lung will develop damage.

The occurrence of the ARDS following simple hypovolemic shock remains a disputed point. Patients with shock lung usually have a combination of risk factors: a history of trauma or ischemic injury (frequently they have been transfused with a large amount of improperly filtered blood); sepsis; and treatment with large amounts of noncolloid fluids. Overzealous fluid replacement may serve to dilute the osmotic effect of blood, but it does not fully explain why these patients are so susceptible to capillary leak with fluid overload.

NEUROGENIC PULMONARY EDEMA

A 32-year-old white female was admitted to the hospital after being involved in an automobile accident. The patient arrived at the accident floor unconscious but responding to painful stimuli, able to move all extremities. Physical examination re-

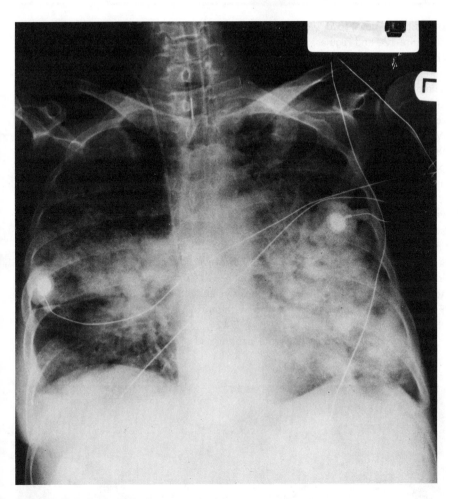

Figure 17–6. Bilateral alveolar edema in shock lung.

vealed a well-developed, well-nourished white female with a blood pressure of 100/60, pulse 120 and regular. Examination of her head showed multiple lacerations about the facial area, especially in the region of the nose, with displacement of the nose to the right. Fresh blood was exuding from both nares. The neck was supple. The pupils were equal and reacted to light and accommodation; the fundi were clear and there was no evidence of papilledema. Neurologically the patient was unresponsive; reflexes were hyperactive with bilateral upgoing toes. Skull x-ray films were negative and bilateral carotid arteriograms were found to be within normal limits, other than the fact that the vessels appeared small, possibly in spasm. The patient, who was supported with intravenous fluids, had a stable cardiorespiratory and renal status.

Approximately 48 hours after admission, the patient became tachypneic and developed respiratory distress. A portable chest x-ray study showed bilateral interstitial edema (Figure 17–7); the central venous pressure was approximately 5 cm H_2O. The arterial oxygen pressure (Pa_{O_2}) was 35 torr; supplemental oxygen was instituted. The arterial oxygen pressure, however, did not improve, and on an inspired oxygen concentration (FI_{O_2}) of 1 was still hovering between 35 and 40 torr. The patient was intubated and positive end expiratory pressure was instituted. Fifteen minutes following intubation, with an FI_{O_2} of 0.6, the Pa_{O_2} was 115 torr, the Pa_{CO_2} was 38 torr, and the pH was 7.42.

Approximately 12 hours later, the patient had a cardiac arrest and was pro-

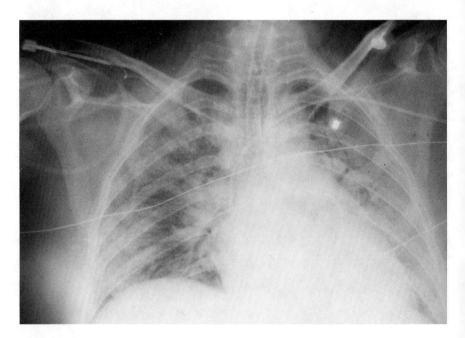

Figure 17–7. Bilateral interstitial edema in neurogenic pulmonary edema.

nounced dead. At autopsy, the patient had a subgaleal hematoma and multiple cerebral hemorrhagic infarcts secondary to trauma; the pathologic examination of the lung showed the findings associated with the adult respiratory distress syndrome. The explanation offered for the clinical syndrome of pulmonary edema following head injury has been related to some malfunction of the left ventricle. However, in most instances, this is not the case, and this pulmonary edema represents another dramatic example of the adult respiratory distress syndrome.

Moss [3], in a series of elegant experiments, elucidated a mechanism of the adult respiratory distress syndrome seen with severe head injury. Furthermore, he speculated that shock lung and high-altitude pulmonary edema shared a common pathophysiologic mechanism. The postulated mechanism notes that head injury may result in brain tissue hypoxia, which triggers a series of derangements in the "brain-lung axis," which is an autonomic malfunction resulting in pulmonary venospasm. This is a complex pathophysiologic disruption, and Moss is quick to point out that the central nervous system derangement is only one of many factors. Nonetheless, lesions in the hypothalamic region of laboratory animals regularly produce a form of pulmonary edema that can be prevented with spinal cord transection. In his experimental design, Moss isolates and perfuses the brain with various levels of hypoxia, attempting to simulate shock brain. Animals so exposed to brain hypoxia showed the lesions of the adult respiratory distress syndrome. Moreover, if one lung was totally denervated, it was spared of any stigma of adult respiratory distress syndrome. Of particular interest is the protective effect the drug phenytoin sodium (Dilantin) has in these animals. If dogs were premedicated with Dilantin, then pulmonary lesions could be prevented in these animals.

In summary, Moss proposes that shock severely alters brain cell function, a result of tissue hypoxia; the subsequent derangement of autonomic function is translated into pulmonary venospasm, and the result is pulmonary vascular congestion, edema, and congestive atelectasis—the adult respiratory distress syndrome.

NARCOTIC OVERDOSE

J. S., a 23-year-old white male, was admitted to the emergency room in extremis. He was without palpable blood pressure and pulse, with only feeble respiratory excursions. The patient had a past history of heroin abuse; however, according to his wife, he had not used heroin for a number of months. After coming home from work on the day of admission, the patient went into the bedroom, and about 15 or 20 minutes later, his wife found him on the bed, comatose. She called an ambulance, and he was brought to the emergency room.

The patient was intubated and resuscitated. The pulmonary wedge pressure at the time of admission was 0; central venous pressure was 1. A chest x-ray study (Figure 17–8) showed bilateral diffuse pulmonary edema. Thick, bubbly edema fluid was aspirated from his endotracheal tube. The diagnosis of narcotic lung was made (urine positive for heroin), and the patient was placed on a volume-controlled respirator with 10 cm H_2O of PEEP. His FI_{O_2} was 0.6, and his Pa_{O_2} was 75 torr.

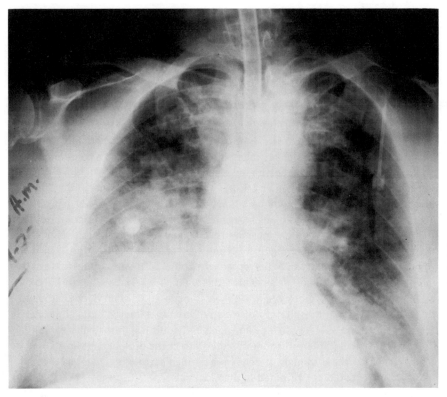

Figure 17–8. Bilateral diffuse pulmonary edema in narcotic overdose.

He remained on positive end expiratory pressure for four days and was gradually weaned from it and, subsequently, from ventilator support. Eventually, he was extubated and discharged.

This case is representative of noncardiac pulmonary edema and adult respiratory distress syndrome that is associated with drug abuse. Various theories have been proposed to explain the occurrence of acute exudative pulmonary edema in patients with narcotic addiction. Of the narcotic agents involved, heroin is by far the most common. Peculiarly, the syndrome generally occurs in addicts who have not used heroin for some time, or, indeed, who are first time users, an observation which would certainly litigate against an allergic type of phenomenon.

The lung of the narcotic addict, when it is examined pathologically, frequently shows a large amount of foreign materials such as talc, quinine, and other crystalline substances that are used to "cut" the heroin. Thus, there is suggestive evidence that debris from such procedures as misuse of syringes results in alteration and injury to the pulmonary microvasculature that can lead to the pulmonary edema.

Other events that are closely associated with drug abuse, such as severe hypoxia from respiratory depression and concurrent aspiration of gastric contents in the obtunded narcotic addict, may play a major role in producing or aggravating the clinical presentation. The picture seen with aspiration may be indistinguishable from other causes of the adult respiratory distress syndrome. This is particularly relevant in the case of the narcotic lung, because many of the reports of acute pulmonary edema with heroin, methadone, barbiturates, meperidine (Demerol), and propoxyphene hydrochloride (Darvon) have occurred in patients who have become obtunded as a result of drug ingestion and who have not been observed for prolonged periods of time, and who subsequently are found with vomitus on their faces or around them, suggesting that they in fact did have an episode of pulmonary aspiration. The role of released mediators such as histamine remains speculative. An awareness and early recognition of the syndrome is mandatory if proper therapeutic intervention is to be instituted.

SUMMARY

The adult respiratory distress syndrome encompasses a group of diseases that share a common clinical, x-ray, and pathologic picture, although there may be diverse etiologies. The common pathophysiologic mechanism revolves around disruption of the integrity of the normal alveolar capillary membrane, and a resultant exudation of fluid with congestive atelectasis. The physiologic consequences are widespread ventilation-perfusion imbalances. Treatment is directed at alleviating the early finding of hypoxemia. If progression of the disease occurs, then respiratory therapy with CPAP or PEEP may be required. Overall mortality with this illness remains at the high level of 50 percent. If conventional therapy is unsuccessful, then recourse to the use of the extracorporeal membrane oxygenator should be considered (see Chapter 23).

REFERENCES

1. Blaisdell, F. W. Pathophysiology of the respiratory distress syndrome. *Arch. Surg.* 108, 1974, p. 44.
2. Clowes, G. H. A., et al. Septic lung and shock lung in man. *Ann. Surg.* 181, 1975, p. 681.
3. Moss, G. The role of the central nervous system in shock; the centroneurogenic etiology of the respiratory distress syndrome. *Crit. Care Med.* 2, 1974, p. 181.
4. Nagaishi, C. *Functional Anatomy and Histology of the Lung.* Baltimore: University Park Press, 1972.
5. Petty, T. L., and Ashbaugh, D. G. The adult respiratory distress syndrome. *Chest* 60, 1971, p. 233.
6. *Taber's Cyclopedic Medical Dictionary* (12th ed.). Philadelphia: Davis, 1970.

Marguerite J. Herschel
Joseph L. Kennedy, Jr.

Recent Advances in the Care of Neonatal Respiratory Disorders

18

The diagnosis and treatment of neonatal respiratory problems continues to be among the more challenging and exciting aspects of modern medicine. Hyaline membrane disease; neonatal asphyxia and resuscitation; meconium aspiration; pulmonary interstitial emphysema, pneumomediastinum, and pneumothorax; apnea; type II respiratory distress syndrome; and finally, persistent fetal circulation are the major areas of interest in the field of neonatal respiratory disorders.

HYALINE MEMBRANE DISEASE

Recent advances in hyaline membrane disease have taken place in the understanding of the etiologic mechanisms, in the prediction of the infant at risk, in the prenatal and postnatal management of the premature infant, and in the prevention of both prematurity and hyaline membrane disease.

The term *idiopathic* can no longer be applied to the respiratory distress syndrome of prematurity, for the etiology has been elucidated. The term *hyaline membrane disease* is now again preferred to distinguish this condition from other causes of respiratory distress.

It is known that hyaline membrane disease is the result of insufficient lung synthesis of a pulmonary surface tension-lowering material, surfactant, whose function is to maintain alveolar volume during spontaneous respiration. Surfactant physiology and pathophysiology have been well reviewed. A deficiency of surfactant results in an increase in surface tension at the alveolus during expiration, requiring by the Laplace equation, $P = 2T/r$, increased pressures to maintain stability. In the absence of increased pressures, alveoli become atelectatic, resulting in shunting of blood from right to left through lung parenchyma as well as through persistent fetal channels, the foramen ovale and the ductus arteriosus.

Pulmonary surfactant is a lipoprotein that includes saturated lecithins and also cholesterol, neutral lipid, and other phospholipids [42]. Its major component, lecithin (phosphatidylcholine) is synthesized in the type II (granular) pneumocyte of the alveolus; it is then secreted so as to form a film over the alveolar surface. Synthesis of lecithin begins in the human fetus as early as 18 weeks in gestation, but secretion may not take place until 28 to 32 weeks, and adequate stores are not usually attained until 35 weeks [29]. Biosynthesis appears to be influenced adversely by perinatal and postnatal factors such as hypoxia, acidosis, reduced pulmonary capillary blood flow, and cold stress, but it may be facilitated by chronic stress in utero [30]. Surfactant utilization may be influenced postnatally by the state of the alveoli during air breathing. With ventilation of the lung from minimal volume as with alveolar collapse, there is destruction of surfactant [78]. Synthesis must then occur at an increased rate to prevent depletion of stores. If synthesis and secretion lag, further atelectasis occurs.

The ability to predict the infant at risk from hyaline membrane disease is based on the following data. In utero, fetal lung fluid, an ultrafiltrate of fetal plasma, contributes to amniotic fluid and can be sampled by amniocentesis. A major advance in the understanding of the development of pulmonary maturity has been the recognition that the lung phospholipid, lecithin, is secreted into amniotic fluid and can be measured there using the fairly rapid technique of thin layer chromatography [29]. Sphingomyelin remains relatively constant in level in the amniotic fluid through the latter part of gestation. A surge of lecithin, variable in timing from infant to infant, occurs in most by 35 weeks of gestational age. When the concentration of lecithin in amniotic fluid becomes at least twice that of sphingomyelin (lecithin-sphingomyelin ratio greater than 2.0), surfactant production is sufficient to support neonatal respiratory adaptation [29].

A simple, more rapid test, the shake test [19], has provided a semiquantitative estimation of surfactant levels. However, results may be erratic and can be depended upon only when positive.

Although there is a general correlation of the results of these tests with length of gestation, biologic variability among infants warrants actual determinations when early delivery of a pregnancy seems likely. Surfactant synthesis may be delayed despite advanced gestational age in certain families [31] and in diabetic pregnancies [77]. Pulmonary maturation appears to be advanced in the fetus of a heroin addict [27], with intrauterine infection [46], and with intrauterine growth retardation secondary to placental insufficiency [28]. When elective delivery is planned, or when nonelective delivery can be postponed, determination of the amniotic fluid lecithin-sphingomyelin ratio will give information on which to base a rational plan of management. Levels of less than 1.0 are associated with a high incidence of severe hyaline membrane disease; levels between 1.0 and 2.0 with a lesser incidence, and often with milder disease; levels over 2.0 are rarely associated with significant disease [29]. When the lecithin-sphingomyelin ratio is less than optimal, measures can be taken (see below) either to prolong the pregnancy or to induce pulmonary maturity.

Optimal obstetric care minimizes factors associated with fetal and neonatal asphyxia. Measurements of placental adequacy, oxytocin stress testing, nonstress testing, fetal monitoring in labor, and the judicious use or omission of analgesic and anesthetic agents in labor and delivery have been helpful.

Hypovolemia is common in infants who develop hyaline membrane disease. The loss of fetal blood in antenatal hemorrhage from placenta previa or abruptio placentae may result in fetal hypotension, hypoxia, and acidosis. Reduced blood volume adversely affects the normal transition from fetal to neonatal circulatory pathways. The systemic pressure fails to rise after occlusion of the umbilical cord. This tends to perpetuate both a right-to-left flow through the foramen ovale and the ductus arteriosus, and a low pulmonary blood flow with secondary exudation of fluid and protein from pulmonary capillaries. With asphyxia, pulmonary artery pressure fails to fall, further impeding flow and leading to right-to-left shunting. These events interfere with surfactant production.

The redistribution of blood at the end of the birth process from the placenta to the infant provides the newborn infant with a greater red blood cell mass and blood volume. It has a beneficial effect on the survival of premature infants with hyaline membrane disease [74]. A delay in cord clamping of 1.5 minutes in the premature infant may minimize the above-mentioned maladaptive processes, particularly after cesarean section, when the placental transfusion is often only minimal [44]. Early correction of volume deficits is beneficial to the infant.

Cesarean section is thought to be a risk factor in the development of hyaline membrane disease, but it has been difficult to identify the particular factors responsible. These may include the reasons for the operative intervention, such as maternal diabetes, the gestational age, the absence of labor, and the amount of placental transfusion.

The finding of evidence of low surfactant in a pharyngeal, tracheal, or gastric aspirate [22] can be helpful in making an early diagnosis of hyaline membrane disease and in distinguishing it from other conditions associated with tachypnea, respiratory effort, diminished air entry, and diffuse roentgenologic reticulogranular densities.

Pressure required to inflate the premature lung at birth is at least 40 cm H_2O and in the absence of surfactant, subsequent breaths require pressures of a similar order because of the small residual volume from which the lung must reinflate. Because of the high compliance of the premature chest wall and the low compliance of the lung, it is difficult for the infant to generate the pressures necessary to expand the lung. Respiratory failure easily ensues as the infant tires.

Oxygen administration is critical in management, for in addition to significant right-to-left shunting there is often some degree of impaired diffusion because of alveolar exudate and interstitial pulmonary edema. With oxygenation pulmonary artery pressure falls, pulmonary blood flow increases, and myocardial function improves, as do tissue perfusion and tissue oxygenation. Aerobic metabolism begins again, the formation of lactic acid ceases, and surfactant synthesis resumes. The goal of oxygen therapy is to maintain the oxygen pressure of arterial blood between 50 and 70 torr. The toxic effect of high oxygen pressure on the retinal vasculature is well known. Increasingly more appreciated are the acute and chronic effects of oxygen on the lung.

The use of constant distending airway pressure has revolutionized the management of hyaline membrane disease [35], particularly because it can be applied in a noninvasive manner [13, 40]. It is now clear that the grunting expiration of the premature infant against a closed glottis serves to maintain intraalveolar pressure at higher levels, enhancing oxygenation by stabilizing alveolar volume and reducing intrapulmonary shunting [38]. Constant distending airway pressure provides the therapeutic equivalent of grunting. It is now common practice to begin constant positive airway pressure (CPAP) shortly after birth in the spontaneously breathing infant with hyaline membrane disease. A nasal piece with two small prongs fitting into the nostrils can maintain pressures up to 10 cm H_2O. The early use of continuous positive airway pressure (or constant negative airway pressure) appears to modify the course of the illness. Early-treated infants need lower levels of ambient oxygen for shorter periods of time than those treated later. Fewer require intermittent positive pressure breathing (IPPB).

The hazards of distending pressure result from overdistention of the lung and include diminished tidal volume, carbon dioxide retention, diminished pulmonary blood flow, interstitial emphysema, pneumomediastinum, and pneumothorax [32, 80]. Decreased venous return and diminished cardiac output have not usually been observed.

Intermittent positive pressure breathing should be used when there is recurrent apnea or when respiratory failure as indicated by hypercapnia, acidosis, or hypoxia ensues (the last is often taken as an arterial oxygen pressure of less than 50 torr with 100% oxygen). Positive end expiratory pressure (PEEP) is continued during ventilation.

The goal of intermittent positive pressure breathing is to achieve proper oxygenation and ventilation while minimizing the chances of pulmonary air leak, a possible precursor of bronchopulmonary dysplasia. This chronic state of pulmonary fibrosis with patchy hyperinflation and recurrent pneumonia appears to be related to intubation, immaturity, and duration and level of pulmonary oxygen exposure as well as to types and levels of ventilating pressure.

Safe management can be achieved by using a positive pressure respirator designed for infants, with low maximum inspiratory pressure (usually 25 cm H_2O or less), respiratory rates of 30 breaths per minute, positive expiratory pressure (5 cm H_2O or less), and an inspiratory-expiratory time ratio of 1:2 or more [39]. The use of negative pressure respirators has not been associated with such high incidences of bronchopulmonary dysplasia or air leak, but the devices are not used on very small infants and supportive nursing care of the infant is difficult. The management of the infant with hyaline membrane disease requires that blood gas measurements using amounts of blood less than 0.3 ml be available at all times, and that these be performed no less frequently than every 2 hours. Umbilical or radial artery catheterization is usually necessary. Skin electrodes have been developed for continuous monitoring of arterial oxygen pressure and should soon become widely available.

Supportive measures are critical. Early and adequate transfusion of the infant who has lost blood or who is hypovolemic (see above) may reduce morbidity. Frequent transfusions should be given to replace the appreciable amounts of blood taken, usually for laboratory determinations. The importance of minimizing oxygen consumption by keeping the infant in a neutral thermal environment is clear. Prompt attention must be given to correcting acidosis and to maintaining normal blood sugar and calcium levels. The use of furosemide has been recommended to improve oxygenation by removal of interstitial pulmonary edema [56]. Improved methods of maintaining nutrition during the acute and recovery phases of the condition include peripheral alimentation, central venous alimentation, and constant gavage feedings. Phototherapy has simplified the management of associated jaundice.

Despite improvements in the identification and management of the patient at risk, premature infants continue to die not only from hyaline membrane disease but also from causes associated with but not clearly attributable to this disease, for example, intraventricular hemorrhage, pulmonary hemorrhage, perinatal asphyxia, and infection. The use of alcohol [81] and beta-sympathomimetic agents [51] can in some instances inhibit labor and prolong pregnancy. When there is at least 24 hours of warning of impending delivery, a situation occurring with perhaps one-third of premature births, the intramuscular administration to the mother of 12 mg of the glucocorticoid betamethasone has been shown to prevent the occurrence of hyaline membrane disease and to reduce mortality [52]. No untoward effects of such treatment on mother or infant have so far been noted [70]. The mechanism of action of such agents has been the subject of a recent review [6].

NEONATAL ASPHYXIA AND RESUSCITATION

Research in mammalian fetal physiology has led to advances in the understanding and management of the asphyxiated newborn infant [2]. Dawes [21] has reviewed the effects of asphyxia on the newborn monkey. A characteristic sequence evolves in the experimentally asphyxiated monkey. After clamping the umbilical cord, a short period of respiratory activity occurs accompanied by a slight increase in heart rate and blood pressure and then a fall, as well as a fall in heart rate to levels of 60 beats per minute (bpm). By this time the arterial oxygen pressure is unmeasurable and the pH is falling because of a combined respiratory and metabolic acidosis. The monkey can be resuscitated easily at this point using external stimuli such as stimulation of the soles of the feet. If asphyxia continues, however, a second period of spontaneous gasping follows; it is variable in duration and associated with a further fall in blood pressure and with persistent bradycardia. The last gasp is followed by secondary (terminal) apnea that persists until death or resuscitation. During terminal apnea there is no response to external stimuli. Correction of acidosis, support of blood pressure, and provision of glucose, in addition to cardiopulmonary resuscitation, are critical to recovery.

The sequence of events in asphyxiated human newborn babies is similar [37]. Resuscitation in primary apnea is usually rapid. The infant has some tone and cries before there is an improvement in skin color. Resuscitation in terminal apnea is prolonged and requires an average of 2 minutes of cardiorespiratory assistance for each minute of preceding asphyxia. The infant is flaccid; his color improves before there is spontaneous respiration.

Two types of brain damage are seen when monkey fetuses which have been subjected to periods of asphyxia are later resuscitated [57]. With prolonged total asphyxia there is brain stem damage. With repeated episodes of partial asphyxia there is bilateral hemispheric injury. Myocardial injury also may be extensive and significant.

The fetus has intermittent irregular respiratory movements in utero. The normal infant breathes and cries within a few seconds of birth. The stimuli to the first breath are multiple and include hypoxia, hypercapnia, and recoil chest expansion following delivery. Fetal asphyxia remains the commonest cause of failure to initiate respiration. Maternal hypnotic, analgesic, and anesthetic agents are well known to depress initial respiratory attempts.

With the first breaths, air replaces lung fluid, which is absorbed into lymphatic channels and the pulmonary capillary bed, and which wells up through the trachea into the oropharynx. On occasion, particularly after cesarean section, an abnormal mixing of air and fluid produces a thick foam that causes respiratory obstruction. After initial lung expansion, about 5 breaths are required before arterial oxygen pressure and pH begin to rise and carbon dioxide pressure to fall [18].

Fetal gas exchange has been well reviewed by Adamsons and Myers [2]. The use of intrapartum fetal monitoring has furthered clinical knowledge in this area [54]. The maintenance of an effective fetal respiratory exchange depends upon the adequacy and integrity of maternal ventilation, maternal circulation, uterine flow, placental flow, placental size and function, umbilical vessel flow, and fetal circulation. Conditions such as maternal hypotension, abnormal uterine contractions, and placental abruption have long been known to interfere with fetal gas exchange and to produce neonatal asphyxia. More recently, maternal hyperventilation leading to decreased uterine blood flow has been recognized as another factor in fetal asphyxia [55]. Administration of catecholamines to the mother, and maternal anxiety, both have the same effect [1].

Hypovolemia is increasingly recognized as a significant factor in neonatal asphyxia. Half of all preterm asphyxiated infants appear to be hypovolemic [33]. Premature placental separation can result in fetal hypovolemia with asphyxia secondary to inadequate fetoplacental circulation [62]. Umbilical cord problems, such as ruptured vasa previa, can also result in fetal hypovolemia [62]. A common, though not often severe, cause of a redistribution of the fetoplacental blood pool into the placenta is partial compression of the cord [14]. Incision of a placenta previa during cesarian section causes hypovolemic neonatal asphyxia when extraction of the infant is at all delayed [58].

The value of allowing a placental transfusion to occur is still debated [79]. It would seem reasonable to give it to the small infant who is likely to be hypovolemic unless a delay in cord clamping would compromise other resuscitative efforts.

Correction of hypovolemia plays a large role in the resuscitation of infants afflicted with this condition. Blood pressure should be measured routinely in the delivery room in sick infants and treatment instituted when indicated, with the rapid infusion of 10 to 15 ml per kilogram of body weight of whole blood, plasma, or 5% albumin; larger amounts are often necessary [33].

Clinical assessment of the newborn infant at birth is accomplished by using the Apgar score, which at one minute correlates well with the need for resuscitation and with early neonatal mortality. The evaluation of the infant's color appears to be the least helpful of the five components of the score and may in fact reduce the discriminating value of the total score [20]. A simplified scoring system using only heart rate and respiratory effort has recently been proposed [15].

Provision of adequate radiant heat to the infant during evaluation and resuscitation is critical. Continuous heart rate monitoring has been effective and practical [67]. Detailed procedures for resuscitation are presented in Gregory's excellent review [33].

After initial recovery from asphyxia the infant should be cared for in an intensive care nursery with adequate provisions for observing and monitoring vital signs and neurologic and metabolic status.

MECONIUM ASPIRATION

Meconium aspiration is a significant cause of morbidity and mortality, particularly in the term and postterm infant. There has been some advance in prevention but little advance in treatment.

Meconium, the greenish-black tenacious material filling the fetal large bowel, derives from the in utero digestion of swallowed amniotic material and desquamated gastrointestinal cells, as well as fetal intestinal secretions. It is rich in mucopolysaccharides and bile pigments [11]. Under the stress of even brief intrauterine asphyxia, meconium may be passed into the amniotic fluid by mechanisms probably involving anoxic stimulation of gut motility and inhibition of anal sphincter tone [54]. The normal infant born without asphyxia does well even though bathed at birth in meconium-stained amniotic fluid. It is only when there is concurrent intrapartum asphyxia producing gasping, irregular respirations, and when the meconium has been recently passed and is thick or particulate, that a problem may develop—the aspiration of this material into the tracheobronchial tree.

Thick meconium causes respiratory distress both by its action as a foreign body causing partial or total respiratory obstruction, and by its action as a chemical irritant producing pulmonary inflammation and edema. In addition meconium appears to be a favorable medium for bacterial growth [23]. Meconium aspiration causes asphyxia and acidosis, right-to-left shunting, atelectasis, and consolidation. It is often complicated by pulmonary air leak caused by overdistention of parts of the lung because of ball-valve air trapping, and because of uneven alveolar expansion [75].

Despite optimal management of meconium aspiration by oxygen, antibiotic agents, mechanical ventilation, and physical therapy, the mortality rate remains high, and the quality of some of the surviving infants is poor [61, 75]. Administration of corticosteroids has been recommended but has not been demonstrated to be helpful in human infants [5]; it has had an adverse effect in animals [25]. Constant distending airway pressure up to 5 to 7 cm H_2O has provided better oxygenation without increasing the risk of pulmonary air leak [24]; intermittent positive pressure breathing when necessary is more often best accomplished with the use of curariform agents because of the size and vigor of these infants and their tendency even when untreated to develop interstitial emphysema. Antibiotic agents are frequently given to prevent bacterial superinfection [65] but they have not been shown to be of value. The high incidence of perinatal asphyxia preceding this syndrome makes hypoglycemia secondary to exhaustion of hepatic glycogen stores a not uncommon phenomenon; as with the premature infant, supportive treatment must include adequate caloric nutrition.

Meconium staining of amniotic fluid occurs in approximately 10 percent of deliveries; in more than half of these occasions meconium can be recovered from the trachea [34]. The absence of the material in the oropharynx does not preclude its presence in the trachea.

It is clear that immediate tracheal aspiration of infants at risk will lower the morbidity rate [34]. Infants at risk include those born through thick or particulate meconium, and those infants who, though born through thin meconium, are asphyxiated at birth. Otherwise healthy infants should not have routine tracheal aspiration. Suction is effected by the rapid insertion, before the first breath if possible, of an endotracheal tube followed by direct suction applied to the tube, removal, and repeated reinsertions until the trachea is clear. Bag and mask ventilation with 40% oxygen should follow. The methods and choices of treatment and the decision-making process have been well reviewed by Gregory [33].

Aspiration of blood, mucus, and possibly amniotic fluid may occur with delivery. In a series of 3,344 live-born deliveries, 50 infants had a clinical aspiration syndrome, only 19 of which could be attributed to meconium [49]. Management is similar.

Pulmonary aspiration of feedings secondary to dysfunctional swallowing or to regurgitation continues to be a problem in the depressed, sick, or premature newborn infant. Aspiration of water is less harmful to rabbit lungs than either 5% dextrose or formula [59]. Continuous gastric [48], nasojejunal [12], and nasoduodenal [76] feedings have been recommended for premature infants in part to avoid this problem.

PULMONARY INTERSTITIAL EMPHYSEMA, PNEUMOMEDIASTINUM, AND PNEUMOTHORAX

Pulmonary air leak may be asymptomatic or a catastrophic event. Its treatment and prognosis depends upon the etiology and presentation as well as on the presence of underlying lung disease. We use the term here to include pulmonary interstitial emphysema, pneumomediastium, and pneumothorax.

The incidence of pneumothorax is by x-ray survey 1 to 2 percent of live births [68]. A substantial percentage of these are spontaneous and not secondary to overvigorous resuscitation. In infants in whom assisted ventilation is used, the incidence of pulmonary air leak is 5 to 40 percent or greater [8].

Overdistention of the alveoli leads to rupture, with dissection of air into perivascular spaces. Gas trapped in the interstitium of the lung (pulmonary interstitial emphysema) is recognized radiologically as linear or cystlike lucent streaks that are more numerous, more irregular, more peripheral, and more lucent than air bronchograms. If the air easily dissects toward the hilum along perivascular planes, then pneumomediastinum formation occurs without x-ray evidence of pulmonary interstitial emphysema. Rupture of a pneumomediastinum into the pleural space is recognized as pneumothorax.

Earlier studies demonstrated that the full-term infant is at highest risk for pulmonary rupture, but with the advent of intensive neonatal respiratory care, the majority of infants with this problem are now premature infants with hyaline membrane disease [71, 80]. In contrast to term or postterm infants with aspiration syndrome who present with respiratory difficulty caused by pneumothorax in the first hour of life, the premature infant with hyaline membrane disease usually sustains pulmonary rupture at the end of the second day of life (range 12 to 140 hours) [80]. The alveoli are more distensible and thus subject to rupture the lower their surface tension and the lesser the lung tissue elastic forces; therefore air leak is more likely to occur in the premature infant with hyaline membrane disease, and in particular during the recovery phase of the disease [3].

The radiologic distribution of abnormal intrathoracic gas can be related to gestational age and to the presence or absence of hyaline membrane disease. Interstitial emphysema occurs almost exclusively in premature infants with hyaline membrane disease. It may progress to pneumomediastinum and pneumothorax. When there is no hyaline membrane disease the presentation is usually extrapulmonary.

The distribution and severity of pulmonary interstitial edema correlates strongly with outcome. Bilateral mild pulmonary interstitial edema in an infant with hyaline membrane disease is invariably associated with progressive respiratory failure and the need for assisted ventilation. This is not necessarily the case when pulmonary interstitial edema involves only a limited area of one lung. When pulmonary interstitial edema is bilateral and severe, survival even with respiratory support is unusual [71].

Pneumomediastinum and pneumothorax are frequently asymptomatic. Diagnosis can be suggested by the increased anteroposterior diameter of the chest, tachypnea, grunting, and retractions. When the infant is not severely distressed and shows no sign of a tension pneumothorax, recommended treatment is with high ambient oxygen concentrations, which accelerate resorption [17]. The prognosis is good but the arterial oxygen pressure must be followed closely to avoid hyperoxemia. The infant with hyaline membrane disease who develops pneumothorax nearly always requires chest tube drainage. The degree of tension in the pneumothorax may not be appreciated on the chest film because the noncompliant lung resists collapse.

The diagnosis of pneumothorax must always be considered in an infant with hyaline membrane disease who suffers sudden deterioration. Rapid diagnosis of pneumomediastinum and pneumothorax by transillumination of the chest with a high-intensity fiberoptic light has recently been described. Total darkness is not required [47]. In life-threatening situations the presence and location of the pneumothorax can be confirmed by this method and treatment begun without delay. Efficacy of tube placement can also be evaluated. In nonemergency situations, x-ray documentation is still preferred.

Emergency chest tube drainage has been simplified by the use of the Heimlich valve, a one-way flutter valve that obviates the need for underwater seals and bottles [9]. This valve is of particular value in the transport of neonates.

An infrequent complication of pulmonary air leak is pneumopericardium, a condition that may be unsuspected or that may produce diminished heart sounds, markedly reduced pulse pressure, bradycardia, and severe distress. If these signs of tamponade are present, needle aspiration of the pericardium must be performed, followed, if indicated, by indwelling catheter drainage. Rarely, air will dissect from a pneumomediastinum to the retroperitoneum and then rupture into the peritoneal cavity. Pneumoperitoneum from this cause must be distinguished from a perforation of the gastrointestinal tract.

Two increasingly recognized causes of pneumothorax presenting immediately at birth are intrauterine needle perforation of the thorax during amniocentesis, and pulmonary hypoplasia associated with absent renal function (Potter's syndrome).

The full-term, otherwise healthy infant who sustains a spontaneous pneumothorax and who is treated appropriately has an excellent prognosis. In contrast, the premature infant with hyaline membrane disease who has pulmonary interstitial edema alone or with pneumothorax has a more guarded outlook. If the infant survives, the pulmonary interstitial edema may evolve into bronchopulmonary dysplasia.

APNEA

Idiopathic apnea of prematurity is a common phenomenon that may result in severe hypoxia and that is associated with significant mortality and morbidity rates. Major advances have taken place recently in its management, and investigations continue into its cause.

Apnea of prematurity is generally defined as repetitive episodes of cessation of breathing of at least 20 seconds' duration, or less if accompanied by a heart rate under 100 beats per minute, and often requiring therapeutic intervention for termination [73]. It is increasingly prevalent with decreasing gestational age, occurring in

84 percent of infants under 1,000 gm [4]. Usually it appears on the third to fourth day of life and may continue for weeks. Other disorders commonly associated with apnea must be ruled out: metabolic disturbance, pulmonary disease, cardiac disease, sepsis, central nervous system infection, or hemorrhage.

Apnea has been associated with rising environmental air temperature in incubators controlled by on-off servomechanisms [60] with decreased environmental humidity [7] and has been attributed to a lack of sensitivity of the respiratory system to carbon dioxide [63] and central depression caused by hypoxia [63, 64]. It is found to occur in rapid eye movement [16] or in quiet [36] sleep states.

Conventional treatment has been to provide increased ambient oxygen because it has been long known that this will eliminate periodic breathing and reduce the frequency of apnea, but this procedure carries with it the risk of retrolental fibroplasia if the arterial oxygen pressure is not carefully monitored. For severe apnea, cutaneous stimulation, bag and mask ventilation, or, often, respirator management have been necessary.

Recently it has been shown that oral theophylline, in a dose of 2 to 4 mg per kilogram of body weight every 6 hours, is effective in reducing or eliminating apneic attacks [66, 73]. Presumably its mechanism of action is a change in sensitivity of the medullary respiratory center to carbon dioxide [45, 53]. Its use has been reserved for severe recurrent apnea.

Other useful modes of treatment are prophylactic sensory stimulation (5 minutes of cutaneous stimulation out of each 15 minutes) or, even more effective, low pressure (2 to 4 cm H_2O) nasal constant positive airway pressure [41].

A preliminary report has been published that suggests that a gently oscillating water bed is effective in reducing the number of apneic attacks [45].

Apnea of prematurity has been linked with the sudden infant death syndrome. Recent research has focused on the apneas associated with sleep states and the possibility of upper airway occlusion in the pathogenesis of this bewildering condition [66, 72].

TYPE II RESPIRATORY DISTRESS SYNDROME

Some prematurely born infants, often with intrapartum depression, have a benign form of respiratory distress commonly called transient tachypnea of the newborn, or type II respiratory distress syndrome. Chest x-ray studies do not show the reticulogranular pattern of hyaline membrane disease, but rather heavy perihilar bronchovascular markings, hyperinflation, fluid in the lobar fissure, and often patchy infiltrates.

Clinically, these infants have signs of a respiratory problem sometimes with retractions, grunting, and cyanosis, but follow a milder course than those with hyaline membrane disease. Their blood volumes are normal; their oxygen pressures respond to 100% oxygen in a near normal fashion. They rarely have metabolic or respiratory acidosis after the first 6 hours of life, and they have an excellent prognosis. Respiratory rates of 100 to 140 breaths per minute are often seen, but they return to normal during the first week of life.

The etiology has been attributed to aspiration of mucus or amniotic fluid, or to delayed resorption of fetal lung fluid [69].

PERSISTENT FETAL CIRCULATION

Most newborn infants with cyanosis and signs of respiratory distress have pulmonary disease, congenital heart disease, or central nervous system disorders. A group of infants has now been recognized in whom there is no demonstrable cardiac or pulmonary disease but who have true right-to-left shunting at the level of the foramen ovale and the ductus arteriosus secondary to persistently elevated pulmonary artery pressure. This entity has been called *persistent fetal circulation*.

This condition occurs most commonly in full-term infants who are often asphyxiated at birth, presents in the first 24 hours of life with cyanosis as the predominant feature, and may resolve within days or weeks or go on to end fatally. The x-ray appearance of the lung is normal; there may be mild to moderate cardiomegaly. Histopathologic examination shows normal pulmonary parenchyma and pulmonary arteriolar medial hypertrophy.

Persistent fetal circulation may be idiopathic, or it may occur in association with other conditions such as the neonatal hyperviscosity syndrome, hypoglycemia, or the atypical respiratory distress syndrome. If these conditions can be ruled out, cardiac catheterization may be necessary to exclude transposition of the great vessels.

REFERENCES

1. Adamsons, K., Mueller-Heubach, E., and Myers, R. E. Production of fetal asphyxia in the Rhesus monkey by administration of catecholamines to the mother. *Am. J. Obstet. Gynecol.* 109, 1971, p. 248.
2. Adamsons, K., and Myers, R. E. Perinatal asphyxia: Causes, detection, neurologic sequelae. *Pediatr. Clin. North Am.* 20, 1975, p. 465.
3. Adler, S. M., and Wyszogrodski, I. Pneumothorax as a function of gestational age: Clinical and experimental studies. *J. Pediatr.* 87, 1975, p. 771.
4. Alden, E. R., et al. Morbidity and mortality of infants weighing less than 1000 gm in an intensive care nursery. *Pediatrics* 50, 1972, p. 40.
5. Avery, M. E., and Fletcher, B. D. *The Lung and Its Disorders in the Newborn Infant.* Philadelphia: Saunders, 1974, p. 238.
6. Avery, M. E. Pharmacological approaches to the acceleration of fetal lung maturation. *Br. Med. Bull.* 31, 1975, p. 13.
7. Belgaumkar, T. K., and Scott, K. E. Effects of low humidity on small premature infants in servocontrol incubator. II. Increased severity of apnea. *Biol. Neonate* 26, 1975, p. 348.
8. Berg, T. J., et al. Bronchopulmonary dysplasia and lung rupture in hyaline membrane disease: Influence of continuous distending pressure. *Pediatrics* 55, 1975, p. 11.
9. Bernstein, A., Waqaruddin, M., and Shah, M. Management of spontaneous pneumothorax using a Heimlich flutter valve. *Thorax* 28, 1973, p. 386.
10. Boddy, K., and Mantell, C. C. Observations of fetal breathing movements transmitted through maternal abdominal wall. *Lancet* 2, 1972, p. 1219.

11. Boune, G. *The Human Amnion and Chorion.* Chicago: Year Book, 1962, p. 143.
12. Caillie, M. V., and Powell, G. K. Nasoduodenal versus nasogastric feedings in the very low birthweight infant. *Pediatrics* 56, 1975, p. 1065.
13. Caliumi-Pelligrini, G., et al. Twin nasal cannula for administration of continuous positive airway pressure to newborn infants. *Arch. Dis. Child.* 49, 1974, p. 228.
14. Cashore, W. J., and Usher, R. H. Hypovolemia resulting from a tight muchal cord at birth. *Pediatr. Res.* 7, 1973, p. 399.
15. Chamberlain, G., and Banks, J. Assessment of Apgar score. *Lancet* 2, 1974, p. 1225.
16. Chernick, V., Heldrich, F., and Avery, M. D. Periodic breathing of premature infants. *J. Pediatr.* 64, 1964, p. 330.
17. Chernick, V., and Reed, M. H. Pneumothorax and chylothorax in the neonatal period. *J. Pediatr.* 76, 1970, p. 624.
18. Chou, P. J., Ullrich, J. R., and Ackerman, B. D. Time of onset of effective ventilation at birth. *Biol. Neonate* 24, 1971, p. 74.
19. Clements, J. A., et al. Assessment of the risk of respiratory distress syndrome by a rapid test for surfactant in amniotic fluid. *N. Engl. J. Med.* 286, 1972, p. 1077.
20. Crawford, J. S., Davies, P., and Pearson, J. F. Significance of the individual components of the Apgar score. *Br. J. Anaesth.* 45, 1973, p. 148.
21. Dawes, G. S. Revolutions and cyclical rhythms in prenatal life: Fetal respiratory movements rediscovered. *Pediatrics* 51, 1973, p. 965.
22. Evans, J. J. Prediction of respiratory distress syndrome by shake test on newborn gastric aspirate. *N. Engl. J. Med.* 292, 1975, p. 1113.
23. Florman, A. L., and Teubner, D. Enhancement of bacterial growth in amniotic fluid by meconium. *J. Pediatr.* 74, 1969, p. 111.
24. Fox, W. W., et al. The therapeutic application of end-expiratory pressure in the meconium aspiration syndrome. *Pediatrics* 56, 1975, p. 214.
25. Frantz, I. D., III, Wang, N. S., and Thach, B. Experimental meconium aspiration: Effects of glucocorticoid treatment. *J. Pediatr.* 86, 1975, p. 438.
26. Gersony, W. Persistence of fetal circulation: A commentary. *J. Pediatr.* 82, 1973, p. 1103.
27. Glass, L., Rajegowda, B. K., and Evans, H. D. Absence of respiratory distress syndrome in premature infants of heroin addicted mothers. *Lancet* 2, 1971, p. 685.
28. Gluck, L., and Kilovich, M. V. Lecithin sphingomyelin ratios in amniotic fluid in normal and abnormal pregnancies. *Am. J. Obstet. Gynecol.* 115, 1973, p. 539.
29. Gluck, L., et al. Diagnosis of the respiratory syndrome by amniocentesis. *Am. J. Obstet. Gynecol.* 109, 1971, p. 440.
30. Gluck, L., et al. Biochemical development of surface activity in mammalian lung. IV. Pulmonary lecithin synthesis in the human fetus and newborn and etiology of the respiratory distress syndrome. *Pediatr. Res.* 6, 1972, p. 81.
31. Graven, S. N., and Misenheimer, H. R. Respiratory distress syndrome and the high risk mother. *Am. J. Dis. Child.* 109, 1965, p. 489.
32. Gregory, G. A. Methods of neonatal respiratory assistance. *Br. J. Anaesth.* 45, (Suppl.), 1973, p. 806.

33. Gregory, G. A. Resuscitation of the newborn. *Anaesthesiology* 43, 1975, p. 225.
34. Gregory, G. A., et al. Meconium aspiration in infants—a prospective study. *J. Pediatr.* 85, 1974, p. 848.
35. Gregory, G. A., et al. Treatment of the idiopathic respiratory distress syndrome with continuous positive airway pressure. *N. Engl. J. Med.* 284, 1971, p. 1333.
36. Guilleminault, C., et al. Apneas during sleep in infants: Possible relationship with sudden infant death syndrome. *Science* 190, 1975, p. 677.
37. Gupta, J. M., and Tizard, J. P. M. Sequence of events in neonatal apnea. *Lancet* 2, 1967, p. 55.
38. Harrison, V. C., Heese, H. deV., and Klein, M. The significance of grunting in hyaline membrane disease. *Pediatrics* 41, 1968, p. 549.
39. Herman, S., and Reynolds, E. O. R. Methods for improving oxygenation in infants mechanically ventilated for severe hyaline membrane disease. *Arch. Dis. Child.* 48, 1973, p. 612.
40. Kattwinkel, J., et al. A device for administration of continuous positive airway pressure by the nasal route. *Pediatrics* 52, 1973, p. 131.
41. Kattwinkel, J., et al. Apnea of prematurity. *J. Pediatr.* 86, 1975, p. 488.
42. Klaus, M. H., Clements, J. A., and Havel, R. J. Composition of surface-active material isolated from beef lung. *Proc. Natl. Acad. Sci. U.S.A.* 47, 1961, p. 1958.
43. Klein, M. Asphyxia neonatorum caused by foaming. *Lancet* 1, 1972, p. 1089.
44. Kleinberg, F., Dong, L., and Phibbs, R. H. Caesarian section prevents placenta to infant transfusion despite delayed cord clamping. *Am. J. Obstet. Gynecol.* 121, 1975, p. 66.
45. Kornet, A. F., et al. Effects of waterbed flotation on premature infants: A pilot study. *Pediatrics* 56, 1975, p. 361.
46. Kotas, R. V. Accelerated pulmonary surfactant after intrauterine infection in the fetal rabbit. *Pediatrics* 51, 1973, p. 655.
47. Kuhns, L. R., et al. Diagnosis of pneumothorax or pneumomediastinum in the neonate by transillumination. *Pediatrics* 56, 1975, p. 355.
48. Landwirth, J. Continuous nasogastric infusion versus total intravenous alimentation. *J. Pediatr.* 81, 1972, p. 1037.
49. Leake, R. D., Gunther, R., and Sunshine, P. Perinatal aspiration syndrome: Its association with intrapartum events and anesthesia. *Am. J. Obstet. Gynecol.* 118, 1974, p. 271.
50. Levin, D. L., et al. Persistence of the fetal cardiopulmonary circulatory pathway: Survival of an infant after a prolonged course. *Pediatrics* 56, 1975, p. 58.
51. Liggins, G. C. Intravenous infusion of salbutamol in the management of premature labor. *J. Obstet. Gynaecol. Brit. Commonw.* 80, 1973, p. 29.
52. Liggins, G. C., and Howie, R. N. A controlled trial of antepartum glucocorticoid treatment for the prevention of respiratory distress syndrome in premature infants. *Pediatrics* 50, 1972, p. 515.
53. Lucey, J. F. The xanthine treatment of apnea of prematurity. *Pediatrics* 55, 1975, p. 584.
54. McCrann, D., Jr., and Schifrin, B. S. Fetal monitoring in high risk pregnancy. *Clinics Perinatol.* 1, 1974, p. 229.
55. Motoyama, E. K., et al. Adverse effect of maternal hyperventilation on the foetus. *Lancet* 1, 1966, p. 296.

56. Moylan, F. M. B., et al. Edema of the pulmonary interstitium in infants and children. *Pediatrics* 55, 1975, p. 783.
57. Myers, R. E. Two patterns of perinatal brain damage and their conditions of occurrence. *Am. J. Obstet. Gynecol.* 112, 1972, p. 246.
58. Neligan, G. A., and Russell, J. K. Anaemia of newborn following anterior placenta praevia. *Br. Med. J.* 1, 1955, p. 164.
59. Olson, M. The benign effects on rabbit lungs of the aspiration of water compared with 5% glucose or milk. *Pediatrics* 46, 1970, p. 538.
60. Perlstein, P. H., Edwards, N. K., and Sutherland, J. M. Apnea in premature infants and incubator air-temperature changes. *N. Engl. J. Med.* 282, 1970, p. 461.
61. Prod'hom, L. S. The Paediatric Aspect of Fetal Asphyxia: The Postasphyxia Syndrome. *Proceedings of the Second European Congress of Perinatal Medicine,* London, 1970, p. 131.
62. Raye, J. R., Gutberlet, R. L., and Stahlman, M. Symptomatic posthemorrhagic anemia in the newborn. *Pediatr. Clin. North Am.* 17, 1970, p. 401.
63. Rigatto, H., Brady, J. P., and de la Torre, V. R. Chemoreceptor reflexes in preterm infants. II. The effect of gestational and postnatal age on the ventilatory response to inhaled carbon dioxide. *Pediatrics* 55, 1975, p. 614.
64. Rigatto, H., de la Torre, V. R., and Cates, D. B. Hypoxia in preterm infants: Evidence for central respiratory depression. *Pediatr. Res.* 8, 1974, p. 450.
65. Schaffer, A. J., and Avery, M. E. *Diseases of the Newborn.* Philadelphia: Saunders, 1971, p. 75.
66. Shannon, D. C., et al. Prevention of apnea and bradycardia in low-birthweight infants. *Pediatrics* 55, 1975, p. 589.
67. Sherline, D. M., and Thompson, J. Continuous cardiac rate monitoring during resuscitation of the newborn infant. *Am. J. Obstet. Gynecol.* 116, 1973, p. 1166.
68. Steele, R. W., et al. Pneumothorax and pneumomediastinum in the newborn. *Radiology* 98, 1971, p. 629.
69. Sundell, H., et al. Studies on infants with type II respiratory distress syndrome. *J. Pediatr.* 78, 1971, p. 754.
70. Taeusch, H. W., Jr. Glucocorticoid prophylaxis for respiratory distress syndrome: A review of potential toxicity. *J. Pediatr.* 87, 1975, p. 617.
71. Thibeault, D. W., et al. Pulmonary interstitial emphysema, pneumomediastinum, and pneumothorax. *Am. J. Dis. Child.* 126, 1973, p. 611.
72. Tonkin, S. Sudden infant death syndrome: Hypothesis of causation. *Pediatrics* 55, 1975, p. 650.
73. Uauy, R., et al. Treatment with orally administered theophylline. *Pediatrics* 55, 1975, p. 595.
74. Usher, R. H., et al. Estimation of red blood cell volume in premature infants with and without respiratory distress syndrome. *Biol. Neonate* 26, 1975, p. 241.
75. Vidyasagar, D., et al. Assisted ventilation in infants with meconium aspiration syndrome. *Pediatrics* 56, 1975, p. 208.
76. Wells, D. H., and Zachman, R. D. Nasojejunal feedings in low-birth-weight infants. *J. Pediatr.* 87, 1975, p. 276.
77. Whitfield, C. R., Sproule, W. B., and Brudnell, M. The amniotic fluid lecithin-

sphingomyelin area ratio (LSAR) in pregnancies complicated by diabetes. *J. Obstet. Gynaecol. Br. Commonw.* 80, 1973, p. 918.

78. Wyszogrodski, I., et al. Release and inactivation of surfactant by hyperventilation: Conservation by end expiratory pressure in anaesthetized cats. *J. Appl. Physiol.* 38, 1975, p. 461.

79. Yao, A. C., and Lind, J. Placental transfusion. *Am. J. Dis. Child.* 127, 1974, p. 128.

80. Yu, V. Y. H., Liew, S. W., and Roberton, N. R. C. Pneumothorax in the newborn: Changing pattern. *Arch. Dis. Child.* 50, 1975, p. 449.

81. Zlatnik, F. J., and Fuchs, F. A controlled study of ethanol in threatened premature labor. *Am. J. Obstet. Gynecol.* 112, 1972, p. 610.

Therapeutic
Agents

4

Maurice S. Segal

Therapeutic Aerosols

19

The respiratory therapist can effectively treat bronchopulmonary disease, achieving both topical and systemic effects. Most therapeutic aerosols, like Janus of ancient Roman mythology, act (look) in two directions: forward, by means of the mucosal surfaces, and, in a sense, backward by means of absorption into the pulmonary circulation. No other organ is so easily disposed to provide comparable direct therapeutic access as the lungs, by means of the airways (ventilation) and the pulmonary blood perfusion relationships $(\dot{V}/\dot{Q})$. The ventilatory surface area of the adult pulmonary apparatus (65 square meters) is approximately 500 times larger than that of the external body surface. The great vascularity of this large area provides a remarkable absorptive and circulatory apparatus. It is thus possible, by means of the inhalatory route, to obtain high mucosal and submucosal concentrations of a drug introduced directly in the areas of pathology with appreciable blood levels for further systemic effects when needed.

Aerosols may be defined as relatively stable suspensions of liquids or solids in air, oxygen, or inert gases. The terms *nebulization therapy* and *aerosol therapy* are often used interchangeably. There are numerous factors involved in the determination of aerosol retention in the respiratory tract and their diffusion into the bloodstream: the particle size, type of nebulizer, type of respiration, degree of bronchospasm, aerodynamic factors, and the stability and surface tension of the aerosols themselves, to name but a few. The selection of the proper nebulizer for the production of aerosols is of primary importance. True nebulization, by a process of baffling, removes from the mist the larger particles, which cannot penetrate the lower respiratory tract. In general, small particles in the range of 0.5 up to 2.0 μ in size are more desirable for small airway effects. Atomizers deliver very large particles that are deposited largely in the oropharynx; hence they should not be used to deliver therapeutic aerosols.

In studies with the metabolic fate of aerosols, it was demonstrated, employing penicillin as a model, that approximately one-third of the nebulized aerosols, non-pressurized, was actually absorbed by the lungs, one-sixth was lost within the apparatus and the oropharynx, and almost one-half was lost into the air [20]. A study by Davies of the metabolic fate of pressurized aerosols of beta-adrenergic broncho-dilator drugs concluded that a large proportion (probably greater than 90 percent of the drug) administered from the canister is eventually swallowed. At least 50 percent of the dose is deposited in the mouth and pharynx, and a small proportion (less than 10 percent) of the dose reaches the airways, producing the rapid bronchodila-tion. The drug that is swallowed is absorbed too slowly to account for this effect. Furthermore, with many preparations, a large proportion of the swallowed drug is conjugated, O-methylated, probably in the lungs and in the gut wall during absorp-tion, and thus enters the circulation in an inactive form. Gut wall conjugation is important, for it permits the more desirable selective local-topical action by admin-istering the drug only into the airways [16].

Undesirable systemic effects with aerosols of isoproterenol and/or isoetharine, a part of any selective pharmacologic actions on beta 1 and/or beta 2 receptors, is avoided, for they (isoetharine to a lesser degree) are metabolized by O-methylation and conjugation in the lungs and gut, in contrast to the newer preparations, meta-proterenol, salbutamol, and terbutaline [16]. These newer drugs resist O-methyla-tion and are actually absorbed through the gut, demonstrating additional systemic beta-adrenergic functions, which may be undesirable. Hence, one advantage of aerosols of isoproterenol and isoetharine is the selective property of almost total airway deposition and effect, with less systemic effect via gastrointestinal absorp-tion [16]. As will be discussed, the most recent pressurized beclomethasone (ste-roid) aerosols are largely topical, and systemic absorption is kept to a minimum; this is a striking advance in steroid therapy.

A general classification of therapeutic aerosols includes the following (see Table 24-1): those employed as enzymes and steroids and as bronchodilator, bronchovaso-constrictor, antimicrobial, sputalytic, and humidifying agents; and those employed to maintain adequate surface tension. Of special interest are the (1) beta-adrenergic agonist, (2) anticholinergic, (3) prostaglandin, (4) cromolyn, and (5) steroid aero-sols. These will be discussed in detail below; see also Chapter 24.

BETA-ADRENERGIC AGONIST CATECHOL
AND NONCATECHOL AEROSOLS
The catecholamines as well as the noncatecholamines stimulate the alpha and/or beta adrenoreceptors. The catecholamines are substrates for catechol-O-methyl transferase (COMT) and hence are inactivated in the lungs and gut, whereas the non-

catecholamines are much longer acting, resisting degradation by COMT or by sulfatase enzymes in the gut.

1. Catecholamines
   a. Norepinephrine is the neurotransmitter of most sympathetic postganglionic fibers, is subject to COMT inactivation, and stimulates the physiologic receptors, mediating bronchovasoconstriction.
   b. Epinephrine, the major hormone of the adrenal medulla, stimulates both alpha and beta receptors, mediating bronchodilation.
   c. Isoproterenol (isoprenaline) stimulates both alpha and beta receptors, mediating bronchodilation.
   d. Isoetharine, a modification of isoproterenol, stimulates both alpha and beta receptors, with more selective (beta 2) bronchodilation.
   e. Rimiterol is similar to isoproterenol (not available in U.S.A.).
2. Noncatecholamines (not subject to COMT inactivation)
   a. A salinogen, salbutamol (Ventolin) (not available in U.S.A.)
   b. A resorcinol, orciprenaline, metaproterenol (Alupent, Metaprel)
   c. A resorcinol, terbutaline (Bricanyl)

These active noncatechol, beta-adrenergic agonists exhibit both beta 1 and beta 2 properties. However, it is believed that the principal effect of terbutaline and salbutamol are by means of their beta 2, bronchoselective properties.

The actual molecular structure determines to which physiologic receptor "hook" the pharmacologic mediator attaches. The larger molecules (orciprenaline, salbutamol, and terbutaline) attach more firmly, are more stable, and—unlike isoproterenol, isoetharine, and rimiterol—resist enzymatic degradation by COMT in the gut; hence they act longer and by mouth as well by aerosol.

Beta 1 receptors mediate the stimulation of cardiac muscle (cardioselective action). Hence, palpitations, tachycardia, and increase in cardiac output may occur as undesirable side effects.

Beta 2 receptors mediate the inhibition of bronchiolar smooth muscle contraction by beta agonists; they produce bronchodilation by means of the second messenger, the chemical cyclic $3'$, $5'$ adenosine monophosphate (cyclic AMP) mechanism. The science of chemical manipulation to alter molecular structures to attach onto the beta 2 receptors is the key in developing newer bronchodilator drugs. Hence, of these pharmacologic mediators, the beta 2 stimulators are the principal bronchodilators; however, other factors should aid the physician in the selection of one aerosol over another. The action of isoproterenol is effective promptly but is short-lived, whereas the action of salbutamol may not come on as rapidly but it lasts longer. Isoproterenol has the advantage, for example, in preventing exercise-induced asthma when administered 5 to 10 minutes before playing tennis or squash. Furthermore, the occurrence of tolerance, with loss of effectiveness, has been noted with the longer acting aerosols with repetitive dosing, e.g., orciprenaline. However,

Paterson et al. [49] also noted tolerance with isoprenaline aerosols, related to the metabolized beta-adrenergic blocking properties of the 3-methoxy-isoprenaline.

Both salbutamol and terbutaline tend to lower the diastolic pressure and also produce some tachycardia [29]. Salbutamol appears to have greater bronchoselectivity than cardioselectivity compared to metaproterenol [7, 57]. Salbutamol also appeared less likely to induce angina in asthmatic patients in the presence of ischemic heart disease [66]. Salbutamol should be employed in the asthma patient more susceptible to cardiac stimulants. The physician must decide what effect he desires and then select the appropriate aerosol. For routine use in asthma, the author finds the short-acting topical therapeutic aerosol isoproterenol preferable.

Recently in comparing the preventive beneficial effects of aerosol versus oral salbutamol, Anderson et al. [3] noted that only the aerosol effectively prevented exercise-induced bronchospasm in most asthma patients. Their patients attained higher values in peak expiratory flow rates (PEFR)15 minutes after 200 μg of aerosol salbutamol than 90 minutes after 4 mg of oral salbutamol. The aerosol apparently provided higher concentrations of salbutamol to the beta receptors on the bronchial smooth muscle, achieving mast cell membrane stabilization and thus preventing mast cell disruption.

The alpha adrenergics (e.g., phenylephrine used in combination with beta adrenergic aerosols) stimulate alpha adrenoreceptors, which mediate bronchovasoconstriction by (1) interfering with the enzyme adenyl cyclase in producing cyclic AMP, and (2) by increasing the production of cyclic guanosine monophosphate (cyclic GMP). The action of the alpha adrenergics is particularly significant when there is a disruption of beta function [4]. There appears to be agreement that the receptor for the beta adrenergics is membrane-bound adenyl cyclase, which mediates cyclic AMP and bronchodilation, whereas the receptor for the parasympathetic, acetylcholine (ACh) (see the following section, Anticholinergic Aerosols) is membrane bound to guanylate cyclase, which mediates cyclic GMP and bronchoconstriction. These two systems may play a see-saw effect in the control of bronchial tone. There is suggestive evidence that alpha adrenergic agonists may play a similar role to unopposed parasympathetic tone (acetylcholine) in mediating bronchoconstriction by means of the cyclic GMP mechanism [1, 48]. The therapeutic use of alpha adrenergic blockers and/or atropine analogues in severe resistive asthma should prove helpful if the latter theories are substantiated. In still another point of view, the maintenance of bronchomotor tone by vagal parasympathetic activity (acetylcholine) appeared greatly increased in asthmatic patients. Hence, beta adrenergic activity is needed to balance the bronchoconstriction. The harmful role of beta blockers would then enable more acetylcholine overactivity and bronchoconstriction [29].

Hazards of the Beta Adrenergic Aerosols

There has been considerable controversy concerning the use of pressurized bronchodilator nebulizers. Most asthma patients prefer the use of pressurized beta-adrenergic aerosol inhalers, for their relief from asthma is usually prompt and immediately available from pocket to hand. Abuse, however, soon may follow this easily developed psychological dependency. An epidemic of deaths in England and Wales between 1959 and 1966 occurred in young asthma patients from 5 to 34 years of age [57]. Most of the patients had used this technique excessively. The inhaler, sold over the counter, was said to deliver 400 µg per puff, several times the dose of most of the isoproterenol inhalers prescribed in the United States [59]. A review of the reports and subsequent studies would indicate (1) that the majority of deaths occurred because of failure of the patients to receive more appropriate medications, namely, theophylline and/or steroids; (2) that the patients were probably of the "asthma risk type," who are very susceptible to increased morbidity and mortality; and (3) that the toxicity from excessive concentrations and amounts of drugs inhaled could be explained by means of any of the following mechanisms:

a. Arrhythmias or cardiac arrest may occur secondary to the effects of the adrenergics or the fluorocarbons acting on a hypoxic myocardium very sensitive to the effects of the catecholamines. With normal usage, Dollery et al. [17] found the arterial concentrations of fluorocarbon to be only 20 percent of that which induced arrhythmias in dogs. However, it is conceivable that with excessive use in hypoxic patients, toxic myocardial levels could be reached [24].

b. Adrenergic aerosols with repeated use may be involved in toxicity. This is more likely to occur with the newer, longer-lasting adrenergics rather than with the short-acting isoproterenol. More severe asthma usually follows in the wake of repeated usage.

c. Actual blockade of the beta adrenergic receptors by a metabolite of isoproterenol, 3-methoxy-isoprenaline, produced in the bronchi, was proposed by Paterson et al. [49].

d. A "locked lung" syndrome, suggesting a form of beta blockade characterized by bronchospasm rather than by relief, has also been observed with excessive amounts of isoproterenol aerosols [52]. This syndrome has been attributed to idiosyncrasy by others [58].

e. Palmer and Diament [47] in 1967 reported that the paradoxical action of isoproterenol, promoting bronchodilation in well-ventilated segments of the lung with increased pulmonary perfusion in the underventilated portions of the lung (slow space), led to intrapulmonary shunting and arterial hypoxemia. A drop in arterial oxygen tension may be observed following administration of beta adrenergic aerosols. The drop in arterial oxygen tension is usually not significant. However, in severe asthma, when there is evidence of hypoxemia, these preparations should be used with great caution and then only with oxygen administration.

It is most likely that any or all of the above mechanisms can be interchangeably involved with the excessive use of any potent beta adrenergic aerosol, and depending on the age and underlying cardiac status of the asthma patient, will lead to increased morbidity or mortality.

ANTICHOLINERGIC AEROSOLS

Bronchial hyperactivity appears to be the common denominator in bronchial asthma. This condition follows exposure to allergens, numerous nonimmunologic factors, as well as an increased cholinergic autonomic activity associated with emotional stress, sleep, and other conditioned responses. Many nonimmunologic factors may trigger direct or reflex bronchoconstriction or act centrally on the efferent nervous pathways to the bronchi [43, 46, 70].

The role that the parasympathetic nervous system and its neurotransmitter acetylcholine might play in mediating bronchial tone, formerly extensively studied, then neglected for many years, has again come under consideration. The local hormonal function of acetylcholine (vagusstoff) has received limited attention: cholinergic impluses result in depolarization in most smooth muscles, leading to contraction [34]. Different pathways have been described for the control of bronchial tone in normal and asthmatic subjects by means of chemical immunologic mediators, beta adrenergic imbalance, the prostaglandins, the parasympathetic neurotransmitter acetylcholine, and reflex, nonreflex, and other (unknown) mechanisms.

The parasympathetic nervous system and reflex involvement in bronchial asthma were extensively studied in the first half of this century. Eppinger and Hess [19] (1909) described bronchial asthma as a condition with abnormal preponderance of vagal tone, "pathologic vagatonia." Kallos and Pagel [31] (1937) produced asthmatic paroxysms in guinea pigs with acetylcholine aerosols. Moll [42] (1940) reported severe bronchospasm, indistinguishable from spontaneous asthma, after subcutaneous injection of methacholine chloride (acetyl-beta-methylcholine chloride) in asthmatic subjects. Similar observations were made by other investigators [6, 13, 53].

Dale and Gaddum [15] (1930), observing isolated muscle contractures when the parasympathetic nerves were stimulated, proposed that the liberation of acetylcholine occurs in an anatomic area so close to the effector tissue that atropine is unable to exert its usual inhibitory effects. Such a mechanism may also be present in the bronchioles of certain types of asthma patients. Alternatively, one could conclude that bronchial asthma is not a phenomenon of parasympathetic imbalance. More recently Altounyan [2] demonstrated the protective effects of atropine aerosols, in what he considered the "reflex component" of histamine-induced bronchoconstriction. However, when asthma was induced by a "viral cold" one of his patients was not protected by atropine aerosols against what he defined as "the intrinsic muscular component."

Nadel [43] indicated that humoral and autonomic interactions play an important role in the regulation of airway smooth muscle tone. Stimulation of airway receptors reflexly results in potent bronchoconstriction by means of vagal nervous pathways. This may be observed following inhalation of such substances as dusts, chemical irritants, anesthetics, and low pH (acid) aerosols, and these manifestations may partially be abolished by vagotomy or by atropine [43, 55].

Vagus blockade with atropine or vagotomy has increased the anatomic dead space, has reduced airway resistance, and has increased the bronchial caliber [40, 41]. Nevertheless, the clinical course of patients with asthma was not improved by this approach. A return of interest in pharmacologic blockade of the parasympathetic nervous system in asthma followed the demonstration that the vagus nerve plays a role in acute antigen-induced asthma in dogs [22].

The relationship of cyclic AMP, the chemical mediator for bronchodilation, and cyclic GMP, the chemical mediator for bronchoconstriction, in influencing bronchial tone has come under extensive study. Cholinergic stimulation at the membrane site by the enzyme guanylate cyclase results in an increase in tissue concentrations of cyclic GMP [35]. Evidence has been presented that cyclic GMP activates cholinergic responses [18, 36]. Patel [48] demonstrated partial inhibition of the prostaglandin PGF_2 aerosol-induced bronchoconstriction by atropine sulfate aerosols in asthma patients. This is additional evidence that the PGF_2 effects are mediated through specific cholinergic receptors in the airways. Tiffeneau [65] had earlier demonstrated that the bronchoconstriction induced by cholinergic or vagal stimulation was grossly exaggerated in asthma.

Impressed by the notable similarities observed in spontaneous asthma and experimentally in methacholine chloride (Mecholyl)-induced asthma, Segal and his associates carried out studies in asthma patients on the effects of a series of anticholinergic drugs, first as protecting agents, and second as therapeutic aerosols, in relieving the bronchospasm and dyspnea of the asthmatic attack. Studies were made with the following alkaloids: atropine sulfate (racemic hyoscine); Bellafoline (mixed belladonna alkaloids); scopolamine hydrobromide (levohyoscine); Banthine (a quaternary ammonium derivative); and finally epoxymethamine bromide (methscopolamine bromide) (Pamine) [6, 25, 52]. These anticholinergic agents, administered by various routes, demonstrated excellent ability to protect against the bronchospastic effects of methacholine; however, they did not protect against the effects of histamine-induced bronchoconstriction.

The aerosols of Bellafoline, scopolamine, and methscopolamine bromide were particularly effective. Recognizing the changing events in the asthma patient, namely, bronchospasm, trapping of secretions, and inflammatory episodes, and the heterogeneity of patient responses, the therapeutic use of anticholinergic aerosols was suggested for the resistant types of bronchial asthma; the wet, sweating, hypotensive asthmatic patient who exhibits a systemic picture of parasympathetic stimulation (pathologic vagatonia); or in the epinephrine fast or beta blockade type of refractoriness. Aerosols of Pamine, 0.33 mg/ml, were particularly effective in demonstrating adequate and prolonged protection against the bronchospastic effects of intravenous methacholine, and in producing subjective relief from bronchospasm, correlated with significant improvement in vital capacity and maximal breathing capacity [52].

Nevertheless, the clinical use in asthma of aerosols of atropine, Bellafoline, scopolamine, and Banthine was limited because of anticholinergic side reactions, principally drying of the oropharynx, changes in sputum characteristics such as increased viscosity and reduced volume, increased heart rate, sedation, and, on rare occasion, blurred vision. They are contraindicated in patients with glaucoma or obstructive uropathy. The only side reactions observed with the aerosols of methscopolamine bromide was slight dryness of the oropharynx. The absence of cardiovascular side effects favored its use in asthma patients with labile vasomotor systems, hypertension, and tachycardia and cardiac disease, and in bronchospasm in patients with chronic pulmonary emphysema. The usefulness of Pamine aerosols for prolonged effects, combined with isoproterenol aerosols for their acute and short-lasting effects, was suggested. Further studies with antigen challenges demonstrated that intravenous atropine also gave significant and prolonged protection against dog and horse antigen in 3 trials in two asthma patients; however, no significant protection was noted against dust allergens in 3 trials in these patients [25].

The significance of the parasympathetic system in the mechanism of asthma received renewed interest by other investigators, demonstrating that atropine can prevent (1) antigen-induced bronchospasm in human subjects [72], (2) methacholine-induced bronchospasm [52], and (3) in some patients, exercise-induced bronchospasm [32]. The bronchodilator effects of atropine were further attributed to the inhibition of cholinergic, vagally mediated bronchospasm in series of animal studies [4, 21, 22, 28]. However, studies by Rosenthal et al. [50] demonstrated that atropine sulfate, though capable of blocking methacholine-induced bronchoconstriction, did not block antigen aerosol-induced bronchoconstriction. A different histamine-mediated pathway may have become involved in these studies.

Recent studies have appeared that focus on the therapeutic usefulness of atropine aerosols and an anticholinergic analogue (SCH 1000) Atrovent N-isopropyl nortropine methyl bromide, with comparisons to the beta adrenergic effects of isoproterenol. Cropp [12], recording physiologic data on large and small airway changes, noted that the therapeutic effects of atropine aerosols in children with perennial asthma were not significantly different from those of isoproterenol aerosols. Undesirable side effects were not observed from the atropine aerosols. Interest in the use of safer and less drying analogues of atropine have also appeared, employing the above-mentioned preparation SCH 1000 [3, 23, 32, 34, 35]. This preparation is said to have equal or greater bronchodilator activity than atropine, without atropine's side effects. The effects of SCH 1000 aerosols appear later and persist longer than those of isoproterenol [23]. The structure and beneficial effects with this atropine analogue appear identical to those reported in our previously discussed studies with methscopolamine bromide [52]. The combined usage of a short-acting beta-adrenergic aerosol with one of these atropine analogues was recommended in this earlier study.

In a recent study Klock et al. [33] found aerosols of 1 mg atropine sulfate useful and as effective as 1 mg isoproterenol aerosols in the improvement of pulmonary function values over a 1-hour period of observation in 15 patients with chronic bronchitis.

The quaternary tropine alkaloids deserve more attention in the control of bronchial asthma. Both scopolamine and atropine belong to a class called *tropane* alkaloids: Dr. Max Tishler stated that "The quaternary salts of atropine and scopolamine (atropine methobromide and scopolamine methobromide) have strikingly different pharmacological properties from those of their parents (atropine and scopolamine) since each is more polar and each has little or no CNS effects" and "it appears that the oxide ring in scopolamine may impart a very subtle (unknown) pharmacologic activity not seen in atropine" [66].

Methascopolamine bromide (Pamine) lacks the CNS actions of scopolamine, and furthermore, though less potent, provides more prolonged action than atropine.

The ideal anticholinergic aerosol should have preferential, acute, bronchoselective effects, be of short half-life and duration to avoid tolerance, and should remain subject to rapid enzymatic degradation to minimize any undesirable systemic effects. There is adequate evidence that such an anticholinergic aerosol would be effective in blocking the cholinergic, vagus-induced types of bronchoconstriction observed in many asthma patients. Furthermore, these aerosols should prove useful prior to endoscopic procedures in reducing secretions, blocking reflex bronchoconstriction, and preventing vagally induced changes in heart rate and rhythm in patients with hemodynamic instability.

PROSTAGLANDIN AEROSOLS

Prostaglandin research has been phenomenal, significant, and rapid: the reader is referred to an extensive critical review for its effects in asthma and other pulmonary disorders [45]. The prostaglandins (PG) are biologically active lipid substances (20 carbon hydroxy fatty acids, derivatives of prostanoic acid) that exert important physiologic roles in health and disease. They were first isolated from the seminal vesicle and plasma in the early 1930s. The lung, in addition to its primary respiratory function of oxygen and carbon dioxide exchange, plays an active metabolic role in the homeostasis of numerous humoral functions; one significant role is its involvement in the formation and inactivation of prostaglandins, albeit to a much lesser degree than semen.

The biologic function of the various prostaglandins varies extensively. The prostaglandins E_1 and E_2 exert vasodilator and bronchodilator actions [14], whereas the prostaglandins F_1 and F_2 are vaso- and bronchoconstrictors. Although controversial, it appears likely that PGE_1 and PGE_2 cause an increase in adenyl cyclase and subsequently the cyclic AMP responsible for bronchodilation, whereas PGF_2 causes a decrease in cyclic AMP, resulting in bronchoconstriction. However, the bronchodilator actions of the E prostaglandins do not appear to be beta receptor-mediated; hence, its "first messenger" route differs from that of the catecholamine isoproterenol. These (simplistically) reduced observations are based largely on small animal studies. In human subjects, the prostaglandins are more effective bronchodilator aerosols than isoproterenol, on a weight basis. However, when administered intravenously they have an extremely short half-life and are rapidly inactivated in the lungs.

The bronchodilator duration of effects of PGE_1 and isoproterenol appear similar; the response, however, is slower and the peak effect later in appearance (30 minutes) with PGE_1 than with isoproterenol. There is no further improvement when one is administered after the other. In view of the potent bronchoconstrictor action of $PGF_{2\alpha}$ and its increased release during the antigen-antibody reaction, it has been postulated that this compound serves as a major chemical mediator in the pathogenesis of bronchial asthma. The lability of the airways in the asthma patient is effected by the release of the prostaglandins.

Although the use of prostaglandin aerosols remains experimental in the United States, these aerosols hold much promise of expanding the therapeutician's armamentarium.

CROMOLYN SODIUM

Cromolyn sodium (Intal, Aarane) presents a significant therapeutic advance in management [11]. The micronized preparation is inhaled as an aerosol by means of a Spinhaler device. It is not an antiinflammatory, antihistamine, bronchodilator, or steroid substance, and furthermore it does not act by means of the cyclic AMP mechanism. It inhibits the disruption of the sensitized granulated mast cell, thus blocking the release of chemical mediators responsible for bronchoconstriction. Cromolyn sodium has proved quite effective in blocking the type I hypersensitivity reaction seen with pollens. Hence, it is an effective preventive in extrinsic (atopic) bronchial asthma, particularly as seen in children and the younger adult. It is of no value in the treatment of the acute attack or in status asthmaticus or in intrinsic nonatopic asthma. A nasal insufflator (Rynacrom) and nasal solution (Lomusol) employed for the prevention of allergic rhinitis in England are not presently available in the United States.

There is potential usefulness of sodium cromoglycate as demonstrated by its inhibitory effects in allergen-induced asthma and in the prevention of exercise-induced asthma.

CORTICOSTEROID AEROSOLS

The therapeutic use of the new steroid aerosols represents a significant advance in the therapy of patients with bronchial asthma. Recent evidence indicates that the use of the halogenated corticoids, beclomethasone dipropionate (Becotide), Vanceril, and betamethasone valerate (Bextasol), and triamcinolone acetonide [71] present selective topical effects with minimal absorption from the respiratory tract. They do not appear to suppress adrenal function, they present minimal hazards, and they provide a means for controlling mild bronchial asthma.

The aerosols can be administered by the nasal route (for allergic rhinitis) and by the pulmonary route for asthma. For the latter, the recommended dose is 100 μg 3 or 4 times a day, which is approximately equivalent to 5 mg prednisone. These aerosols also enable safe steroid withdrawal (weaning) programs and smaller (basic) oral doses in steroid-dependent asthma. Pulmonary function improvements have been observed in the second week of continuous steroid aerosol therapy. However, hoarseness, sore throat, and mouth, pharyngeal, and laryngeal *Candida albicans* or *Aspergillus niger* infections may occur, particularly with high dosages and continued use, but these may be prevented by strict oral hygiene, proper inhalation, the use of antifungal lozenges and/or amphotericin B gargles, and reduced daily dosages of 100 or 200 μg. Their excessive use must be avoided, for some systemic absorption may occur by swallowing, or through mucosal absorption mechanisms. Caution must be employed in patients susceptible to fungus infections such as those with bronchiectasis and blood dyscrasias.

The steroid aerosols may be ineffective during upper respiratory infections. McAllen et al., in careful studies in 120 patients with asthma followed for 12 months, obtained long-term control of asthma with maintenance dosages of 300 µg daily, in most instances. The incidence of oral candidiasis was 45 percent with the lower (400 mg) and 77 percent with the higher (800 µg) daily dosages [37]. Hodson et al. recorded the successful transfer of steroid-dependent patients receiving 10 mg (or the equivalent) or less of daily prednisone to beclomethasone dipropionate aerosols [27].

The use of betamethasone valerate (100 µg per puff), one puff every 6 hours, made it possible for one of us (M. S. S.) to very slowly change two patients from a program that had required daily steroids for several years. The patients had demonstrated severe steroid sequelae with cushingoid manifestations, cataracts, glaucoma, and purpura; several previous attempts at very gradual changeover to alternate-day therapy (ADT) with oral prednisolone had failed.

The use of steroid aerosols may be advisable for support on the "off" steroid days in the difficult alternate-day steroid patient. Enthusiasm for any new form of treatment must always be tempered with restraint, for there are very few miracle drugs. Nonetheless, steroid aerosols are assuming a proper and a prominent role in the treatment of stubborn asthma.

SUMMARY

It is clear that aerosol therapy (the inhalatory route) is a safe, effective method of drug delivery providing the advantage of selective local deposition and action with minimal or no systemic effects when given in proper dosage and properly employed. Pharmacologic manipulation, such as fluorinated steroids, allows for increased topical drug utilization. Continued exploration of this method of inhalation therapy holds much promise.

The principal pharmacologic agents presently employed for the relief of bronchospasm (namely, the adrenergics, xanthines, and steroids, as well as the newer E prostaglandins) accomplish this directly or indirectly via the production of cyclic AMP. The *adrenergics* act directly by stimulating the enzyme adenyl cyclase, which increases the intracellular cyclic AMP; the *methylxanthines* act indirectly, by inhibiting the enzyme phosphodiesterase and thus preventing the destruction of cyclic AMP; the *steroids* act indirectly, ultimately via methylation of norepinephrine to epinephrine in the adrenal medulla; and the *E prostaglandins* also act by stimulating the enzyme adenyl cyclase and the formation of cyclic AMP.

REFERENCES

1. Alston, W. C., Patel, R. K., and Kerr, J. W. Response of leucocyte adenyl cyclase to isoprenaline and effect of alpha-blocking drugs in extrinsic bronchial asthma. *Br. Med. J.* 1, 1974, p. 90.
2. Altounyan, R. E. C. Discussion of Howell, J. B. L. Asthma: A Clinical View.

Porter, R., and Birch, J. (eds.), *Identification of Asthma.* Ciba Foundation Study Group No. 38. Edinburgh and London: Churchill Livingstone, 1971. P. 160.

2a. Anderson, S. D., et al. Inhaled and oral salbutamol in exercise-induced asthma. *Am. Rev. Resp. Dis.* 114, 1976, p. 493.

3. Austen, K. R., et al. Generation and Release of Chemical Mediators of Immediate Hypersensitivity. In Brent, L., and Holborrow, J. (eds.), *Progress in Immunology.* Amsterdam: Excerpta Medica, 2, 1972, p. 61.

4. Aviado, D. M., and Salem, H. Basic Mechanisms of Bronchodilator and Antiasthmatic Drugs. In Weiss, E. B., and Segal, M. S. (eds.), *Bronchial Asthma: Mechanisms and Therapeutics.* Boston: Little, Brown, 1976, Chapter 50.

5. Axelrod, J., and Weinshelboum, R. Catecholamines. *N. Engl. J. Med.* 287, 1972, p. 237.

6. Beakey, J. F., et al. Evaluation of therapeutic substances employed for the relief of bronchospasm. III. Anticholinergic agents. *Ann. Allergy* 7, 1949, p. 113.

7. Brittain, R. T., Jack, D., and Ritchie, A. C.   Recent B-Adrenoceptor Stimulants. In Harper, N. J., and Simmonds, A. B. (eds.), *Advances in Drug Research.* London and New York: Academic, 1970.

8. Brown, H. M., Storey, G., and George, W. H. S.   A new steroid aerosol for the treatment of allergic asthma. *Br. Med. J.* 1, 1972, p. 585.

9. Claman, H. N. How corticosteroids work. *J. Allergy Clin. Immunol.* 55, 1975, p. 145.

10. Collins, J. V., et al. Intravenous corticosteroids in treatment of acute bronchial asthma. *Lancet* 2, 1970, p. 1047.

11. Cox, J. S. G. Disodium Cromoglycate (Cromolyn Sodium) in Bronchial Asthma. In Weiss, E. B., and Segal, M. S. (eds.), *Bronchial Asthma: Mechanisms and Therapeutics.* Boston: Little, Brown, 1976, Chapter 56.

12. Cropp, G. J. Effectiveness of atropine sulfate as a bronchodilator in asthmatic children. *J. Allergy Clin. Immunol.* 55, 1975, p. 98.

13. Curry, J. J. The action of histamine on the respiratory tract in normal and asthmatic subjects. *J. Clin. Invest.* 25, 1946, p. 785.

14. Cuthbert, M. F. Bronchodilator activity of aerosols of prostaglandins E_1 and E_2 in asthmatic subjects. *Proc. R. Soc. Med.* 64, 1971, p. 15.

15. Dale, H. H., and Gaddum, J. H. Reactions of denervated voluntary muscle and their bearing on the mode of action of parasympathetic and related nerves. *J. Physiol.* 70, 1930, p. 100.

16. Davies, D. S. Pharmachokinetics of Inhaled Drugs. In Burley, P. M., et al. (eds.), *Evaluation of Bronchodilator Drugs.* The Trust for Education and Research in Therapeutics. Folkestone, England: Parsons, 1974, p. 151.

17. Dollery, C. T., et al. Arterial blood levels of fluorocarbons in asthmatic patients following use of pressurized aerosols. *Clin. Pharmacol. Ther.* 15, 1973, p. 59.

18. Eichorn, J. H., Salzman, E. W., and Silen, W. Cyclic GMP responses in vivo to cholinergic stimulation of gastric mucosa. *Nature,* 248, 1974, p. 238.

19. Eppinger, H., and Hess, L. On the pathology of the vegetative nervous system. *Z. Klin. Med.* 67, p. 345; 68, p. 205; both 1909.

20. Gaensler, E. A., Beakey, J. F., and Segal, M. S. Pharmacodynamics of pulmo-

nary absorption in man. I. Aerosol and intratracheal penicillin. *Ann. Intern. Med.* 31, 1949, p. 582.

21. Gold, W. M. Cholinergic Pharmacology in Asthma. In Austen, K. F., and Lichtenstein, L. M. (eds.), *Asthma: Physiology, Immunopharmacology and Treatment.* New York: Academic, 1973.

22. Gold, W. M., Kessler, G. F., and Yu, D. Y. C. Role of vagus nerves in experimental asthma in allergic dogs. *J. Appl. Physiol.* 33, 1972, p. 719.

23. Gross, N. J. Sch 1000: A new anticholinergic bronchodilator. *Am. Rev. Respir. Dis.* 112, 1975, p. 823.

24. Harris, W. S. Toxic effects of aerosol propellants on the heart. *Arch. Intern. Med.* 131, 1973, p. 162.

25. Herschfus, J. A., et al. Evaluation of therapeutic substances employed for the relief of bronchial asthma. A review. *Int. Arch. Allergy Appl. Immunol.* 2, 1951, p. 97.

26. Herschfus, J. A., Bresnick, E., and Segal, M. S. Pulmonary function studies in bronchial asthma. I. In the control state. *Am. J. Med.* 14, 1953, p. 23; II. After treatment. *Am. J. Med.* 14, 1953, p. 34.

27. Hodson, M. E., et al. Beclomethasone dipropionate aerosol in asthma: Transfer of steroid-dependent asthmatic patients from oral prednisone to beclomethasone dipropionate aerosol. *Am. Rev. Respir. Dis.* 110, 1974, p. 403.

28. Islam, M. S., Melville, G. N., and Ulmer, W. T. Role of atropine in antagonizing the effect of 5-hydroxytryptamine on bronchial and pulmonary vascular systems. *Respiration* 31, 1974, p. 47.

29. Jack, D. Adrenoreceptors and bronchial asthma. *Scand. J. Respir. Dis.* (Suppl.), 89, 1974, p. 29.

30. Jones, R. S. Significance of effect of beta blockade on ventilator function in normal and asthmatic subjects. *Thorax,* 27, 1972, p. 572.

31. Kallos, P., and Pagel, W. Experimentelle Untersuchungen uber Asthma bronchiale. *Acta Med. Scand.* 91, 1937, p. 292.

32. Kiviloog, J. Bronchial reactivity to exercise and methocholine in bronchial asthma. *Scand. J. Respir. Dis.* 54, 1973, p. 347.

33. Klock, L. E., et al. A comparative study of atropine sulfate and isoproterenol hydrochloride in chronic bronchitis. *Am. Rev. Respir. Dis.* 112, 1975, p. 371.

34. Koelle, W. A., and Koelle, G. B. The localization of external or functional acetylcholinesterase at the synapses of autonomic ganglia. *J. Pharmacol. Exp. Ther.* 126, 1959, p. 1.

35. Kuo, J., et al. Cyclic nucleotide-dependent protein kinases. X. An assay method for measurement of guanosine $3',5'$ monophosphate in various biological materials and a study of agents regulating its levels in heart and brain. *J. Biol. Chem.* 247, 1972, p. 16.

36. Lewis, H. A., Douglas, J. S., and Bouhuys, A. Biphasic responses to guanosyl nucleotides into smooth muscle preparations. *J. Pharm. Pharmacol.* 25, 1973, p. 1011.

37. McAllen, M. K., Kochanowski, S. J., and Shaw, K. M. Steroid aerosols in asthma. An assessment of betamethasone valerate and a 12-month study of patient on maintenance treatment. *Br. Med. J.* 1, 1974, p. 171.

38. Melby, J. C. Systemic corticosteroid therapy: Pharmacology and endocrinolog-

ic considerations. *Ann. Intern. Med.* 81, 1974, p. 505.

39. Melby, J. C. Pituitary-Adrenal Function: Considerations in Asthma. In Weiss, E. B., and Segal, M. S. (eds.), *Bronchial Asthma: Mechanisms and Therapeutics.* Boston: Little, Brown, 1976, Chapter 52.

40. Middleton, E., Jr. The anatomical and biochemical basis of bronchial obstruction in asthma. *Ann. Intern. Med.* 62, 1965, p. 695.

41. Middleton, E., Jr., and Coffey, R. G. In Heinzelman, R. V. (ed.), *Annual Reports on Medicinal Chemistry.* New York: Academic, 1973.

42. Moll, H. H. The action of parasympathetic-mimetic drugs in asthma. *Q. J. Med.* 9, 1940, p. 229.

43. Nadel, J. A. Factors Influencing Airway Smooth Muscle. In Burley, P. M., et al. (eds.), *Evaluation of Bronchodilator Drugs.* The Trust for Education and Research in Therapeutics. Folkestone, England: Parsons, 1974, p. 11.

44. Nadel, J., and Widdicombe, J. G. Reflex effects of upper airway irritation on total lung resistance and blood pressure. *J. Appl. Physiol.* 17, 1962, p. 861.

45. Nakano, J., and Rodgers, R. L. The Prostaglandins: Biochemistry, Pathophysiology, and Clinical Pharmacology in Asthma and Other Lung Disorders. In Weiss, E. B., and Segal, M. S. (eds.), *Bronchial Asthma: Mechanisms and Therapeutics.* Boston: Little, Brown, 1976, Chapter 15.

46. Paintal, A. S. Vagal sensory receptors and their reflex effects. *Physiol. Rev.* 53, 1973, p. 159.

47. Palmer, K. H. V., and Diament, M. L. Hypoxemia in bronchial asthma. *Lancet,* 1, 1969, p. 318.

48. Patel, K. R. Atropine, sodium cromoglycate, and thymoxamine in PGF_2-induced bronchoconstriction in extrinsic asthma. *Br. Med. J.* 2, 1975, p. 360.

49. Paterson, J. W., et al. Isoprenaline resistance and the use of pressurized aerosols in asthma. *Lancet* 2, 1968, p. 426.

50. Rosenthal, R. R., et al. Effect of atropine on antigen-mediated bronchospasm. *J. Allergy Clin. Immunol.* 53, 1974, p. 73.

51. Roy, P., Day, L., and Sowton, E. Effect of new B-adrenergic blocking agent, atenolol (Tenormin), on pain frequency, trinitrin consumption, and exercise ability. *Br. Med. J.* 3, 1975, p. 195.

52. Salomon, A., Herschfus, J. A., and Segal, M. S. Aerosols of epoxytropine tropate methylbromide for the relief of bronchospasm. *Ann. Allergy* 13, 1955, p. 90.

53. Segal, M. S. *The Management of the Patient with Severe Bronchial Asthma.* Springfield, Ill.: Thomas, 1950.

54. Segal, M. S. Death in Bronchial Asthma. In Weiss, E. B., and Segal, M. S. (eds.), *Bronchial Asthma: Mechanisms and Therapeutics.* Boston: Little, Brown, 1976, Chapter 73.

55. Simonsson, B. G., Jacobs, F. M., and Nadel, J. A. Role of autonomic nervous system and the cough reflex in the increased responsiveness of airways in patients with obstructive airway disease. *J. Clin. Invest.* 48, 1967, p. 12.

56. Spector, S., and Ball, R. E., Jr. Bronchodilating effects of aerosolized Sch 1000 and atropine sulfate in asthmatics. *Chest* 68, 1975, p. 3.

57. Speizer, S. E. Epidemiology, Prevalence, and Mortality in Asthma. In Weiss, E. B., and Segal, M. S. (eds.), *Bronchial Asthma: Mechanisms and Therapeutics.* Boston: Little, Brown, 1976, Chapter 4.

58. Stanescu, D. C., and Teculescu, B. B. Exercise and cough-induced asthma. *Respiration* 27, 1970, p. 377.

59. Stolley, P. D. Asthma mortality. Why the United States was spared an epidemic of deaths due to asthma. *Am. Rev. Respir. Dis.* 105, 1972, p. 883.

60. Storms, W. W., et al. Aerosol Sch 1000, an anticholinergic bronchodilator. *Am. Rev. Respir. Dis.* 111, 1975, p. 419.

61. Sutherland, E. W., Robison, G. A., and Butcher, R. W. Some aspects of the biological role of adenosine 3′,5′-monophosphate (cyclic AMP). *Circulation* 37, 1968, p. 279.

62. Szentivanyi, A. The beta adrenergic theory of the atopic abnormality in bronchial asthma. *J. Allergy Clin. Immunol.* 42, 1968, p. 203.

63. Szentivanyi, A., and Fishel, C. W. The Beta-Adrenergic Theory and Cyclic AMP-Mediated Control Mechanisms in Human Asthma. In Weiss, E. B., and Segal, M. S. (eds.), *Bronchial Asthma: Mechanisms and Therapeutics.* Boston: Little, Brown, 1976, Chapter 10.

64. Thorn, G. W., and Lauler, D. P. Treatment Schedules with Steroids. In Weiss, E. B., and Segal, M. S. (eds.), *Bronchial Asthma: Mechanisms and Therapeutics.* Boston: Little, Brown, 1976, Chapter 53.

65. Tiffeneau, R. Hypersensibilité cholinergique histaminique pulmonaire de l'asthmatique. *Acta Allergol.* (Kbh) 12 (Suppl. 5), 1958, p. 187.

65a. Tishler, M. Personal Correspondence, Wesleyan University, June 24, 1976.

66. Turnbull, F. W. A. The treatment of asthma in the presence of ischaemic heart disease. *Postgrad. Med. J.* (Suppl.) 47, 1971, p. 81.

67. Ulmer, W. T. Inhalation therapy with atropine derivatives. *Med. Klin.* 66, 1971, p. 326.

68. Van Metre, T. E., Jr., and Lopez, A. Possible adverse effects of chlorpromazine and excessive isoproterenol in status asthmaticus. *J. Allergy Clin. Immunol.* 39, 1967, p. 109.

69. Vlagopoulos, T., et al. Abstract 74, American Academy of Allergy, Annual Meeting, Feb. 15–19, 1975, San Diego, Calif. Comparison of the onset of action and bronchodilation effects of the anticholinergic agent SCH 1000 with Isoproterenol. *J. Allergy Clin. Immunol.* 55, 1975, p. 99.

70. Widdicombe, J. G., and Sterling, G. M. The autonomic nervous system and breathing. *Arch. Intern. Med.* 126, 1970, p. 311.

71. Williams, M. H., Kane, C., and Shim, C. S. Treatment of asthma with triamcinolone acetonide delivered by aerosol. *Am. Rev. Respir. Dis.* 109, 1974, p. 538.

72. Yu, D. Y. C., Galant, S. P., and Gold, W. M. Inhibition of antigen-induced bronchoconstriction by atropine in asthmatic patients. *J. Appl. Physiol.* 32, 1972, p. 823.

Maurice S. Segal   **Methylxanthines**
                                    20

The group of drugs classified as the methylxanthines constitute the cornerstone of therapy in patients suffering from bronchospasm. Thus, all those involved in the care of patients with reversible airways obstruction must have an understanding of the metabolism, degradation, toxicity, and pharmacokinetics of the methylxanthines. If the respiratory therapist or nurse is able to recognize a toxic effect of aminophylline (e.g., tachyarrhythmia), then appropriate steps may be taken and a potentially life-threatening situation avoided.

Although the methylxanthines aroused initial clinical interest in the late nineteenth century, it was their use for the management of allergic reactions and status asthmaticus in the mid-1930s that gradually led to their present popularity. Many chemical derivatives of theophylline have been synthesized to alter or selectively improve certain properties, but none has shown significant advantages over aminophylline in producing the same biologic response as epinephrine in overcoming bronchospasm, by means of the cyclic AMP mechanism.

METABOLISM

The metabolism, degradation, and excretion of theophylline are very complex processes, with the liver largely responsible for its metabolism. Based on quantification of theophylline and metabolites after oral aminophylline, Jenne and associates suggested that 1-demethylation to 3-methylxanthine may be the principal metabolic determinant of ultimate serum theophylline. Of considerable interest, they also found significantly shorter serum half-lives of theophylline after bolus injection in healthy young smokers as compared with healthy nonsmokers, probably because of induction of theophylline metabolism by polycyclic hydrocarbons [22]. Thus variable theophylline metabolism makes it difficult to determine the exact dose requirements based on the predicted serum theophylline levels per dosage employed.

The metabolism of theophylline is also affected by common drugs, such as phenobarbital and allopurinol, that reduce the hepatic content of the oxidative microsomal enzymes essential to its degradation [65]. Furthermore, tolerance to theophylline will vary depending on metabolic rates that in turn change from time to time within the same individual. The therapeutic effect of the drug is generally closely related to its blood level.

AMINOPHYLLINE INTERACTIONS

Interactions of aminophylline with other drugs commonly used in asthma occur. These effects become accentuated, particularly in children and in the infirm, elderly, or cardiac patient [69]. Currently, studies are appearing on interactions between the methylxanthines and a number of hormones and other drugs. In vitro studies have demonstrated a synergistic relaxing effect of theophylline when administered with beta agonist catecholamines, and also a potentiation of the latter by some steroids [27].

Aminophylline potentiates the diuretic action of furosemide [37] and of the thiazides [9], and the cardiac effect of digitalis glycosides [9]. The author has observed severe cardiovascular effects (tachyarrhythmias) with the combined intravenous administration of mercurial diuretic agents and aminophylline in cardiac failure. Care should be taken to avoid the rapid reduction in serum potassium, with resulting weakness, cardiac arrest, or arrhythmias, that may occur when this drug is used with diuretics, a synergistic effect. The normal serum potassium and chloride levels must be maintained.

Antagonism may be observed with the beta-adrenergic receptor-blocking agents such as propranolol or the phenothiazines, with ganglionic blocking agents such as hexamethonium chloride, or with reserpine on the chronotropic actions of theophylline [57]. Serum lithium levels were decreased to ineffective ranges by the action of aminophylline in increasing the ratio of clearance of lithium-creatinine [8].

ACTIONS OF THEOPHYLLINE

Sutherland and his co-workers in 1957 discovered a new molecule, cyclic AMP, the intracellular mediator of the first messenger, epinephrine, as well as of other hormones. The highly beneficial bronchodilation effected by aminophylline in asthma patients probably occurs by means of the following actions: by an increase in the active cyclic $3', 5'$ adenosine monophosphate (cyclic AMP), by the smooth muscle relaxing substance (SMRS) [58, 59], and by inhibiting histamine release by the mast cells [40, 46].

Aminophylline inhibits phosphodiesterase, the enzyme responsible for converting the active $3', 5'$ cyclic AMP to the inactive cyclic AMP, thus indirectly increasing the concentration of the SMRS in the cells. The method of action of the xanthine pharmacologic mediators thus differs somewhat from the direct stimulation of the regulating agent cyclic AMP by such hormones as the catecholamines (beta agonists) and the newer E prostaglandins by means of beta-receptor adenyl cyclase interaction as well as from the more complex and indirect action of the steroids by means of the adrenal glands; thus it is believed that these pharmacologic mediators ultimately act by increasing intracellular levels of the common "second messenger" cyclic AMP. Although their routes in accomplishing relief in the asthma patient are different, they can be used in combination, and with potentiating effects. The comparable and synergistic biochemical mechanisms of the methylxanthines and catecholamines may be responsible for the potentiation of the cardiac inotropic and chronotropic effects of the catecholamines by means of the cyclic AMP mechanism [44].

TOXICITY

Theophylline has narrow margins of safety, particularly in small children, the infirm, and the elderly. Its half-life differs in children and adults; it is short, ranging from around 1.5 to 9.5 hours (mean, 3.6 hours) in children, and from 3.0 to 9.5 hours (mean, 4.5 hours) in adults [43], depending upon the number of doses administered, the variability of absorption and excretion, and other complex metabolic factors [12, 13, 20].

Because the potential of theophylline for toxicity is great, the patient's age, weight, and tolerance must be considered in order to individualize dosages, which may need to be changed from time to time in the same patient. Determination of blood and/or saliva theophylline levels is advisable to maintain proper therapeutic ranges when the patient does not respond to physiologic doses or if toxicity is manifested.

Side effects occur readily in those patients who tend to hyperreact even to minimal dosages. The more commonly observed side effects are anorexia, nausea, abdominal distress, vomiting, diaphoresis, excessive bronchorrhea, palpitations, tachycardia and a range of central nervous system effects such as irritability, hyperawareness, agitation, insomnia, and inability to concentrate. The production of mucus, with notable bronchorrhea, may be observed with high or increasing doses, indirectly as a result of its bronchodilatory effects mobilizing the trapped secretions.

Gastric and upper intestinal erosion with hematemesis, bleeding into stool, and hematuria have been observed as signs of severe toxicity that result more usually from intravenous overdosage. Aspiration, hypotension and collapse, cerebral seizures [72], respiratory arrest, circulatory failure, and acute dilatation of the heart may precede death [61]. Hyperventilation, mild hypoxemia, and cardiac irregularities and arrest have also been observed. With prolonged high dosages, the xanthines in general are nephrotoxic, particularly when administered with other potentially nephrotoxic drugs [8]. Aminophylline also increases coronary and renal blood flow and cardiac output, but decreases cerebral blood flow by constricting cerebral blood vessels [67]. Deaths have been observed in cardiac patients after rapid, intravenous, overconcentrated infusions of aminophylline [5, 50]. To fully understand the potential toxicity of aminophylline, one must also realize that it is a direct stimulator of the respiratory center [24], increasing its responsiveness to carbon dioxide [11, 16]. In the presence of hypoxemia, and particularly when associated with respiratory alkalosis, the respiratory-stimulating effects of intravenous aminophylline may result in cerebral seizures and contribute to mortality [20, 21, 38, 61, 72]. High theophylline concentrations, above 25 μg/ml, were observed in patients who developed grand mal seizures during intravenous theophylline therapy; these high levels were related to the following factors: high dosages; acutely ill patients with underlying severe pulmonary or cardiovascular disease, or both; and associated liver dysfunction slowing the rate of theophylline clearance [20, 21, 39, 72]. *In addition to the above factors, prior theophylline therapy must be considered before a loading dose is indiscriminately administered.*

PHARMACOKINETICS

In general, theophylline is well absorbed (unless compounded for slow release) and presents no bioavailability problems. About 60 percent is protein bound at therapeutic concentrations [25]. Its ultimate activity at the receptor site depends directly on distribution of the free drug into the interstitial fluid [68]. In patients with normal hematocrits, the whole blood concentration of theophylline is usually 55 percent of the serum or plasma concentration; 10 μg/ml in serum or plasma equals 5.5 μg/ml in whole blood [38].

The determination of serum-saliva levels of theophylline has confirmed the clinical impressions of the narrow margins of safety of theophylline, elucidated the reasons for therapeutic failures, and led to advisable guidelines for use of this drug. Unfortunately, fixed dosages cannot be used as exact guidelines for the individual tolerances or to achieve desirable blood levels. A rapid, specific measurement of serum theophylline, without concern about interference from other medications, was presented by Weinberger and Chidsey [71]. This procedure utilizes high pressure cation exchange chromatography, less cumbersome than the traditional Shack and Waxler methods [55]. High-pressure liquid chromatography assays have also been reported by others as specific and most accurate [56, 62].

As early as 1950, Truitt et al. noted that optimal therapeutic effects were achieved with blood levels of 5 μg/ml of theophylline [64], confirming the therapeutic dosage observations made by Segal and co-workers in their protection studies the previous year [48, 53]. More recently several investigators have correlated theophylline blood levels with intravenous dosages and suggested adequate and safe dosage regimens for short- and long-term therapeutic effects [21, 23, 26, 35, 36, 38].

In practice, it was recommended that adults receive an initial loading dose of 375 mg of aminophylline, followed by 1 gm intravenously every 24 hours, given intermittently or by slow continuous infusion, thus combining safety with optimum blood levels [38]. A dose of 5.6 mg per kilogram of body weight followed by infusion of 0.9 mg/kg/hour (21.6 mg/kg/24 hours) to achieve a blood level of 10 μg/ml is advised for moderately severe asthma; the recommended blood level may range up to 20 μg/ml for additional bronchodilation [23, 35, 36].

The periodic measurement of serum theophylline levels is very helpful in determining the bioavailability of the drug and the patient's individual pharmacokinetic pattern. The use of saliva theophylline levels, involving a noninvasive procedure easy to obtain (particularly in small children) and readily reproducible, has been suggested as a means of monitoring the patient on aminophylline [13, 14, 25, 29]. Both measures make it possible to avoid or minimize toxicity as an added hazard in the critically ill patient and others who are not responding adequately to conventional dosages.

Recently, Weinberger pointed out that at the frequently recommended pediatric dosage of 7 mg/kg, 25 percent of children can be expected to have peak serum concentrations in excess of 20 μg/ml and thus may be at risk of toxicity [68]. Eney and Goldstein also demonstrated the importance of serum and saliva theophylline levels in determining the reasons for therapeutic failures in ambulatory asthmatic children [14].

EFFECT ON PULMONARY FUNCTION

It is now recognized that the asthma patient in a relatively stable, asthma-free state of remission will nonetheless demonstrate pulmonary function abnormalities [4, 6, 28, 30, 48]. By means of pulmonary function studies the presence of latent bronchoconstriction in the completely recovered asthma-free state has been frequently demonstrated. Such patients usually benefit from a prophylactic regimen of oral and/or rectal aminophylline solutions [51, 54].

McFadden et al. demonstrated that objective and subjective signs of asthma, usually present when the one-second forced expiratory volume (FEV_1) was 30 percent of normal, were largely cleared when the FEV_1 improved to 50 percent of normal [30]. This is usually accomplished with the synergistic use of one or two inhalations of an effective beta-adrenergic bronchodilator aerosol, followed shortly by an intravenous dose in adults of 0.5 gm of aminophylline in 40 ml of distilled water, administered over a 20-minute period. However, a slow continuous (2 ml/min) infusion of 0.5 gm in 1 liter over an 8-hour period may be necessary in some patients.

Numerous studies have demonstrated significant improvement in pulmonary function parameters related to the concentration of theophylline in the plasma [32, 36, 38]. A linear relationship was observed between the degree of improvement of pulmonary function and the logarithm of theophylline plasma concentration in the 5 to 20 μg/ml range [36]. In 17 patients with chronic bronchial asthma, in a state of moderate bronchoconstriction, aminophylline 0.5 gm given intravenously produced marked improvement in pulmonary function. There was a decrease in residual volume and an increase in functional residual volume and inspiratory capacity; vital capacity and maximal breathing capacity improved, and intrapulmonary gas mixing became more effective [51].

In a more detailed study of a patient during an asthma-free interval, physiologic recording of intraarterial and intravenous pressures, esophageal pressures (for pulmonary compliance), and pneumotachograms of inspiratory and expiratory flow rates recorded a further and significant improvement when aminophylline 0.5 gm was given intravenously after recording the initial improvement from broncho-dilator aerosols [51].

In 20 patients with chronic pulmonary emphysema with known bronchospastic defects, intravenous administration of 0.5 gm of aminophylline produced an average improvement of 21 percent in vital capacity; an increase of 25 percent in the maximal breathing capacity; and decreases of 9 percent in the residual volume, 8.5 percent in the ratio of the residual volume to total lung capacity, and 39 percent in the index of intrapulmonary gas mixing. The improvement noted was comparable to that observed after inhalation of a bronchodilator aerosol [52].

Weinberger and Bronski [69] studied the effects of oral ephedrine and amino-phylline, alone and combined, in "low" and "high" doses, in 12 chronic asthmatic children. High oral doses of aminophylline (6.3 to 10.7 mg per kilogram of body weight) were associated with significant elevations in the pulmonary function values of peak flow rate (PFR), maximal flow rate (MFR), 1 second forced expiratory volume, (FEV_1), and forced vital capacity (FVC).

Palmer and Kelman [41] recently concluded that simple recording of values above 70 percent for FEV_1 and FEV_1-FVC ratio is not sufficient evidence for the absence of latent defects in asymptomatic asthmatics: they demonstrated arterial hypoxemia, hypocapnia, and lung hyperinflation in 35 patients with normal FEV_1-FVC ratios. This is not surprising, since air trapping, compliance, hyperinflation, and $\dot{V}\dot{Q}$ (ventilation-perfusion relationships) occur in the peripheral airways and their alveoli.

The simple spirometric studies of lung function, such as the FEV_1, reflect changes primarily in the caliber of the larger airways, whereas changes in the smaller peripheral airways (less than 2 mm in diameter)—which are responsible for less than one-fifth of the total airway resistance and conductance, or loss of contiguous lung parenchyma elastic recoil—can only be detected by more sophisticated techniques [41].

The physiologic reversibility of small airway disease (an early manifestation of chronic obstructive lung disease) is best recognized by employing tests that detect early involvement, as, for example, closing lung volumes, flow-volume loops, compliance studies, body plethysmography, gas exchange, forced expiratory flow rates, and maximal midexpiratory flow rates (MMEF) at selected time intervals.

In studies designed to detect the effect of theophylline on both central and peripheral airways, some effects on peripheral airways were noted at low dosage levels, and the investigators believed that low dosages given over a long period of time would be as effective as high dosages administered within a short time [26]. Nicholson and Chick [38], among others, demonstrated the beneficial effects of low dosages in 7 patients; airway response varied directly with plasma theophylline values. Bronchodilator effects were first observed at plasma levels as low as 4 μg/ml.

Piafsky and Ogilvie [43] correlated plasma theophylline concentrations and changes in FEV_1 function after administration of adequate amounts of oral and intravenous aminophylline. They noted improvement in adults of 17 percent (3 mg/kg every 6 hours) and 28 percent (6 mg/kg every 6 hours), respectively, with peak plasma levels of 7 and 14 μg/ml after oral dosages, and improvement of 29 to 85 percent with levels of 5 to 20 μg/ml after intravenous administration. These observations would confirm the desirability of around-the-clock aminophylline both orally and/or rectally in many patients with chronic bronchial asthma.

A mild reduction in the arterial oxygen tension has frequently been observed after the use of such pharmacologic agents as the beta adrenergic bronchodilator aerosols, subcutaneous epinephrine, and intravenous aminophylline. However, these reductions are usually insignificant, and are easily correctable with appropriate oxygen therapy.

EFFECT ON CIRCULATORY FUNCTION

Aminophylline has been employed for the management of patients with congestive heart failure, coronary artery disease, and cor pulmonale. Because of its direct action on the heart, it increases coronary blood flow, cardiac work, and output. However, its action is most remarkable in lowering peripheral resistance (more markedly in the pulmonary circulation than in the systemic) and in diminishing right atrial pressure. Aminophylline can also serve as a means of evaluating the degree of reversibility of pulmonary hypertension, with lack of response to this drug indicating a poor prognosis. Parker et al. [42] conducted a detailed study of the hemodynamic effects of aminophylline in chronic obstructive lung disease, and postulated that the decrease seen in pulmonary artery and systemic pressures was due to pulmonary and peripheral arteriolar dilatation.

It must be kept in mind that aminophylline has a direct effect on the cardiac pacemaker, as well as on releasing catecholamine from the adrenal glands [1, 2]. As a result, tachycardia and/or arrhythmias are fairly common, and arrest may occur with toxicity or in patients with underlying heart disease [7]. Recently, Scher and associates [47] studied the effects of bronchodilator agents in patients with chronic obstructive pulmonary disease and known cardiac arrhythmias. They observed no adverse effect on the arrhythmias after two puffs of isoproterenol aerosols. However, they noted worsened arrhythmias after administering intravenous as well as oral aminophylline compounds. As previously pointed out, there is a similarity between the cardiac effects (positive inotropic action) of the xanthines and of the catecholamines, probably by means of the cyclic AMP mechanism [44, 60]. Hence cardiac monitoring is advisable in such patients.

On the other hand, the same category of patients may benefit from the direct action of aminophylline upon the kidney. Renal plasma flow and glomerular filtration rate may be increased because of the hyperemia resulting both from the larger cardiac output and from direct kidney stimulation [15]. Furthermore, by inhibiting tubular resorption of sodium, aminophylline is a valuable physiologic tool in improving diuresis [66].

Severe side reaction and sudden death have been reported occasionally with use of theophyllines [5, 17, 31, 33, 34], probably because of direct cardiac stimulation and possibly too rapid injections with consequent local precipitation of alkaloids [46]. Camarata et al. [7] retrospectively implicated intravenous aminophylline administered over a 3-to-5 minute period (probably too rapidly) as the precipitating factor in 36 percent of cardiac arrests noted in their cardiovascular units.

METHODS OF ADMINISTRATION AND DOSAGES

The methylxanthines are best administered orally, rectally, or intravenously. Other routes—aerosol and intramuscular—are unreliable and not effective [50].

The aim with aminophylline is to achieve maximal therapeutic bronchodilation without severe side effects. The narrow safety margins, particularly in small children, elderly patients, and the infirm, must be respected. The author has observed the best effects in the chronic adult asthma patient, weighing relief against toxicity and its own therapeutic demands, when plasma theophylline levels 5 to 10 μg/ml were achieved with oral preparations or with solutions of rectal aminophylline administered largely around the clock. Because of variable absorption and excretion rates and brief but changing half-lives, therapeutic effectiveness, principally with intravenous aminophylline, is usually notable with the plasma theophylline level ranging between 10 and 20 μg/ml. Toxicity is usually noted above 20 μg/ml and becomes prominent above 25 μg/ml. Nevertheless, some side effects may be noted with levels above 10 μg/ml and in "sensitive" patients even below 10 μg/ml. Toxicity occurs more commonly in patients with underlying hepatic or cardiac disorders, delaying the metabolic degradation of theophylline. Careful pharmacokinetics are advisable with continuous intravenous therapy or when therapeutic "failures" with other routes are present. The author prefers in the 70-kg weight adult status asthmaticus patient, dosages of 0.25 to 0.5 gm per 1 liter of intravenous fluid, with slow flow rates of 2 ml/min, after a bolus of 0.25 in 20 ml has been delivered over a 20-minute period.

Oral Aminophylline

There are more than 100 oral medications containing the methylxanthines, their analogues, or similar derivatives, prepared alone or in combination with barbiturates, hydroxyzine, ephedrine, iodides, glyceryl guaiacolate, antihistamines, ethanol, etc. The exact amount (mg and/or %) of anhydrous theophylline base in the preparation should determine the specific dosage recommended as milligram per kilogram of body weight. Tablets of aminophylline usually contain 85% anhydrous theophylline and 15% ethylenediamine. With oral dosages of 4 to 10 mg/kg/6 hours (mean dose about 7 mg/kg), serum theophylline levels of 10 to 20 μg/ml were noted in children, probably indicating erratic variations of dose relationships to serum theophylline levels among patients [69, 70]. Similar observations previously made by Jenne and colleagues [23] in adults, demonstrating greater dosage requirements (up to 600 mg per dose every 6 hours), were explained as being caused by individual variations in metabolic degradation rates rather than to variable absorption rates of theophylline. *The margin between optimal dosage and toxicity may be narrow; periodic serum levels may be helpful during long-term therapy, but such determinations are not a practical substitute for sound clinical judgment.*

The value of barbiturates to offset the central nervous system- and cardiac-stimulating effects of the xanthines and/or ephedrine has also been questioned. One must remain suspect of toxic, allergic, and idiosyncratic reactions or drug interactions with combined preparations, caused by such substances as excipients, buffers, coloring dyes, and chemical preservatives. Nevertheless, the physician may find one or more of these preparations administered around the clock useful for the relief or prevention of mild or chronic, recurring simple bouts of bronchospasm. The problems noted with oral preparations have encouraged many physicians to employ the more effective technique of administering solutions of aminophylline rectally [3, 54].

Intravenous Aminophylline

Intravenous aminophylline is employed for severe paroxysms of coughing or wheezing, when relief has not been obtained by conventional epinephrine injection, beta adrenergic aerosols, and/or solutions of rectal aminophylline. For the acute attack that has persisted for less than 12 hours, 0.25 gm in 20 ml of distilled water administered over 10 minutes usually brings prompt relief. For the more protracted attack, the dose should be 0.5 gm in 200 ml distilled water administered slowly at a rate of 2 ml/min. These injections may be repeated at intervals of 8 or 12 hours. However, the continuous infusion technique is advisable for the status state. The exact dosages should be based on the patient's weight, previous response to aminophylline (manifestations of intolerance), and underlying cardiac disorders, particularly evidence of myocardial irritability or hepatic disease. In general for continuous infusions the author prefers to employ 0.25 to 0.5 gm aminophylline per liter of 5% dextrose in water or in half-strength normal saline solution [20, 50]. The choice of water, glucose, and/or saline infusion fluids depends on the serum electrolyte, cardiac, and renal status of the patient. The intravenous solution should be monitored at a 2 ml/min flow rate, thus assuring delivery of 1 liter every 8 hours or 3 liters in 24 hours. Initially, aminophylline 0.25 to 0.5 gm in 20 to 40 ml solution (priming dose), may be injected over 10 to 20 minutes, directly intravenously just as the continuous infusion is started.

Rectal Aminophylline

Suppositories of aminophylline are usually unreliable, because of variable absorption rates, rectal irritation and rejection, and toxicity to additives, particularly in infants and children. Furthermore, pediatric suppositories, in 250-mg doses, do not allow for accurate adjustment according to age/weight and individual tolerances, a critical need in view of the high incidence of toxicity in infants and small children. Many pediatricians recommend a dosage of 7 mg per kilogram of body weight every 8 hours. Effective theophylline blood levels were seldom reached after 0.5 gm suppository [10]. On the other hand, rectal solutions of aminophylline are readily absorbed via the rectal vascular plexus, reaching the pulmonary circulation [13, 43, 49]. The aminophylline does not enter the upper gastrointestinal tract and initially short-circuit the liver; thus it avoids some of the unpleasant GI tract side effects observed after oral aminophylline. The dosages can be accurately controlled and easily changed from time to time by dilution with water. This is particularly helpful in the management of infants, children, and others subject to aminophylline side effects.

Barach [3] recommended a rectal instillation of diluted aminophylline solution (300 mg/15 ml). The solutions can be administered at 5-, 8-, or 12-hour intervals, maintaining a continuous effective therapeutic level whenever indicated, with minimal patient discomfort. Many of our patients have been kept on similar programs with rectal aminophylline solutions, once or twice a day, for as long as 20 years with no demonstrable ill effects and with freedom from severe recurrent attacks. Other investigators have also reported effective clinical results with disposable plastic rectal units, employing similar dosages but in larger volumes — 25 to 38 ml [19, 45]. Considerable amounts may remain in these disposables. The large volumes are not well tolerated by some patients; retention failure and rectal distension, on occasion, may cause troublesome vagal reflex stimuli.

In an attempt to minimize the technical and aesthetic disadvantages of rectal administration the author has extensively studied the clinical effects of concentrated forms of aminophylline, correlating them to plasma blood levels; initially, with a compact plastic disposable unit, Rectalad (100 mg/ml) [63]; and more recently with Somophyllin, a solution form (60 mg/ml) [54]. Significant theophylline blood levels were achieved with 300-mg aminophylline dosages within 15 minutes, persisting for 6 hours and peaking at 5.6 μg/ml in 1 hour, thus explaining the clinical effectiveness of this valuable therapeutic aid for patients with bronchospasm, particularly when given at 6- to 12-hour intervals [54]. Bronchospastic crises have frequently been minimized and prevented. The patients soon become aware of their own dose requirements and acquire an added sense of personal security, with the assurance of an effective therapeutic agent on hand. The physical activities of many chronic asthma patients may be enhanced and exercise tolerance improved.

REFERENCES

1. Atuk, N. O. Intravenous aminophylline. *Lancet* 1, 1974, p. 1056.
2. Atuk, N. O., et al. Effect of aminophylline on urinary excretion of epinephrine and norepinephrine in man. *Circulation* 35, 1967, p. 745.
3. Barach, A. L. Rectal instillation of aminophylline in intractable asthma. *J.A.M.A.* 128, 1945, p. 589.
4. Beale, H. D., Fowler, W. S., and Comroe, J. H., Jr. Pulmonary function studies in 20 asthmatic patients in the symptom-free interval. *J. Allergy* 23, 1952, p. 1.
5. Bresnick, E., Woodard, W. K., and Sageman, C. G. Fatal reactions to intravenous administration of aminophylline. *J.A.M.A.* 136, 1948, p. 397.
6. Cade, J. F., and Pain, M. D. F. Pulmonary function during clinical remission of asthma. How reversible is asthma? *Aust. N. Z. J. Med.* 3, 1973, p. 545.
7. Camarata, S. J., et al. Cardiac arrest in the critically ill. I. A study of predisposing causes in 132 patients. *Circulation* 44, 1971, p. 688.
8. Cohen, S. N., and Armstrong, M. F. *Drug Interactions.* Baltimore: Williams & Wilkins, 1974, pp. 134, 307.
9. D'Arcy, P. F., and Griffin, J. P. *Iatrogenic Diseases.* London: Oxford University Press, 1972, pp. 16–18.
10. Dennison, A. D., Jr. Aminophylline suppositories effective? *Circulation* 12, 1955, p. 693.
11. Dowell, A. R., et al. Effect of aminophylline on respiratory-center sensitivity in Cheyne-Stokes respiration and in pulmonary emphysema. *N. Engl. J. Med.* 272, 1965, p. 1148.

12. Ellis, E. F. Bioavailability of theophylline. Presented at the 31st Annual Meeting of the American Academy of Allergy, San Diego, February 1975.

13. Ellis, E. F., Yalte, S. J., and Levy, G. Pharmacokinetics of theophylline in asthmatic children. *J. Allergy Clin. Immunol.* 53, 1974, p. 79.

14. Eney, R. C., and Goldstein, E. O. Compliance of chronic asthmatics with oral theophylline as measured by serum and salivary levels. Presented at the 31st Annual Meeting of the American Academy of Allergy, San Diego, February 1975.

15. Escher, D. J. W., et al. The effect of aminophylline on cardiac output and renal hemodynamics in man. *Fed. Proc.* 7, 1948, p. 31.

16. Galdston, M., and Myles, M. G. The use of aminophylline in respiratory depression and carbon dioxide retention induced by oxygen in patients with pulmonary emphysema. *Am. J. Med.* 33, 1962, p. 852.

17. Heaf, P. F. Deaths in asthma: A therapeutic misadventure? *Br. Med. Bull.* 26, 1970, p. 245.

18. Hirsch, S. Klinischer und experimentaller Beitrag zur krampflosenden Wirkung der Purindervate. *Klin, Wochenschr.* 1, 1922, p. 615.

19. Isaksson B., and Lindholm, B. Blood plasma level of different theophylline derivatives following parenteral, oral and rectal administration. *Acta Med. Scand.* 171, 1962, p. 33.

20. Jacobs, M. H., and Senior, R. M. Theophylline toxicity due to impaired theophylline degradation. *Am. Rev. Respir. Dis.* 110, 1974, p. 342.

21. Jacobs, M. H., Senior R. M., and Kessler, G. Clinical experience with theophylline: Relationships between dosage, serum levels and toxicity. *Am. Rev. Respir. Dis.* 109, 1974, p. 715. Abstract.

22. Jenne, J. W., et al. A possible metabolic basis for variation in serum theophylline concentrations and the effect of cigarette smoking on theophylline half-life. *Am. Rev. Respir. Dis.* 111, 1975, p. 898.

23. Jenne, J. W., et al. Pharmacokinetics of theophylline: Application to adjustment of the clinical dose of aminophylline. *Clin. Pharmacol. Ther.* 13, 1972, p. 349.

24. Jezek, V., et al. The effect of aminophylline on the respiration and pulmonary circulation. *Clin. Sci.* 39, 1970, p. 549.

25. Koysooko, R., Ellis, E. F., and Levy, G. Relationship between theophylline concentration in plasma and saliva of man. *Clin. Pharmacol. Ther.* 15, 1973, p. 454.

26. Lampton, L. M. Is a dose formula adequate to predict physiologic effects of intravenous theophylline? From text of presentation at the American Thoracic Society meeting, Cincinnati, May, 1974.

27. Lefcoe, N. M., Toogood, J. H., and Jones, T. In vitro pharmacologic studies of bronchodilator compounds, interactions and mechanisms. Presented at the 31st Annual Meeting of the American Academy of Allergy, San Diego, February 1975. Abstract.

28. Levine, G., Housely, E., MacLeod, P., and Macklem, P. T. Gas exchange abnormalities in mild bronchitis and asymptomatic asthma. *N. Engl. J. Med.* 282, 1970, p. 1277.

29. Levy, G., Ellis, E. F., and Koysooko, R. Indirect plasma-theophylline monitoring in asthmatic children by determination of theophylline concentration in saliva. *Pediatrics* 53, 1974, p. 873.

30. McFadden, E. R., Jr., Kiser, R., and DeGroot, W. J. Acute bronchial asthma. Relations between clinical and physiologic manifestations. *N. Engl. J. Med.* 299, 1973, p. 221.

31. McKee, M., and Haggerty, R. J. Aminophylline poisoning. *N. Engl. J. Med.* 256, 1957, p. 956.

32. Maselli, R., Casal, G. L., and Ellis, E. F. Pharmacologic effects of intravenously administered aminophylline in asthmatic children. *J. Ped.* 76, 1970, p. 777.

33. Merrill, G. A. Aminophylline deaths. *J.A.M.A.* 123, 1943, p. 115.

34. Messer, J. W., Peter, G. A., and Bennett, W. A. Causes of death and pathologic findings in 304 cases of bronchial asthma. *Dis. Chest* 39, 1960, p. 616.

35. Mitenko, P. A., and Ogilvie, R. I. Rapidly achieved plasma concentration plateaus, with observations on theophylline kinetics. *Clin. Pharmacol. Ther.* 13, 1972, p. 329.

36. Mitenko, P. A., and Ogilvie, R. I. Rational intravenous doses of theophylline. *N. Engl. J. Med.* 289, 1973, p. 600.

37. Moissev, V. S., Poliantseva, L. R., and Ermolenko, V. M. Klinicheskoe Izuchenie Novogo diuretika furzemida. (Clinical study of new diuretic furosemide.) *Soviet Med.* 30, 1967, p. 83. In Russian.

38. Nicholson, D. P., and Chick, T. W. A re-evaluation of parenteral aminophylline. *Am. Rev. Respir. Dis.* 108, 1973, p. 241.

39. Nicholson, D. P., and Chick, T. W. Theophylline toxicity due to impaired theophylline degradation. *N. Engl. J. Med.* 111, 1974, p. 240.

40. Orange, R. P., Austen, W. G., and Austen, K. F. Immunological release of histamine and slow-reacting substance of anaphylaxis from human lung. I. Modulation by agents influencing cellular levels of cyclic 3',5'-adenosine monophosphate. *J. Exp. Med.* 134 (Suppl.), 1971, p. 136.

41. Palmer, K. H. V., and Kelman, G. R. Pulmonary function in asthmatic patients in remission. *Br. Med. J.* 1, 1975, p. 485.

42. Parker, J. O., Kumar, K., and West, R. O. Hemodynamic effects of aminophylline in chronic obstructive lung disease. *Circulation* 35, 1967, p. 356.

43. Piafsky, K. M., and Ogilvie, R. I. Dosage of theophylline in bronchial asthma. *N. Engl. J. Med.* 393, 1975, p. 1218.

44. Rall, T. W., and West, T. C. The potentiation of cardiac inotropic responses to norepinephrine by theophylline. *J. Pharmacol. Exp. Ther.* 139, 1963, p. 269.

45. Ridolfo, A. A., and Kohlstaedt, K. G. A simplified method for rectal instillation of theophylline. *Am. J. Med. Sci.* 237, 1969, p. 585.

46. Ritchie, J. M. Central Nervous System Stimulants. II. The Xanthines. In Goodman, L. S., and Gilman, A. (eds.), *The Pharmacological Basis of Therapeutics.* (5th ed.). New York: Macmillan, 1975, p. 367.

47. Scher, S., Shim, C., and Williams, M. H., Jr. Effect of bronchodilation agents on arrhythmia. *Am. Rev. Respir. Dis.* 111, 1975, p. 897

48. Segal, M. S. *The Management of the Patient with Severe Bronchial Asthma.* Springfield, Ill.: Thomas, 1950, pp. 49–51.

49. Segal, M.S. The acute asthma attack. *Compr. Therapy* 2, 1976, p. 36.

50. Segal, M. S. Death in Bronchial Asthma. In Weiss, E. B., and Segal, M. S. (eds.), *Bronchial Asthma: Mechanisms and Therapeutics.* Boston: Little, Brown, 1976, Chapter 73.

51. Segal, M. S., and Attinger, E. O. Bronchial Asthma. Pathophysiology, Pulmo-

nary Function Tests and Therapeutic Aspects. In *Clinical Cardiopulmonary Physiology.* New York: Grune & Stratton, 1957.

52. Segal, M. S., and Dulfano, M. J. *Chronic Pulmonary Emphysema. Physiopathology and Treatment.* New York: Grune & Stratton, 1953.

53. Segal, M. S., et al. Evaluation of therapeutic substances employed for the relief of bronchospasm. VI. Aminophylline. *J. Clin. Invest.* 29, 1949, p. 1182.

54. Segal, M. S., and Weiss, E. B., with technical assistance of Cecilia Carta. Rectal aminophylline (blood levels with concentrated solutions). *Ann. Allergy* 29, 1971, p. 135.

55. Shack, J. A., and Waxler, S. H. An ultraviolet spectrophotometric method for the determination of theophylline and theobromine in blood and tissues. *J. Pharmacol.* 97, 1949, p. 283.

56. Sitar, D. S., et al. Analysis of plasma theophylline concentrations by high pressure liquid chromatograph. *Clin. Res.* 22, 1974, p. 726A.

57. Strubelt, O. The influence of reserpine hexamethonium, propranolol and adrenalectomy on the chronotropic actions of theophylline and caffeine. *Naunyn Schmeidebergs Arch. Pharmacol.* 261, 1976, p. 1968.

58. Sutherland, E. W., and Rall, T. W. The relation of adenosine-3′,5′-phosphate and phosphorylase to the action of catecholamines and other hormones. *Pharmacol. Rev.* 12, 1960, p. 265.

59. Sutherland, E. W., Robison, G. A., and Butcher, R. W. Some aspects of the biological role of adenosine 3′,5′-monophosphate (cyclic AMP). *Circulation* 37, 1968, p. 279.

60. Szentivanyi, A. The beta adrenergic theory of the atopic abnormality in bronchial asthma. *J. Allergy Clin. Immunol.* 42, 1968, p. 203.

61. Thiemes, C. H., and Haley, T. J. *Clinical Toxicology* (4th ed.). Philadelphia: Lea & Febiger, 1964.

62. Thompson, R. D., Nagasawa, H. T., and Jenne, J. W. Determination of theophylline and its metabolites in human urine and serum by high-pressure liquid chromatograph. *J. Lab. Clin. Med.* 84, 1974, p. 584.

63. Traverse, N., and Segal, M. S. Rectal aminophylline. *Ann. Allergy* 20, 1962, p. 182.

64. Truitt, E. G., Jr., McKuskick, V. A., and Krantz, J. C., Jr. Theophylline blood levels after oral, rectal and intravenous administration and correlation with diuretic action. *J. Pharmacol.* 100, 1950, p. 309.

65. Vessell, E. S., Passananti, G. T., and Greene, F. E. Impairment of drug metabolism in man by allopurinol and nortriptyline. *N. Engl. J. Med.* 283, 1970, p. 1484.

66. Vogl, A., and Esserman, P. Aminophylline as a supplement to mercurial diuretics in intractable congestive heart failure. *J.A.M.A.* 147, 1951, p. 625.

67. Wechsler, R. L., Kleiss, L. M., and Kety, S. S. The effects of intravenously administered aminophylline on cerebral circulation and metabolism in man. *J. Clin. Invest.* 29, 1950, p. 28.

68. Weinberger, M. Theophylline. Presented at Symposium on Asthma and Allergy, Denver, May 28–30, 1975.

69. Weinberger, M. M., and Bronsky, E. A. Evaluation of oral bronchodilator therapy in asthmatic children. *J. Ped.* 84, 1974, p. 421.

70. Weinberger, M. M., and Bronsky, E. A. Interaction of ephedrine and theophyl-

71. Weinberger, M., and Chidsey, C. Rapid specific measurement of serum theophylline. Presented at the 31st Meeting of the American Academy of Allergy, San Diego, February 1975.
72. Zwillich, C. W., et al. Theophylline-induced seizures in adults. *Ann. Intern. Med.* 82, 1975, p. 784.

Nursing
Care

5

Marsha Goodwin
Ellen Moloney Bergeron

Nursing Care of the Patient with Respiratory Disease

21

It is essential to utilize a coordinated team approach in the care of individuals with acute or chronic respiratory insufficiency. The physician, nurse, pulmonary therapist, and physical therapist must continuously assess the individual's status, confer on data, and together plan, implement, and evaluate the effectiveness of therapeutic measures.

The person's physical condition is the primary concern, but other factors must also be considered when formulating an individualized plan of care. One factor is anxiety, which is a common response to stress. Easily detectable signs of an anxiety reaction include diaphoresis, increased blood pressure, rapid pulse and respiratory rates, and dilatation of the pupils. Discrete effects of anxiety include increased release of epinephrine from the adrenal glands and increased peristaltic activity, producing anorexia, nausea, and abdominal cramps. Resistance to stress is reduced in the physically ill person, and exhaustion is imminent unless measures are taken to relieve the cause and/or effects of anxiety.

Another factor for consideration applies primarily to the individual with chronic respiratory disease. The chronicity of a disease has a definite impact on the life-style of the affected person. Certain activities of daily living may become increasingly difficult to perform. This situation can result in frustration and despair for the individual. Relationships with family members can become strained, and the person's frustration level can increase further. These psychological aspects of chronic disease will be of primary concern to the health team when establishing long-term plans for rehabilitation of the individual.

Quality nursing care is dependent on three assets of the nurse: (1) knowledge of the pathophysiologic changes that occur with acute or chronic pulmonary disease; (2) knowledge of scientific principles related to specific nursing approaches; and (3) ability to systematically assess the patient's status, and to plan, implement, and evaluate nursing care measures.

ASSESSMENT

Assessment is an essential step in the planning of both medical treatment and nursing care. The utilization of data obtained is the main difference between the two assessments. A medical diagnosis is derived from the assessment done by the physician. The focus of the nursing assessment is on patient needs. Is the patient able to meet his needs for food, activity, or self-esteem independently, or is satisfaction of one or more of these needs interfered with by his illness or hospitalization? The nursing diagnosis formulated from analysis of assessment data includes functional abilities and disabilities exhibited by the patient in activities of daily living. It is inevitable that overlap will occur in the medical and nursing assessments, but it should be kept to a minimum so that the patient does not become unduly fatigued.

Areas of priority in the nursing assessment will depend upon the patient's physical status on admission to the hospital. The initial assessment of the patient with acute respiratory failure will include vital signs, neurologic status, and respiratory function. Immediate medical and nursing intervention will follow until the patient's status has stabilized. A more extensive assessment will then be indicated.

The following method is appropriate for the patient with chronic pulmonary disease who is in no acute distress on admission to the hospital. The first part of the nursing assessment is concerned with obtaining data related to past history and present problems experienced by the patient. It is beneficial to identify the person, either patient or family member, from whom one is obtaining information in the initial interview, in the event that data obtained on subsequent interviews differs.

Questions regarding past history would derive the following data: (1) reason and length of any previous hospitalizations; (2) the person's reactions to hospitalizations, and (3) relationships between present illness and past illnesses. The nurse can help prevent some problems that have occurred during previous hospitalizations once he or she is aware of their nature. The nurse can also draw some conclusions concerning the chronicity of the patient's disease and his perceptions regarding his level of health.

The individual's perceptions of the present problem is the focus of the remaining interview. How does the patient's state of illness affect his life-style? What problems have resulted from the need to be hospitalized at the present time? Answers to these questions can give the nurse information regarding the degree of psychological stress the individual may be experiencing because of his illness and hospitalization. The individual with chronic lung disease often must adjust his life-style in order to deal with any limitations that have resulted from pathophysiologic changes. Knowledge of the patient's performance in each activity of daily living can give the nurse clues to determine whether or not the person is limited and, if so, whether he is coping with his disability. The nurse can also utilize the patient's pattern of daily living in planning nursing care to meet the individual's needs during hospitalization and upon discharge.

The nurse must be aware of the patient's priorities as the patient himself perceives them to ensure formulation of realistic goals for the patient. The patient's chief complaint may be a persistent cough that interferes with his activity level, whereas the nurse may perceive the problem as a persistent cough interfering with the patient's ability to sleep for an adequate period of time at night. This individual patient may very well be at least partially meeting his need for rest by modifying his daily routine to include periods of sleep.

A list of complaints expressed by the patient will be included in the nursing interview, and each complaint will be qualified. For example, the patient's complaint may be a cough. The nurse must inquire into the type of cough, i.e., productive, dry, constant; appearance and amount of sputum if the cough is productive; and precipitating factors. If the patient complains of shortness of breath, the nurse must determine if it occurs at rest, during sleep, or during activities of daily living. It is also important to know the effects of exercise on the degree of shortness of breath. The plan of care formulated for the patient will revolve around his tolerance of activity and need for rest. Aggravation of common symptoms may indicate need for revision of the nursing care plan.

The final part of the nursing interview directs questions concerning the patient's personal history as it relates to his disease. The information obtained will aid the nurse in identifying areas of correlation between past medical problems, environmental factors, and present condition requiring hospitalization. Factors such as smoking habits, known allergic reactions, exposure to pollutants in the work environment, history of tuberculosis, and previously diagnosed heart disease can have a bearing on the patient's present respiratory condition.

It is essential to know specific medications that the patient may have been taking at home and any form of pulmonary therapy such as intermittent positive pressure breathing or supplemental oxygen that he may have been utilizing prior to hospitalization. The individual may be quite familiar with pulmonary regimen, and he may have developed preferences that should be honored whenever possible while he is in the hospital. Conversely, the nurse may discover that the individual has incorrect information regarding medications or pulmonary therapies, identifying on admission an area for teaching and discharge planning.

Unusual behaviors exhibited by the individual can be detected by the observant nurse during the interview session. Increased use of facial muscles during respirations, creasing of the forehead with each breath, and telegraphic speech are three behaviors exhibited by the moderately dyspneic individual in his effort to compensate for low serum oxygen levels.

The patient's family can be very resourceful to the nurse in completing the behavioral assessment. It is important to ask the family members if they have noted any recent changes in the patient's behavior. Discrete, gradual changes in behavior can have a psychological or physiologic basis. Psychological reactions to real or perceived disability associated with a chronic illness are manifested in such behaviors as withdrawal or hostility. Physiological effects of hypoxia on brain tissue also manifest themselves in behavioral changes such as poor judgment and inappropriate responses to stimuli.

A record of the data obtained from the nursing interview should be a part of the patient's record and a summary included in the nursing record file.

The next area of the nursing assessment deals with essential data from physical examination of the patient. The lungs and thorax are thoroughly assessed by utilizing methods of inspection, palpation, percussion, and auscultation. Inspection of the chest includes observation of the patient's breathing rate, rhythm, depth, and symmetry of chest movements. Abnormalities in any or all of these areas may indicate need for immediate medical intervention.

Observing the degree of respiratory excursion, muscles used on inspiratory and expiratory phases of respiration, and the presence of retractions or splinting can give the nurse clues regarding the acuteness or chronicity of the patient's respiratory problem. The nurse also observes the patient for voluntary control of breathing. These data are important in analyzing the patient's need to learn breathing exercises.

Data obtained from palpation and percussion of the chest mainly give the nurse indications of pathophysiologic changes. For example, asymmetry of the chest noted on palpation can indicate pleural effusion or pneumothorax. Decrease in vocal fremitus over any area of either lung indicates decreased transmission of airway sounds. Pain experienced by the patient as one palpates each area of the chest may be indicative of inflammation or infection involving underlying structures. A dull or flat percussion note is heard over areas of the lung with atelectasis, pneumonia, pleural effusion, or a tumor mass.

Auscultation of the lungs requires knowledge of the location and characteristics of normal and of adventitious breath sounds, and the ability to discriminate between the two. Normal breath sounds include vesicular, bronchial, and bronchovesicular sounds. Vesicular sounds are heard normally over the entire lung surface except at areas of bone density. The inspiratory phase is louder and longer than the expiratory phase, which is almost silent. Bronchial sounds can be heard over the trachea near the suprasternal notch. Inspiration is short and expiration is louder and longer. Bronchial breath sounds heard over the lung fields may be indicative of consolidation. Bronchovesicular sounds may be heard in the major airways of the lungs such as the anterior second interspaces and in the posterior interscapular area. Inspiratory and expiratory sounds are loud and almost equal in duration.

Adventitious breath sounds include rales, rhonchi, and pleural friction rub. Fine rales heard at the very end of inspiration are indicative of moisture in smaller airways, whereas coarse rales heard at the beginning of inspiration are produced by accumulation of secretions in larger airways. Rhonchi result from the passage of air through a narrowed airway. They may be heard during both inspiration and expiration, but they are more noticeable on expiration. A pleural friction rub is heard during inspiration and expiration but is more prominent during inspiration. This sound is indicative of pleuritis.

Priority will be given to the affected areas of the patient's lungs when positioning him for maximum ventilation and when administering prescribed pulmonary therapy. Comparison of breath sounds before and after pulmonary therapy aids in evaluating the effectiveness of the treatment. Data obtained from this area of the assessment can be readily validated by conferring with the physician and respiratory therapist.

The heart, kidneys, brain, and skin are other body organs most frequently affected by pathophysiologic changes in the lungs. Specific abnormalities of these organs will be discussed in the remainder of the physical assessment.

Cardiac arrhythmias may occur concomitantly with an acute hypoxic state, and right-sided heart failure and cor pulmonale may develop as complications of chronic lung disease (see Chapter 15). Consequently, the patient's apical heart rate and rhythm, peripheral venous return, and fluid balance need to be assessed.

The patient's kidney function is assessed by monitoring his fluid intake and output and determining if any weight gain or loss has occurred. It is important to know if the person has been on diuretic therapy, which may predispose him to dehydration and deterioration of renal function. Decreased urinary output and elevated specific gravity of the urine can be indicative of dehydration.

Changes in blood gas levels can be noted in the assessment of the patient's neurologic status. Restlessness, agitation, anxiousness, and muscle irritability may be exhibited by the hypoxic patient. Increased carbon dioxide retention may severely alter behavioral patterns and judgment. Any change in neurologic status indicates the need for immediate nursing intervention for the safety and protection of the patient.

The patient's skin is thoroughly inspected for texture and turgor. Extreme dryness and loss of turgor, inconsistent with normal changes occurring with the aging process, are signs of dehydration. The nail beds and mucous membranes are assessed for the presence of cyanosis secondary to hypoxia. It should be noted that cyanosis is a late sign of the hypoxic state. Last, the patient's fingers are inspected for the presence of clubbing, which may be indicative of such conditions as bronchiectasis or cancer of the lung or of the pleura.

Any available diagnostic test results should be reviewed by the nurse and related to the signs and symptoms presented by the patient during the interview or physical examination. The physician ordering the diagnostic tests will usually include pulmonary function tests, chest radiography, arterial blood gas studies, complete blood count, serum electrolyte and blood urea nitrogen tests, electrocardiography, and the tuberculin skin test.

The serial blood gas study is the most discriminative test for diagnosing hypoxia and identifying the degree of respiratory insufficiency. Chest radiography and pulmonary function tests are very useful for planning pulmonary hygiene for the patient and for evaluating the effectiveness of therapy and medications. Abnormally increased hemoglobin and hematocrit can indicate the presence of secondary poly-

cythemia in the chronic patient, whereas increased hematocrit and normal hemoglobin levels can indicate dehydration. Increased eosinophil count would be
consistent with an atopic allergic reaction. Cardiac and renal involvement noted on
an electrocardiogram and by abnormalities in serum electrolytes and kidney function
tests are main considerations in planning the patient's diet, fluid intake, and
activity level.

The nurse analyzes the assessment data and formulates nursing diagnoses. A list
of patient problems is recorded in the nursing record file and in the nurse's progress notes. Appropriate nursing measures are then formulated for each patient
problem.

Continuation of the assessment process throughout hospitalization, along with
accurate recording, analyzing, and communicating of data obtained from that
assessment, are two of the most important responsibilities of the nurse. It is therefore obvious that a tool should be devised in obtaining essential data on a daily or
more frequent basis. Table 21-1 illustrates an assessment checklist designed with
three considerations in mind: (1) the inclusion of all areas essential to the nurse in
identifying changes in the patient's respiratory status and/or secondary complications; (2) a tool that will aid the nurse in systemic and efficient assessment of the
patient on a continuing basis; and (3) a record conducive to clear and concise documentation of assessment data and formulation of a patient profile.

PATIENT PROBLEMS AND PLANNED INTERVENTIONS

A patient problem can be defined for the purpose of planning nursing care as any
physical or psychosocial state that interferes with the individual's ability to meet
his universal needs independently and that necessitates therapeutic intervention.
In order to effectively utilize the patient problem approach, the nurse first must
have a clear understanding of the physical and behavioral characteristics of good
health, the universal needs of the individual, and the adaptive means used by the
individual in fulfilling these needs for the attainment and/or maintenance of
optimum health. Utilizing this basic, but broad, scientific knowledge as a standard
of reference, the nurse can analyze specific data obtained in the assessment of the
patient and accurately identify potential or actual patient problems.

In Table 21-2, a list is given of common problems occurring in the patient with
respiratory disease, the cause or predisposing factors, and the signs and symptoms
of each problem. Although the patient may not exhibit indications of any of these
problems during the initial assessment, the nurse needs to formulate a plan of care
that meets the objective of preventing such potential problems during hospitalization and after discharge. Systematic assessment of the patient and his condition
while in the hospital will aid the nurse in detecting early signs and symptoms of
actual problems that may occur despite preventative measures.

The nursing care plan is formulated by recording each identified problem, the
universal needs affected by the problem, and the nursing interventions that will
effectively correct the problem by reducing or eliminating interferences with need

Table 21-1. Daily Assessment Checklist

Name:			Date:			
				Time		
	8 a.m.	12 p.m.	4 p.m.	8 p.m.	12 a.m.	4 a.m.
Specific Respiratory Care						
Oxygen percentage						
Room air						
24%						
28%						
35%	✓	✓				
40%			✓		✓	
Above 40%						
Method						
Nasal	✓	✓				
Face mask			✓	✓		
Ventilator					✓	
Endotracheal tube					✓	
Tracheostomy						
Ventilator						
Rate					Assist	
Volume					900	
FIO_2					40%	
O_2 flow						
Initial peak pressure					30	
Nebulization						
Heated						
Unheated					✓	
Chest Physical Therapy						
Breathing exercises	✓	✓				

Table 21-1 *(continued)*

	8 a.m.	12 p.m.	4 p.m.	8 p.m.	12 a.m.	4 a.m.
			Time			
Postural drainage						
Percussion	√					
Frequency						
Tracheostomy care						
Suction						
Deflate cuff						
Deep breaths						
Change dressing						
Clean inner cannula						
Reposition endotracheal tube						
Respiratory Status						
Chest excursion						
Normal, full						
Limited	√					
Asymmetrical						
Cough						
Absent						
Productive	√					
Nonproductive		√				
Hacking						
Sputum: quantity						
Minimal						
Moderate	√					
Copious						
Sputum: color						

Table 21-1 *(continued)*

	Time					
	8 a.m.	12 p.m.	4 p.m.	8 p.m.	12 a.m.	4 a.m.
Clear						
Purulent	√					
Green						
Blood-tinged						
Sputum: consistency						
Thick	√					
Thin						
Breath sounds (P = present; A = absent)						
Rales (F = fine; M = medium; C = coarse)						
Rhonchi	√					
Pleural friction rub						
Laboratory Work (R = results obtained; D = test done)						
Chest film			D			
ECG		D				
Hematocrit		D	R			
Hemoglobin		D	R			
Na						
K						
Cl						
CO_2						
BUN						
Pulmonary functions						
Vital capacity		D				
FEV_1						

Table 21-1 *(continued)*

	Time					
	8 a.m.	12 p.m.	4 p.m.	8 p.m.	12 a.m.	4 a.m.
Sputum						
Urine						
Arterial blood gases	D	R				
Nursing Observations						
Daily weight	110 lb					
Bowel elimination				√		
Guiac hematest				+		
Fluid intake	⟶			1500 ml		
Fluid output	⟶			700 ml		
Diet						
Tolerated well	√		√			
Tolerated fairly well		√				
Tolerated poorly						
Vital signs						
Blood pressure	90/60					
Apical pulse	110					
Temperature (rectal)	99.6°F					
Respirations	28					
Neurologic Status						
Pupils	R					
Handgrasps	Good					
Footpress	Good					
Alert	√					
Oriented	√					
Semicomatose						
Comatose						

Table 21-2. Potential Problems of Patients with Respiratory Illness

Patient Problem	Causes or Predisposing Factors	Signs and Symptoms
Hypoxia, with or without hypercapnia, leading to respiratory failure.	Impaired ventilation Chronic airways obstruction Restrictive defects Neuromuscular defects Respiratory center damage or depression Impaired diffusion and gas exchange Ventilation-perfusion abnormality and venous admixture	PaO_2, 50 torr; $PaCO_2$, 50 torr; pH, 7.35 if condition is acute, near normal pH if condition is chronic *Early symptoms and signs:* restlessness, slight confusion, headache, hyperventilation, hypertension, tachycardia *Symptoms and signs of chronic hypoxia:* increased respiratory rate, increased red blood cell production (secondary polycythemia)
Extracellular fluid volume excess leading to circulatory overload	Excess infusion of saline solution Steroid therapy with sodium retention Cardiac failure, chronic kidney failure, liver disease, or cerebral damage	Weight gain; pitting edema; dyspnea; cough with production of frothy, pink-tinged sputum; sweating
Intracellular fluid deficit leading to dehydration	Inability to ingest adequate quantities of water Water loss from hyperventilation Hyperosmolar, high-protein feedings by mouth or tube without adequate water intake Impaired renal function	Normal or elevated serum sodium; specific gravity of urine > 1.030; hypoalbuminemia Thirst, poor skin turgor, dry skin and mucous membranes; pale, cool skin, elevated temperature; apprehension, restlessness
Protein and vitamin deficiency leading to malnutrition	Anorexia caused by aesthetic factors Psychological depression Gastric ulcer secondary to stress of illness	Hypoalbuminemia, low hemoglobin, weight loss, fatigue, anorexia, dehydration, nervous irritability, poor wound healing
Interruption in or lack of sleep, leading to deprivation	Constant auditory and visual sensory stimulation in immediate environment Symptomatology of respiratory disease (i.e., coughing, shortness of breath, paroxysmal nocturnal dyspnea) Psychological attitude toward disease manifested by fear, anxiety, or depression	Fatigue, emotional irritability, irrational behavior if awakened during rest periods, disorientation, decreased ability to concentrate
Loss of independence, leading to anxiety and depression	Addiction to modes of pulmonary hygiene Loss of productivity caused by effects of disease on life-style Need for frequent hospitalizations	Overdependence on hospital staff, uncooperative in rehabilitation process, angry or hostile if plan of care is altered or not carried out at scheduled time

fulfillment. Table 21-3 identifies general nursing interventions that may be implemented in assisting patients to meet their own needs, and provides the rationale for each nursing measure.

The following section is devoted to the nursing responsibilities involved in the implementation of an individualized plan of care for the patient with the identified problems resulting directly or indirectly from his respiratory pathophysiology.

NURSING RESPONSIBILITIES IN THE CARE OF THE PATIENT WITH RESPIRATORY FAILURE

The patient problem of respiratory failure challenges the basic and advanced practical skills of the professional nurse. Such nursing care centers around providing an optimal environment for external and internal respiration. Such an environment is based on (1) maintaining a patent airway, (2) oxygenation, (3) humidification, (4) ventilation, (5) communication, and (6) prevention of infection.

The Patent Airway

Maintenance of the patent airway is essential to life. Body defense mechanisms in the healthy person effectively remove mucous or foreign bodies from the tracheo-bronchial tree by means of coughing and deep breathing. When these mechanisms are depressed because of illness, the nurse must intervene to maintain airway patency.

The clinical condition of the patient indicates which technique to employ to prevent airway occlusion. A semicomatose and/or comatose patient may need only to be properly positioned on his side, with his head hyperextended to prevent the tongue from falling back into the oropharynx. An oropharyngeal airway may be implemented if necessary to keep the tongue in the proper position. Continuous assessment of this patient for adequate chest movement, auscultation of breath sounds, and examination of blood gas levels are necessary to evaluate the effectiveness of this method of treatment.

Despite the presence of a mechanical airway, abnormal breath sounds and abnormal blood gas levels indicate that further therapy is necessary. Because of depression of the cough and gag reflex, all mechanical means of stimulating coughing may fail, and the patient may have to be suctioned to clear the airway. Pharyngeal suctioning is necessary to remove accumulated secretions from the back of the throat. The procedure is done by inserting a suction catheter through the nose or the mouth and intermittently applying suction to remove the cause of obstruction. Oxygen should be administered after each attempt at suctioning. The need for deep tracheal suctioning is indicated by the presence of rhonchi on auscultation of breath sounds. Discretion must be used before, during, and after suctioning, for oxygen is removed from the lungs and vagal stimulation may cause arrhythmias and cardiac arrest.

Oxygen depletion and damage to the mucous membranes of the respiratory tract can be avoided by the use of proper equipment and technique. The maximum time for a single suction attempt is 5 to 8 seconds to avoid excess removal of oxygen. Patients having an arterial blood gas tension of less than 70 torr should not be suctioned without the availability of emergency equipment and supplemental

Table 21-3. Planned Nursing Interventions for Patient Problems

Patient Problem and Needs Affected	Objectives of Care and Nursing Interventions	Rationale

Respiratory failure affecting need for oxygen and carbon dioxide exchange in alveoli, cellular and tissue oxygenation, and acid-base balance	Maintain a patent airway
	  Schedule deep breathing and coughing exercises
	  Insert oropharyngeal airway if patient is not alert
	  Assist with endotracheal intubation, if indicated, and implement care (suctioning, oxygenation, etc.)
	  Tracheostomy care when indicated
		Obstruction of upper airway or tracheobronchial tree must be prevented or treated immediately to allow air to enter the lungs and carbon dioxide to be removed from the body

	Reestablish normal levels of blood gases and pH balance Selective administration of oxygen therapy according to arterial blood gases	Indiscriminate administration of oxygen to a patient who is hypoxic and is retaining carbon dioxide could worsen the patient's condition if respiratory center function is dependent on the hypoxic state
	Humidification of supplemental oxygen	Drying effect of oxygen can cause damage to the mucous membrane lining of the respiratory tract
Circulatory overload affecting need for fluid and electrolyte balance	Reestablish fluid and electrolyte balance Accurately monitor all prescribed infusion rates, with special attention to solutions with saline solution	Saline infusions must be given in amounts determined by laboratory electrolyte data and at a predetermined flow rate; the rate should be monitored very closely at night, when kidney function is decreased
	Assess effectiveness of prescribed diuretic therapy by recording daily weight and observing grossly visible fluid retention in body tissues	Weight gain is the most apparent indication of fluid retention, hence it should be observed at the same time each day and recorded for comparison purposes
	Maintain prescribed fluid and/or sodium dietary restrictions	Maintenance and patient teaching with regard to therapy are essential for treatment and prevention of recurrent fluid retention
	Reposition hourly, elevating dependent extremities and keeping head of bed elevated	To prevent skin breakdown resulting from retention of fluid in tissues; elevating head of bed reduces pulmonary congestion secondary to edema
Dehydration affecting need for fluid and electrolyte balance	Reestablish fluid and electrolyte balance Accurate observation and recording of fluid intake and output	The nurse must see that nasogastric or parenteral feeding is instituted immediately if the patient is unable to take fluids by mouth

Table 21-3 *(continued*

Patient Problem and Needs Affected	Objectives of Care and Nursing Interventions	Rationale
Malnutrition affecting need for tissue and organ integrity maintained by the ingestion, absorption, and metabolism of essential nutrients	Plan diet and scheduling of meals to ensure optimum nutrition Accurate dietary assessment and discussion of information with dietitian	Physical, cultural, and psychosocial factors influence one's dietary habits; by means of a diet history the patient's habits and his need for education can be identified
	Plan pulmonary treatments at least 1 hour before meals and follow therapy with mouth care	Effective therapy should improve the patient's respiratory status and thus reduce coughing and other, similar interferences with eating. Good oral hygiene will eliminate foul taste of expectorated sputum. Some mucolytic agents utilized in inhalation therapy are known to have a foul taste and odor, frequently a cause of nausea in the patient. Good oral hygiene, including rinsing the mouth with a fresh-tasting mouthwash, can reduce the aftereffect of treatment with these agents
	Record types and amounts of nutrients ingested at each meal	Record utilized to evaluate patient's nutritional status and need for supplemental feedings
	Create an environment that will enhance the patient's desire for food: Remove all distasteful distractions in the patient's immediate environment (e.g., soiled tissues, bedpans, spilled food on the tray)	An aesthetic environment is essential in preventing or eliminating such feelings as anorexia or nausea, which interfere with ingestion of food
Sleep deprivation affecting need for biologic rhythm of sleep activity to prepare the body and mind for waking activity	Provide environment conducive to sleep Plan care with alternating periods of rest and activity Coordinate therapies with other health care team members in order to allow for longer periods of uninterrupted sleep during the night	During each cycle of sleep, five distinct stages have been identified: stages I, II, III, IV, and rapid eye movement (REM) sleep. Certain bodily and psychic activities, including hormone release and dreams, occur during each stage. Each activity is felt to be essential in preparing the body and mind for functions of daily living. If sleep is interrupted or lost, the individual is unable to function adequately during waking hours

Table 21-3 (continued)

Patient Problem and Needs Affected	Objectives of Care and Nursing Interventions	Rationale
	Promote relaxation of the patient Assist with personal hygiene in evening before sleep Massage the patient's back Position in correct body alignment Tighten bedding under patient and loosen top bedding Provide warm beverage (e.g., milk or weak tea) Encourage patient to vent feelings	Measures that may be effective in reducing muscle tension and psychological tension in the patient
Anxiety and depression affecting need for independence in activities of daily living as well as the need for the self-actualizing process	Encourage optimal independence in the activities of daily living Plan activities such as hygiene and ambulating in accordance with the patient's tolerance for exercise Encourage the patient to identify and discuss, as he perceives, the limitations of his disease and his capabilities in activities of daily living Reinforce patient's participation in activities of daily living	It is necessary for the nurse to accept a patient's disability as he perceives it and to identify all capabilities as a basis for encouraging and reinforcing his rehabilitation toward an optimal state of well-being

oxygen. Use of intermittent suction prevents tearing of the membranes during catheter withdrawal. Following the suctioning procedure, breath sounds should be auscultated to determine the efficacy of the procedure. After elimination of loud rhonchi by suctioning, the presence of rales indicating fluid problems and the need for further therapy may be determined. Failure to clear the airway or improve arterial blood gases may indicate the need for intubation and perhaps mechanical ventilation. In order to avoid disaster, necessary equipment should be available at the bedside. Equipment should be checked at least every 8 hours to ensure that it is in good working order.

Nursing responsibilities during intubation include proper positioning of the patient, maintaining a patent airway through suction, and monitoring the patient's vital signs. Assistance of the respiratory therapist or another nurse will be necessary to assure that the patient is adequately oxygenated before, during, and after intubation. Following intubation, the nurse should listen for bilateral, equal breath sounds and observe the patient for adequate bilateral chest expansion to locate the position of the endotracheal tube. These clinical indications of a successful intubation should be immediately confirmed by chest x-ray picture. Nursing care of the patient following intubation revolves around maintenance of the tube in the proper position and maintenance of patency through proper suctioning technique. Particular attention must be paid to oral hygiene and the care of the skin so as to avoid the development of decubiti at the sides of the mouth.

Repositioning of the endotracheal tube should be done at least every 8 hours, or more frequently if pressure areas have developed. Assisted by another person, the nurse suctions the patient. After adequately evacuating the upper airway, the cuff is deflated. The tube is then moved to the opposite side of the mouth and the cuff reinflated. Tincture of benzoin may be used on the skin beneath the tube to keep the skin from breaking down. The tube must be securely tied in place and breath sounds checked before the procedure is considered completed.

An area of pressure not so apparent, but of utmost importance, is the area of contact between the trachea and the endotracheal balloon. Necrosis of the trachea at this site leads to postintubation tracheal stenosis and malacia (see Chapter 13).

The endotracheal balloon, or cuff, should be inflated with the least amount of air required to achieve desired results. Cuff pressures should be maintained at well below 25 torr. The cuff should be deflated at least once an hour and the same amount of air reinserted as is withdrawn. A record of the amount of air required to seal the trachea should be kept from hour to hour. A need for an increase in the amount of air should be investigated, for it could indicate leakage in the balloon or damage to the trachea. Particular attention to the endotracheal tube and the routine of care is needed to provide safe, uncomplicated recovery of the patient.

Because of certain medical conditions, or at the discretion of the physician, a tracheotomy may be performed to gain access to the airway. This strictly sterile procedure is usually performed in the operating room, but it may be done at the bedside in an emergency situation. Because of the presence of a surgical incision, and the insertion of a foreign body into the sterile airway, utmost care must be taken to observe the principles of asepsis during suctioning and changing of the tracheostomy tube and dressing. The complications of tracheal stenosis and malacia are related to infection and necrosis of the trachea, and they can be effectively avoided by proper care of the tracheostomy tube and stoma site.

The routine of tracheostomy care, especially cuff inflation and deflation, should be strictly and uniformly adhered to. Unless the patient requires positive pressure ventilation, the cuff may remain deflated at all times. Once inflated, however, it should be deflated at least once an hour. If the oropharynx is properly suctioned prior to deflation of the cuff, it may or may not be necessary to suction by means of the tracheostomy tube. Suctioning should be done only when secretions are present so as to minimize trauma to the tracheobronchial tree.

At least every 4 hours, and as necessary, the inner cannula should be removed and cleaned. At this time, also, the tracheostomy site should be cleaned with a sterile solution and a sterile gauze dressing applied. Redness or drainage at the stoma site should be immediately reported.

Patient and understanding care is the key to helping the patient cope with the inherent frustrations of intubation. Inability to communicate basic needs gives rise to feelings of anxiety and frustration. With the cooperation of the nurse and other team members, the patient can devise effective methods of communication. Careful explanation of procedures and, in the case of tracheotomy, constant reinforcement of the ideas that this tube is a temporary situation, and that upon removal of the tube the patient will assume normal functions of talking and eating, are helpful both to the patient and to his family.

Oxygenation
Once the patent airway is established, it must be decided if the patient needs supplemental oxygen and in what specific concentrations. These decisions are based upon results obtained by means of arterial blood gas tests and examination of the clinical condition of the patient. Prior to establishing the patient's premorbid status and receiving definitive blood gas results, oxygen should be administered only in controlled low-flow rates to prevent complications of hypercapnia and acidosis occurring in some patients who are sensitive to oxygen.

The efficacy of the oxygen concentration in use must be checked frequently through serial arterial blood samples. The inspiratory oxygen concentration can be adjusted until the results closely approximate those considered normal or therapeutic for the patient. Disturbances in the oxygen transport system, as in anemia or perfusion and/or diffusion abnormalities, will become apparent if increasing concentrations of oxygen have little or no effect on blood gas levels. Efforts must then be taken to correct the primary problem and then adjustments made of the oxygen concentration accordingly. Increasing percentages of oxygen should never be given indiscriminately.

Nurses and others concerned with the oxygen needs of the patient must have a sound understanding of the physiology and the pathophysiology of respiratory disease in order to effectively administer oxygen therapy. Constant checking of oxygen settings on the machinery to prevent mechanical errors is the responsibility of nurses and therapists. Proper care demands intelligent observation and prompt reporting of effects and side effects of therapy to provide safe, expeditious care.

Humidification
Compressed room air, or oxygen, should be humidified before being directly administered to the patient. This procedure is especially important in the intubated patient with either an endotracheal or a tracheostomy tube, as normal humidifying passageways of the nose and mouth are bypassed. Prevention of drying of the mucous membranes of the nose and the throat is necessary to prevent cracking and infection of the membranes of the respiratory tract. Adequate humidification also prevents crusting of secretions, which leads to occlusion of the airway.

The nurse maintains a moist environment by providing close-fitting face or tracheostomy masks as well as making certain that water reservoirs are full and equipment is functioning properly. A constant, fine mist emanating from a humidifier confirms proper functioning of the machinery. The humidifier chamber must always be kept full above the warning line and functioning properly, for the introduction of dry, pressurized air to the lungs can cause inspissation of secretions.

Ventilation

Despite medical and nursing interventions to provide adequate pulmonary ventilation, there are instances when mechanical devices will necessarily be employed to establish adequate oxygenation and alveolar ventilation. There are various types of mechanical ventilators. The physician chooses the type of ventilator most suited to the needs of the patient. Individual needs are continually assessed and the machinery adjusted accordingly. Serial arterial blood gas tests will determine the efficacy of treatment or indicate need for changes.

The psychological needs of the patient requiring mechanical ventilation are as great as his independence and ability to communicate his basic needs are limited. Meeting the psychological needs, primarily by means of adequate and supportive explanation, will gain the confidence of the patient and eliminate mechanical problems that arise because of anxiety. Fear of the machinery can render the machine ineffective by causing the patient to breathe "out of phase."

Comprehensive nursing care and meticulous attention to basic nursing skills preclude preoccupation with machines. The nurse who is secure in the environment of machines uses them merely as tools to provide complete and safe care. The whole patient must be nursed or the machine will have little or no effect.

The routine care requires that the patient be turned hourly to provide adequate ventilation of all lung fields. Suctioning, deflation of the cuff, monitoring of vital signs, and checking of equipment must be done on at least an hourly basis. An intelligent, organized approach should be implemented to provide both maximum care and comfort for the patient.

Communication

Because of the patient's limited ability to express his feelings and anxieties, the nurse must take great care to anticipate his needs and reinforce the fact that the medical procedures undertaken are helping him to get well. A pad of paper or a drawing board can be used so the patient can write out his requests. Various signals can be devised to minimize frustration for both the patient and the nurse. It is amazing how little time it takes to communicate with these patients once rapport has been established and the patient feels relaxed and confident with those who are caring for him.

Prevention of Bronchopulmonary Infection

Seriously ill and debilitated patients must be protected from incurring infections while in the hospital. Because of decreased resistance, they are particularly susceptible to the many pathogens in the hospital environment. Careful personal hygiene and proper use of equipment minimizes the transmission of infection through cross-contamination. The nurse must see that all personnel are aware of hospital infection control procedures and that they follow these procedures strictly. Aseptic technique should be constantly enforced in the areas of suctioning, dressing change, and isolation.

Proper collection of specimens for laboratory examination must be done on a routine basis, especially after antibiotic therapy is begun. Positive cultures should be immediately reported to the physician.

NURSING RESPONSIBILITIES IN THE CARE OF THE PATIENT WITH A PROBLEM OF FLUID AND ELECTROLYTE IMBALANCE

The two imbalances occurring most frequently in the patient with chronic pulmonary disease are circulatory overload and dehydration. The nursing responsibilities in both of these problems can be discussed concurrently, because the plan of care for each patient is formulated to meet a unified objective.

In order to effectively implement the interventions listed in Table 21-3, the nurse must (1) accurately assess the patient, including review of his serum electrolyte levels; (2) closely monitor the type and amount of all fluid intake; and (3) analytically compare the patient's total daily fluid intake and fluid output.

The nurse's responsibility in this ongoing process, assessment-monitoring-evaluation, is emphasized for two reasons. First, the chronicity of the patient's respiratory condition, the pathophysiologic changes that result, and the aspects of the treatment necessary for maintenance of optimal health together predispose the patient to the complication of fluid and electrolyte imbalance. Second, it can be difficult to rid the body of excess water in conditions of fluid overload without causing a fluid deficit and electrolyte imbalance. The reverse of this is also true. In essence, the effective management of the problem is dependent on several factors, including adequate cardiac, renal, and endocrine function.

The key members of the health team responsible for the detection and effective treatment of fluid and electrolyte imbalances are the physician and the nurse, who should cooperatively assess, plan, implement, and evaluate the patient and his condition.

NURSING RESPONSIBILITIES IN THE CARE OF THE PATIENT WITH NUTRITIONAL DEFICIENCIES

Nutritional problems or deficiencies are not always apparent in the hospitalized patient. It is in the taking of a nursing or dietary history that many problems are brought to light. The physical, emotional, and psychosocial aspects of nutrition must be understood to properly tailor nutritional care to the individual patient.

Because tissue and organ integrity is essential to combat skin breakdown, decubitus ulcers, infection, and negative nitrogen balance, immediate diet therapy must be instituted to restore or maintain optimal nutritional status. Continual assessment of the patient's physical condition will determine the type of diet that the patient requires. Rapid progression from intravenous feedings to a normal complete diet is best for the physical and emotional wellbeing of the patient. In every category of feeding—parenteral, nasogastric, or oral—there are different types of feedings and foods that are suitable to the needs of the patient (Table 21-4). The specific needs of the patient as regards calories, nutrients, vitamins, fluid, and

Table 21-4. Progressive Nutritional Plan

Feedings	Nutritional Content	Comment
Intravenous Feedings		
5% dextrose	Lacks large amounts of nitrogen, vitamins, calories, and minerals	Should not be on this alone any longer than needed
Hyperalimentation solutions	Contains large amounts of nitrogen, vitamins, calories, and electrolytes	Fluid intake and oxygen, daily weights, electrolytes, glucose levels, urine sugars, and infusion must be controlled exactly to prevent hyperosmolar overload. Aseptic technique is essential to prevent fungal infections
Nasogastric Tube Feedings		
Compleat-B (Doyle) Ensure (Ross)	All contain 1,000 cal/1,000 ml; lowest in sodium and potassium	All are nutritionally balanced diets available in liquid form
Isocal Complete Liquid Diet (Mead Johnson) Meritene (Doyle)	Highest in protein: 60 gm; high in sodium and potassium.	
Oral or Nasogastric Supplemental Feedings		
Citrotein (Doyle) Controlyte (Doyle) Ensure (Ross)	Low fat; high calorie; low protein, sodium, and potassium	These feedings may be given between meals to supplement what is missing in the diet. Some may be chosen for high calorie, low fluid, low electrolyte content
Hi/Cal (Beecham-Massengill) Meritene (Doyle)	Hi-Cal 2,458 cal/1,000 ml; no protein or fat; minimum sodium and potassium; limited liquid	
Polycose (Ross) Sustacal (Mead Johnson)	High carbohydrate, low protein, low fat, high sodium and potassium	
Elemental Feedings		
Vivonex (Eaton) (regular and high nitrogen) Flexical Elemental Diet (Mead Johnson)	Completely balanced; combination of purified amino acids, vitamins, and minerals	Regular may be used up to 12 months; high nitrogen 2 months
Precision Feedings Low residue Moderate nitrogen High nitrogen		

electrolytes should be specified by the physician and should be provided in the diet.

It is the nurse who "administers" the diet to the patient, either directly or indirectly. Therefore, the nurse must be the one to create the atmosphere for eating. Minimizing distasteful noises, odors, and distractions in the room may help the patient to relax and enjoy his meal. The patient's physical needs must be met before he is likely to feel like eating. Aesthetic needs such as a clean environment, clean utensils, and attractive meals are important. Anything that prevents the patient from effectively enjoying his food, such as loose-fitting dentures, shortness of breath, or foul taste in his mouth, should be attended to before food is introduced.

The nurse must be convinced that good nutrition is vital to regaining and maintaining health so that he or she can communicate this fact to the patient. With this conviction in mind, great care will be taken to create the optimum environment and to take the time to properly administer the diet.

An accurate history on admission will point out the patient's needs. Accurate record-keeping of the nutritional status of the patient while in the hospital will provide a basis for habits that must be continued at home and that will ensure that the patient's needs are being met. The diet must be complete when it comes to the patient, but to be therapeutically effective, it must also be consumed.

NURSING RESPONSIBILITIES IN THE CARE OF THE PATIENT WITH SLEEP DEPRIVATION

It is important for the nurse to understand why sleep is essential to health, how the different bodily systems function during sleep, and the purposes of dream activity. A great deal of research has recently been done on sleep activity utilizing electroencephalography and electrical devices to monitor the individual's blood pressure, pulse, respiration, temperature, and hormone levels. As a result of this research, five distinct stages of sleep have been identified.

Stage I is identified by alpha waves seen on the electroencephalogram. This stage produces muscle relaxation and a feeling of drifting off to sleep. Respirations are very regular; the pulse slows and is also regular. The person can be easily awakened and would become as coherent as he was before going to sleep in a short period of time after being aroused.

When a person enters stage II of sleep, spindles appear on his electroencephalogram. Dissociated dream activity begins during which one can observe the person's eyes slowly rolling from side to side. It is more difficult to awaken the person in this stage, but he is not in a deep sleep.

Stage III is entered about 20 minutes after falling asleep when the person is very relaxed. Large, slow waves are seen on the electroencephalogram pattern. Body temperature and blood pressure start decreasing.

During stage IV of sleep activity, the person is very difficult to arouse. Electroencephalogram tracings reveal delta waves for the 10-to-20 minute duration of this stage. Biological function occurring during this stage will be of significant interest to the nurse. The growth-stimulating hormone is released from the anterior pituitary gland to stimulate body processes responsible for growth, tissue and bone healing, and lowering of blood cholesterol.

After stage IV sleep is completed, the individual starts retracing stages back to stage II. At this time, the fifth stage, rapid eye movement (REM) sleep, is initiated. The electroencephalogram tracing is similar to that of the person while he is awake but very pensive. It is this stage of sleep that has led to much research into dreams and their effects on a person's individual well-being. Dreams during REM sleep seem to serve the purpose of affording time for an individual to solve problems of his daily activities and adapt to stresses that may have affected him during his wakeful hours. Consequently, a certain peace of mind is felt to result from these dreams, the content of which the individual does not usually remember.

The physiologic aspects of REM sleep include increased metabolism, autonomic nervous system activity, and release of adreno-cortical hormones. There is a sudden spurting release of adrenal hormones into the bloodstream during periods of REM sleep, thought to serve the function of preparing the body for activities of the new day by recharging the metabolic processes, the natural body defenses against infection and the transmitter of nerve impulses.

After the first REM sleep period is completed, the individual goes back through stages III and IV. This entire cycle from stage I through stage IV and then back up to REM sleep takes approximately 1.5 hours, and is repeated four to five times during a regular night's sleep. As the morning hours approach, stage IV sleep is very brief and REM sleep dominates the cycle. Prior to waking up in the morning, stage I is reentered.

It is understandable then why a person feels physically fatigued and emotionally irritable when deprived of sleep over a period of time. It is also obvious that a person who is suddenly awakened during different stages of sleep may behave irrationally. For example, dreams are predominant during REM sleep, some of which are bizarre, and this may contribute to irrational waking behavior. If awakened during this stage, a person may have difficulty distinguishing between the dream and reality, and he may consequently appear disoriented. The nurse can be instrumental in identifying factors in the patient's environment during the night and eliminating or reducing interferences with sleep.

The physician will prescribe the necessary pulmonary therapy, including medications and their frequency as needed by the individual patient. The nurse's responsibility is then to plan the specific times in a 24-hour period for the treatments and coordinate the implementation of the plan with the other health team members. This aspect is probably the most difficult because of hospital routine, number of personnel working with the patient, and the fact that several needs of the patient must be considered simultaneously.

An example of treatment ordered for the patient with respiratory problems could include the following:

IPPB treatment	every 4 hours
Chest physical therapy	3 times a day
Aminophyllin	250 mg rectally 4 times a day
Robitussin	10 ml orally every 4 hours
Ampicillin	500 mg orally every 6 hours

In addition to prescribed medical treatments, there are nursing treatments, such as coughing and deep breathing and turning, which must be done on a routine basis. The nurse can organize the total plan with consideration of the patient's condition and arrange logical sequencing of treatments and medications. Implied in the administration of antibiotic agents is the necessity to administer the medication at regular intervals over a 24-hour period. The time interval between each dose must be even.

Robitussin	12pm — 4pm — 8pm — 12am — 4am — 8am
Aminophyllin	12pm — 6pm — 12am — 6am
Ampicillin	12pm — 6pm — 12am — 6am
Chest PT	3pm — 9pm — 9am
IPPB	12pm — 4pm — 8pm — 12am — 4am — 8am
Turning, deep breathing, and coughing (alternating with pulmonary therapies)	8am — 12pm — 4pm — 8 pm when awake

With this type of plan, the time between 12 midnight and 4 A.M. would be allotted for a fairly long period of sleep.

The nurse, in assisting the patient with respiratory disease to meet his need for sleep, must use discretion in administering drugs that enhance sleep. Respiratory depressants, such as barbiturates, are prescribed with caution in the acutely or chronically hypoxic patient, because these drugs may decrease the sensitivity of the respiratory center and cause further depression of respiration. For the patient who does not respond to the nursing measures specified in Table 21–3, the use of antihistamines and diphenhydramine hydrochloride can prove effective in producing drowsiness in the patient and enhance relaxation necessary for sleep activity.

NURSING RESPONSIBILITIES IN THE CARE OF THE PATIENT WITH A PROBLEM OF ANXIETY AND DEPRESSION

It is at times frustrating for the nurse to work with the patient who is not psychologically ready to participate in his care because of inability to cope with the effects of chronic pulmonary disease. The goals of the nurse and the patient initially may be disparate—the nurse striving for the patient to attain optimal health, and the patient feeling worthless and indifferent because he can perceive only his limitations and not his capabilities.

In addition to the problem of establishing realistic goals essential for the planning and implementing of care, it is difficult to record the patient's behavioral response to his illness for clear interpretation by all health team members involved in the situation. Each person's perception and interpretation of verbal and nonverbal cues from the patient can vary widely.

The first responsibility of the nurse in planning care for the individual is to establish a nurse-patient relationship based on trust. Skillful use of communication techniques is one method of establishing a therapeutic relationship. The nurse also needs to recognize and accept the patient's immediate need for dependence while encouraging his optimal independence through gradual participation in self-care.

The psychological assimilation of a disability resulting from chronic illness takes time and consequently demands patience on the part of the nurse. The skillful use of positive reinforcement in situations where the patient exhibits independent behavior is essential in assisting the patient to develop a feeling of self-worth.

The nurse assesses the patient's readiness for learning, but it is important to involve the patient in the development of the goals for the learning process. Implementation of a teaching care plan then becomes the nurse's responsibility in the rehabilitation of the patient.

Primary nursing is the preferred method of planning and implementing patient care for the following reasons: (1) the creation and maintenance of rapport and trust is enhanced by consistent interaction between the patient and the primary nurse responsible for his care; and (2) continuity of patient care is established from the time of the patient's admission, throughout his hospitalization to discharge, and on future readmission, when a primary nurse is responsible for the ongoing assessment, the planning, the implementing, and the evaluation of the patient's nursing care needs.

The nursing responsibilities in the care of the patient affected by chronic pulmonary disease are many, and the attainment of immediate and long-range goals is a real nursing challenge.

EVALUATION OF NURSING CARE PLAN

The final step in the nursing process is the evaluation of the patient's response to the planned nursing interventions.

Ongoing evaluation will result in one of the following conclusions: (1) the patient's problem could be corrected, terminating the present need for the specific nursing intervention; (2) the patient's problem may not have been affected by the nursing intervention, necessitating revision of the plan; (3) the patient's problem may be improving, but continued nursing intervention is indicated; or (4) the patient may have developed a new problem that necessitates an additional plan of nursing care.

The nursing interventions for common problems occurring in patients with chronic pulmonary disease have been discussed previously as separate entities. Each problem is an interference with the patient's needs and is the result of the pulmonary pathophysiology or its effect on other systems. Consequently, more than one of these problems can occur simultaneously. It is important for the nurse to always view the patient as an integrated whole and formulate a comprehensive plan to meet the immediate and long-range goals of the patient.

In conclusion, many variables are considered in planning care for patients with pulmonary disease. These include the effects of the disease on the patient's life-style, the ability of the patient to cope with his disease, and the unique characteristics of each patient.

Two of the main constants that aid the nurse in effectively assisting each patient reach optimal health are the nursing process and the scientific principles upon which it is based.

BIBLIOGRAPHY

Barstow, R. Coping with emphysema. *Nurs. Clin. North Am.* 9, 1974, p. 137.

Baum, G. *Textbook of Pulmonary Diseases* (2nd ed.). Boston: Little, Brown, 1974.

Beland, I., and Passos, J. *Clinical Nursing* (3rd ed.). New York: Macmillan, 1975.

Bushnell, S. *Respiratory Intensive Care Nursing.* Boston: Little, Brown, 1973.

Grant, D., and Klell, C. For goodness sake—let your patients sleep. *Nursing* 11, 1974, p. 54.

Johns, M. *Pharmacodynamics and Patient Care.* St. Louis: Mosby, 1974.

Kalish, R. *The Psychology of Human Behavior.* Belmont, Calif.: Wadsworth, 1966.

Lagerson, J. Nursing care of patients with chronic pulmonary insufficiency. *Nurs. Clin. North Am.* 9, 1974, p. 165.

Levis, E., and Browning, M. *Nursing in Respiratory Diseases.* New York: American Journal of Nursing Company, 1972.

Luckmann, J., and Sorensen, K. *Medical-Surgical Nursing.* Philadelphia: Saunders, 1974.

Marram, G., Schlegel, M., and Bevis, E. *Primary Nursing: A Model for Individualized Care.* St. Louis: Mosby, 1974.

Marriner, A. *The Nursing Process.* St. Louis: Mosby, 1975.

Wade, J. *Respiratory Nursing Care.* St. Louis: Mosby, 1973.

On the Horizon

6

Armand A. Lefemine

Lung Transplantation

22

The American College of Surgeons Organ Transplant Registry, as of January 1975, recorded 36 clinical lung transplants with no patients now living; the longest survival to date is 10 months. The lung has been considered a particularly difficult organ to transplant successfully because of the likelihood of postoperative infection, the doubtful early functional capacity of the lungs after transplantation, and the difficulty of sustaining life without infection or other organ dysfunction before transplantation is accomplished. The rejection problems are similar to those posed by other organs. Comparative data for other organs testify to the difficulty encountered in clinical lung transplantation. According to the Registry, 44 of 257 heart recipients are alive and the longest functioning graft has been in place for more than 6 years. Of 220 liver graft recipients, 20 are surviving, the longest for 5 years. One of 36 pancreas recipients is alive and he has survived nearly 3 years. With the improvement in life support systems such as extracorporeal membrane oxygenation in organ preservation and in the control of the rejection phenomenon, we can expect a renewed interest and a rekindling of activity in this field as time goes on. The success of respiratory support programs will depend on the ability to replace lungs that have no hope for restoration of function.

HISTORICAL NOTES
Carrel [11] performed a heart and lung transplant in a cat in 1905. Demikhov [15] and Rabinovitch et al. [41] transplanted a lobe in 1947 in a series of experiments marred by technical problems related to disruption of bronchus and arterial and

venous thromboses. Staudacher et al. [43] in 1950, and Lanari et al. in 1951 [35], reported an experience with a series of homografted and reimplanted lobes. The re-implanted lobes functioned for an average period of 12 days, whereas the homo-grafted lobes functioned for only 7 days because of rejection. Juvenelle et al. [33] reported reimplantation of the right lung in dogs in 1951, with bronchospirometric studies 35 months later that revealed only a moderate loss of pulmonary function. The Hering-Breuer reflex of the replanted lung was lost. The first clinical transplant was performed by Hardy et al. [27] in 1963.

LUNG AUTOTRANSPLANTS

The adequacy of an immediately reimplanted autologous lung to sustain the life of an animal deprived of its opposite lung is limited because of the immediate appear-ance of increased pulmonary arterial pressure, high vascular resistance, and an edematous hemorrhagic lung [3, 28]. Studies of autologous transplantation are im-portant because the problems of rejection are removed. Rabinovitch et al. [41] col-lected data on 948 lung autotransplants reported before 1972. Attempts at removal of the contralateral lung either in the early or late postoperative period usually re-sulted in the animal's death within a few days of the operation, though about 14 percent survived a maximum of 3.5 years. Of three long-term survivors subjected to removal of the contralateral lung, two dogs survived with progressive improvement in ventilation and respiration to normal by the fifteenth postoperative day. One dog followed for 3¼ years after removal of the contralateral lung revealed normal ven-tilation and gas exchange. There was histologic evidence of hypertrophy of the autotransplant, thickening of the intima of small veins, and a regeneration of ner-vous structures.

Present evidence indicates that the high rate of failure in autotransplantation of lobes [40, 50] or lungs [36, 51] is related to anastomotic stenosis, both vascular and bronchial, that create ventilation-perfusion imbalances. After eliminating the animals with anatomic defects, evidence indicates that a small number of animals can function normally [41] even with removal of the contralateral lung. There is, however, evidence using xenon 133 and iodine 131 macroaggregates of human serum albumin (MAA) that normal perfusion, as judged by preoperative levels, is not achieved. Pulmonary hypertension is a response to venous anastomotic defects or to an intrinsic increase in vascular resistance, and this will vary with whether the right or left lung is replanted. Conducting the entire cardiac output through the right lung will increase its blood flow by 70 percent, whereas diverting the whole cardiac output to the left lung will increase the flow to that lung by 150 percent. Thus, arterial pressure will rise after ligation or occlusion of the right pulmonary artery about twice as much as after ligation of the left pulmonary artery. The occur-rence of high pulmonary vascular resistance in reimplanted lung varies with the techniques of measurement by various investigators [14, 39, 50]. A slow but pro-gressive increase in vascular resistance has been seen in the replanted lung that tends to appear after the first year of survival of contralateral pneumonectomy [51]. The reason for this rise, in the absence of anastomotic narrowing, is unclear and leads to speculation of the effect of interruption of lymph drainage and neural fibers and possibly of bronchial stenosis and chronic bronchopneumonitis with induration of the lung. A few dogs have survived a left-lung autotransplantation and allotransplantation and simultaneous contralateral pulmonary artery ligation [21].

Experimental evidence indicates that the dog is not a good model for lung transplantation and that baboons are more closely related to human subjects [20]. Joseph and Morton [32] performed left lung autotransplants in 16 baboons with immediate contralateral pulmonary artery ligation. Twelve survived for long periods, indicating that the autotransplanted lung is capable of providing immediate and total respiration support without a significant increase in pulmonary artery pressure as seen in the dog. Transient decreases in oxygen tension and elevation of pulmonary artery pressure returned to normal in 2 weeks. Similar results were obtained by Castaneda et al. [12], performing cardiopulmonary autotransplantations in primates.

LUNG ALLOGRAFTS
The most common cause of death in allografted lungs during the first 2 months after transplantation is rejection combined with infection of the graft and/or contralateral lungs. Late deaths are related to sepsis in the graft, liver failure, and loss of function of the graft, but without graft rejection [22]. Technical problems such as vein thrombosis and arterial and bronchial stenosis also account for a high percentage of loss in the early days and hours after allotransplantation [30]. Thrombosis of the pulmonary veins immediately after transplantation may be related to poor graft preservation during the period of surgery [8]. The pulmonary venous outflow obstruction that is seen late is probably due to stenosis and contracture at the anastomosis, although microvascular obstruction related to rejection has been implicated [45].

It is difficult to evaluate venous outflow obstruction by angiography. Evaluation of the transplanted lung in the absence of technical problems reveals a number of functional defects that occur with time and that are principally related to the rejection phenomenon. Chronic survivals after allotransplants with simultaneous contralateral pulmonary artery ligation show that allografted lungs are capable of providing total pulmonary function for up to 3 months [49]. Longer survivals and late studies indicate normal resting pulmonary artery pressures within the first 6 months following transplantation and pulmonary hypertension at the 8 and 10 month period [37]. Pulmonary hypertension seen early in the posttransplant period may be reversible [19]. Angiographic studies and blood gas analyses tend to confirm the occurrence of progressive damage to the graft associated with decreased flow to that side. If rejection is controlled, the allotransplanted lung will have a respiratory function profile in terms of lung compliance, diffusion capacity, a functional reserve capacity, and a pulmonary artery pressure that is close to normal and similar to reimplanted lungs [22]. When obvious rejection is found, pulmonary hypertension and increased total vascular resistance are found. The limits to survival seem to be the limits of immunosuppressive therapy, and in the dog it is rare that allotransplanted animals survive longer than 1 year.

FACTORS OF SURVIVAL AND FUNCTION

The lung is always subjected to ischemia in the process of transplantation, and this period will vary with the technical difficulties encountered. Cooling prolongs the period of safe ischemia. There is a significant body of experimental evidence that the dog lung will survive 4 hours of ischemia with satisfactory function [4, 9, 13, 25]. Periods longer than this result in a high mortality rate from pulmonary edema and intolerable diffusion gradients. If ischemic time is less than 4 hours, the lung will have reasonable function immediately and return to normal in 2 weeks [25]. The importance of bronchial circulation in the survival of the allograft is not determined, though it is theoretically ideal. It is probably safe to say that most of the laboratory and clinical transplants have been accomplished without restoring anatomic flow in the bronchial part of the circulation, depending on collateral pathways to prevent ischemic damage to the major bronchi.

Disruption of the bronchial suture line, bronchial ulceration, bronchial stenosis, abnormal mucus production, ciliary action, and cough reflex are recognized causes of pulmonary allograft failures [38]. The major cause of these complications has been thought to be interruption of normal vascular and lymphatic pathways. Such bronchial complications have been reported after human as well as animal single-lung allotransplantation. There is experimental evidence that a large percentage of bronchial complications in the dog can be prevented by reconstituting bronchial artery circulation [38]. A review of human lung allotransplants reveal that approximately 50 percent had bronchial complications. The bronchial circulation was reestablished in one human case with a normal donor bronchus found at postmortem examination [38]. The bronchial complications may be one of the reasons for the high incidence of postoperative pneumonia.

The functional capacity of the lung to respond reflexly and adjust ventilation and perfusion to the requirements of the moment is an important requirement for survival immediately after transplantation and may be an important way of detecting rejection in the late transplant. The response to regional hypoxia is lost immediately after reimplantation but returns after the second or third month [46]. This is important because arterial hypoxemia may result by the inability to shift flow from hypoxic areas. Studies with intravenous xenon 133 reveal a dramatic reduction of perfusion in the transplanted allograft after the fourth day that progresses to death of the animal. The autograft reveals a similar reduction of perfusion index for the first 2 to 3 weeks but returns to normal. A similar return to normal is seen for oxygen uptake and carbon dioxide excretion after 3 to 4 weeks. Full functional recovery of lung autografts does not occur until after several months. Thus, scanning of the lungs with xenon 133 may be used as a rapid estimate of effective alveolar ventilation and perfusion and the progress of rejection [5, 31].

HISTOLOGY

The cellular response to autotransplants reveals pulmonary congestion and edema, occasional histocytic proliferation, intravascular thrombi, and leukocytic agglutinations. In allotransplants, acute rejection was seen in 4 to 6 days [21] characterized by an infiltration and clusters of mononuclear cells around the small vessels and bronchi, often progressing to intravascular thrombus formation and infarction necrosis [23]. In the first week of rejection, the mononuclear infiltrate consists of reticulumlike cells, macrophages, lymphocytes, and plasma cells. After the first week there are increasing numbers of mononuclear cells around bronchi and vessels with an infiltration or migration of inflammatory cells into the intraalveolar spaces, along with exudation of red cells and proliferation of endothelial cells.

In the animals subjected to immunosuppression immediately after transplantation, pulmonary infection is the most common finding. Rejection is delayed for 3 to 5 weeks but then follows a pattern similar to those without suppression. In the late stages of survival (4 to 5 weeks), we may find destruction of small vessels and alveolar patterns with infarction necrosis and fibrosis. The alveolar exudates unaffected by immunosuppression may prevent transplant ventilation and aeration, predispose to infection, and contribute to the ventilation-perfusion imbalance during rejection [6]. This proteinaceous exudate may precede the cellular phase [48]. These changes are found transiently in autografts as well as allografts, and thus may be related to the transplant procedure rather than rejection. Studies of lung allografts in calves and baboons reveal a histology of rejection and of progressive ventilation-perfusion imbalance that is similar to that of the dog [44].

BILATERAL TRANSPLANTATION

Bilateral lung reimplantation [1] and allotransplantation [2] have been studied as a means of overcoming the technical problems of unilateral lung transplants, such as thrombosis and stenosis of the atrial anastomosis and bronchial stenosis or leak. Examination of long-term survivors reveals that neural connections with the respiratory center are not essential for continued activity and survival. Pulmonary edema, the most common cause of early death, was reversible if graft preservation, using time-limited cold ischema, was adequate. Bilateral lung reimplantation allowed a significant long-term survival with a return of normal lung scans, pulmonary angiograms, pulmonary arterial pressures, and arterial blood gas studies to normal several months after the procedure.

In the allotransplant group there were few long-term survivors irrespective of immunosuppression. Dogs without immunosuppression did not survive more than 5 days. These dogs died of pulmonary insufficiency rather than the usual hemorrhagic necrosis seen in unilateral allotransplantation. Dogs with immunosuppression died within 21 days, though one lived as long as 338 days. Autopsies revealed a solid, poorly aerated, wet lung. Bronchi always revealed necroses of the mucosa distal to the suture line. Occasionally, the necroses involved the entire bronchial wall [34]. Immunosuppression contributed only some prolongation of life and an increased incidence of complications such as bronchopneumonia, perforation of the bronchus, intestinal bleeding, pneumothorax, and atrial thrombosis. Dogs surviving the operation of bilateral replacement for periods up to 15 weeks usually revealed a significant rise in mean pulmonary artery pressure and pulmonary vascular resistance, a reduced cardiac output, and mean arterial pressure. In some animals the pulmonary artery pressure, cardiac output, and blood gases return to normal in 8 to 15 weeks [20].

HUMAN ALLOTRANSPLANTATION

Allogenic transplantation of the lung in man remains as a potential approach to the management of various clinical problems characterized by respiratory insufficiency, in spite of the fact that none of the 36 lung transplants in patients are functioning today. The first clinical lung transplant was performed in 1963 by Hardy [29]. This patient died 18 days later of renal insufficiency, a preoperative problem, without evidence of gross or microscopic rejection of the transplanted lung. The transplanted lung functioned immediately and contributed to the respiratory support of the patient. The first successful lung transplant in man was performed in 1968 at the University of Ghent by Derom and associates [16], with survival of the patient for 10 months. This patient was 23 years old, suffering from the terminal stages of micronodular silicosis with pulmonary infection, right ventricular strain, and elevated carbon dioxide tension and reduced oxygen tension on assisted ventilation, for a period of 7 months. The right lung was transplanted from a 40-year-old woman who died from cerebral thrombosis and hemorrhage. Preoperative tissue typing showed a reasonable match of 12 HL-A antigens (4 mismatches in the Van Rood system).

Thoracotomy of the donor was performed first to confirm the suitability of the lung. The right lung was selected for technical advantages of anastomosis and possible cardiopulmonary bypass. Temporary clamping of the pulmonary artery demonstrated that the patient would tolerate transplantation without cardiopulmonary bypass. Heparin was administered to the donor, and the right lung was transplanted with its blood content. The donor lung was not cooled, perfused, or ventilated. The technique used was the standard atrial cuff with continuous and interrupted sutures for bronchus, veins, and artery. Postoperatively, the patient was extubated after 13 hours. The lung functioned well with an oxygen tension of 102 torr and a carbon dioxide tension of 53 torr on 10 liters of oxygen through a face mask. Signs of right ventricular strain disappeared in 24 hours, and oxygen therapy was discontinued on the 27th postoperative day. Drug therapy consisted of antilymphocyte serum, azothioprine, prednisone, actinomycin C, penicillin, and streptomycin. The patient was in a sterile room for 4 months without complications. The patient was able to live a normal life at home from the fifth to the eighth month. Though he recovered from two acute rejections in the early phase of his recovery, a third rejection in the ninth month failed to respond, and he died of pneumonia and sepsis on the 300th day. Ventilation xenon and lung scan studies showed that the left autologous lung was nonfunctional and the transplanted lung was responsible for respiration. There was no perfusion-ventilation imbalance between the two lungs.

A survey of 24 lung transplants by Hardy et al. [26] reveals that most of the patients received a lung for respiratory insufficiency, though pulmonary hypertension was the reason in 2 patients. Most of the recipients as well as donors were men. Living donors were used in 4 cases of lobar transplantation, usually from the uninvolved portions of lungs resected for cancer. Half of the lungs were salvaged postmortem, whereas the others were obtained from neurologically dead donors. The ischemia time for lungs varied from 32 minutes to more than 24 hours. Veith and Blumenstock [48] in a review of 16 patients who survived over 2 days found that all patients had a proteinaceous exudate in their transplanted lungs that contained sloughed alveoli-lining cells and some round cells. Only 5 patients had the classic rejection with perivascular round-cell infiltration.

Orthotopic heart-bilateral lung transplantation was performed in 1969 by Lillehei. The recipient was a 43-year-old man with terminal obstructive emphysema and right ventricular failure. The donor was a woman 50 years of age, who died following a cerebral hemorrhage. She was a D tissue match with the recipient, and she had been on the respirator for 72 hours. Anastomoses were performed in order of trachea, aorta, and venae cavae with a pump time of 1 hour and 50 minutes. Coronary perfusion was carried out through the innominate artery. Postoperatively, this patient was alert, extubated, maintained an arterial pO_2 of 85 to 89 torr on 40% oxygen by mask. Tidal volume was 500 ml. On the fifth postoperative day, an infiltrate began to involve both lungs. Overwhelming *Pseudomonas* infection occurred, and the patient died on the ninth postoperative day without evidence of cardiac rejection.

The moral and ethical decisions in this field are still as difficult as they were 10 years ago. The indications will undoubtedly change when the rejection process comes under reasonable control. It is evident from present experience that clinical lung transplantation can be accomplished technically, that a homotransplanted lung can support life for a prolonged period, and that immunologic rejection can be controlled for periods as long as 10 months. Unfortunately, the success rate to date makes this procedure highly experimental and one that requires further study and refinements.

REFERENCES

1. Alican, F., et al. Surgical technique of one stage bilateral lung reimplantation in the dog. *J. Thorac. Cardiovasc. Surg.* 61, 1971, p. 847.
2. Alican, F., Isin, E., and Cockrell, J. V. One-stage allotransplantation of both lungs in the dog. *Ann. Surg.* 177, 1973, p. 193.
3. Allgood, R. J., Ebert, P. A., and Sabiston, D. C., Jr. Immediate changes in pulmonary hemodynamics following lung autotransplantation. *Ann. Surg.* 167, 1968, p. 352.
4. Ardekarni, R. G., Faber, L. P., and Beattie, E. J. Pulmonary function after various periods of ischemia on the canine lung. *J. Thorac. Cardiovasc. Surg.* 59, 1970, p. 607.
5. Aviado, D. M., Ling, J. S., and Schmidt, C. F. Effects of anoxia on pulmonary circulation: Reflex pulmonary vasoconstriction. *Am. J. Physiol.* 179, 1957, p. 253.
6. Becker, N. H., et al. Fine structure alterations in canine lung transplants. *J. Thorac. Cardiovasc. Surg.* 63, 1972, p. 81.

7. Blades, B., et al. Ischemia of the lung. *Ann. Surg.* 135, 1952, p. 56.
8. Brownle, R. T., and Couves, C. M. Factors concerned in the maintenance of viability in pulmonary transplants. *Ann. Thorac. Surg.* 5, 1968, p. 112.
9. *Bulletin of the American Cancer Society,* March, 1975; vol 60, no. 3, pp. 24–26.
10. Bücherl, E. S., Nasseri, M., and von Prondzynski, B. J. Lung function studies after homotransplantation, autotransplantation, denervation of the left lung, and ligature of the right pulmonary artery. *J. Thorac. Cardiovasc. Surg.* 47, 1964, p. 455.
11. Carrel, A. The surgery of blood vessels. *Bull. Hopkins Hosp.* 18, 1907, p. 26.
12. Castaneda, A., et al. Cardiopulmonary autotransplantation in primates (baboons): Late functional results. *Surgery* 72, 1972, p. 1064.
13. Counaughton, P. J., Bauth, J. J., and Lewis, F. J. Lung ischemia up to six hours, influence of local cooling in situ on subsequent function. *Dis. Chest* 41, 1962, p. 404.
14. Davies, L. G., Rosser, T. H. L., and West, L. R. Autotransplantation of the lung in sheep. *Thorax* 20, 1965, p. 481.
15. Demikhov, V. P. *Experimental Transplantation of Vital Organs.* New York: Plenum, 1962.
16. Derom, F., et al. Ten-month survival after lung homotransplantation in man. *J. Thorac. Cardiovasc. Surg.* 61, 1971, p. 835.
17. Edmunds, L. H., et al. Mucus transport in transplanted lungs of dogs. *Surgery* 66, 1969, p. 15.
18. Eraslan, S., Turner, M. D., and Hardy, J. P. Lymphatic regeneration following lung reimplantation in dogs. *Surgery* 56, 1964, p. 970.
19. Fonkalsrud, E. W., et al. Physiologic evaluation of allogenic canine lung transplants from living donors. *J. Thorac. Cardiovasc. Surg.* 57, 1969, p. 607.
20. Fujimura, S., et al. Hemodynamic alterations after staged and simultaneous bilateral lung autotransplantation in dogs. *J. Thorac. Cardiovasc. Surg.* 63, 1972, p. 937.
21. Fujimura, S., et al. Cellular characteristics of the rejection response to canine lung allotransplants. *J. Thorac. Cardiovasc. Surg.* 65, 1973, p. 183.
22. Garzon, A. A., et al. Functions of canine lung allografts. *J. Thorac. Cardiovasc. Surg.* 65, 1973, p. 76.
23. Gondos, B., White, P., and Benfield, J. R. Histologic changes associated with rejection of canine lung transplants. *J. Thorac. Cardiovasc. Surg.* 62, 1971, p. 183.
24. Haglin, J. J. A comparative study of reimplantation of the lung in the dog and Kenya baboon. Unpublished Ph.D. thesis, University of Minnesota, 1964.
25. Hankington, H. W., and Edwards, F. F. The effect of pulmonary ischemia on lung function. *Thorax* 14, 1959, p. 122.
26. Hardy, J. D., et al. A case of clinical lung allotransplantation. *J. Thorac. Cardiovasc. Surg.* 60, 1970, p. 411.
27. Hardy, J. D., Eraslan, S., and Dalton, M. L., Jr. Lung homotransplantation in man. Report of the initial case. *J.A.M.A.* 186, 1963, p. 1065.
28. Hardy, J. D., Eraslan, S., and Dalton, M. L., Jr. Auto-transplantation and homotransplantation of the lung; further studies. *J. Thorac. Cardiovasc. Surg.* 46, 1963, p. 606.

29. Hardy, J. D., et al. Lung transplantation in man. Report of the initial case. *J.A.M.A.* 186, 1963, p. 1065.
30. Hill, P. M., and Shaw, K. M. Long-term survival of dogs after experimental pulmonary reimplantation and staged contralateral pneumonectomy. *Thorax* 23, 1968, p. 408.
31. Hutchin, P., et al. Ventilation and perfusion after transplantation of the lung. Studies with intravenous xenon-133. *J. Thorac. Cardiovasc. Surg.* 61, 1971, p. 476.
32. Joseph, W. L., and Morton, D. L. Immediate function with survival after left lung autotransplantation and contralateral pulmonary artery ligation in the baboon. *J. Thorac. Cardiovasc. Surg.* 60, 1970, p. 859.
33. Juvenelle, A. A., et al. Pneumonectomy with replantation of the lung in the dog for physiologic study. *J. Thorac. Cardiovasc. Surg.* 31, 1951, p. 111.
34. Kondo Yoshio, et al. One-stage bilateral allotransplantation of canine lungs: Further studies. *J. Thorac. Cardiovasc. Surg.* 65, 1972, p. 897.
35. Lanari, A., Molins, M., and Croxatto, O. Homoinjertos de Pulmon en perros: Technica y resultados funcionales y anatomicos. *Medicina* 11, 1951, p. 12.
36. Lincoln, J. C. R., et al. Serial perfusion and ventilation studies following reimplantation of the lung using xenon 133, pulmonary angiography, and bronchography. *J. Thorac. Cardiovasc. Surg.* 60, 1970, p. 108.
37. Linde, L. M., et al. Physiologic studies following canine lung homotransplantation. Long-term survival of dogs. *J. Thorac. Cardiovasc. Surg.* 57, 1969, p. 607.
38. Mills, N. L., Boyd, A. D., and Gheranpong, C. The significance of bronchial circulation in lung transplantation. *J. Thorac. Cardiovasc. Surg.* 6, 1970, p. 866.
39. Nigro, S. L., et al. Physiological alterations of cardiopulmonary function in dogs living one and one-half years on only a reimplanted lung. *J. Thorac. Cardiovasc. Surg.* 46, 1963, p. 598.
40. Perelman, M. I., and Rabinovitch, J. J. Methods and technique of experimental autotransplantation of a lung lobe. *J. Thorac. Cardiovasc. Surg.* 59, 1970, p. 275.
41. Rabinovitch, J. J., et al. The possibility of prolonged survival of animals with an autotransplanted lung after removal of the intact, contralateral lung. *J. Thorac. Cardiovasc. Surg.* 67, 1974, p. 744.
42. Sabanayagam, P., et al. A correlation of radiographic, functional, and morphological changes in baboon lung allografts. *J. Thorac. Cardiovasc. Surg.* 66, 1973, p. 573.
43. Staudacher, V. E., et al. Su tentativi di reimplanti autoplastici e di traplanti emnoplastici di lobi polmonari. *Chiro. Pat. Sper.* 5, 1950, p. 223.
44. Strandbert, J. D., PioRoda, C. L., and Baker, R. R. Lung allografts in calves. *Arch. Surg.* 106, 1973, p. 196.
45. Suzuki, C., et al. Experimental studies of canine lung allotransplantation. *J. Thorac. Cardiovasc. Surg.* 55, 1968, p. 200.
46. Valenca, L. M., et al. Pulmonary vascular response of the reimplanted dog lung to hypoxia. *J. Thorac. Cardiovasc. Surg.* 61, 1971, p. 857.
47. Veith, F. J. Discussion 16. *Surgery* 66, 1969, p. 22.
48. Veith, F. J., and Blumenstock, D. A. Lung transplantation. *J. Surg. Res.* 11, 1971, p. 33.

49. Veith, F. J., Richards, K., and Lalezari, P. Protracted survival after homo-transplantation of the lung, and simultaneous contralateral pulmonary artery ligation. *J. Thorac. Cardiovasc. Surg.* 58, 1969, p. 829.
50. Wagner, O. A., Cowan, G. S., and Edmunds, L. H. Lobar pulmonary arterial blood flow in reimplanted canine lungs. *J. Thorac. Cardiovasc. Surg.* 65, 1973, p. 171.
51. Wildevuur, C. R. H., et al. Long-term observation of the changes in pulmonary arterial pressure after reimplantation of the canine lung. *J. Thorac. Cardiovasc. Surg.* 56, 1968, p. 799.

Armand A. Lefemine

Respiratory Assistance Using the Artificial Lung

23

The use of an artificial lung to supplement or replace the function of a patient's lungs for a prolonged period is a currently available technique. The indications for the use of such an instrument are not completely detailed, nor are the criteria for discontinuing such use as a hopeless procedure. The logistics of accomplishing an assisted respiration with an extracorporeal device requiring constant observation and trained staff are formidable, and represent reasons for being selective and strict before undertaking this procedure as a long-term commitment.

The modern respiratory intensive care unit has improved the salvage rate in all forms of respiratory insufficiency to such an extent that it is only the rare patient who is considered for artificial lung support. Improvements in respirators, tubes, monitoring, and in the techniques of positive pressure have materially reduced the number of possible candidates for extracorporeal support.

The usual scenario for considering this modality of support is a patient on a ventilator not responding to positive end expiratory pressure, with a Pa_{O_2} below 50 torr and falling [43]. The number of potential clinical conditions that could produce this situation with the possibility of reversal are large. In the infant, hyaline membrane disease is the most reversible condition. In the child or adult, acute respiratory insufficiency may result from trauma, viral pneumonia, aspiration pneumonia, bacterial pneumonia, pump lung, fat emboli, pulmonary embolism, and oxygen toxicity.

Progressive atelectasis or consolidation as well as pulmonary hyperinflation [2] are often seen in patients on respirator therapy, resulting in a low arterial oxygen pressure and a large right-to-left shunt. It is unusual that such a state cannot be handled for hours or even days before considering the artificial lung. In most instances, it is likely that the patient has been supported for weeks before reaching a state that is not only completely unresponsive but that is perhaps also completely unreversible because of lung consolidation and sepsis.

BACKGROUND

The concept of extracorporeal circulation and oxygenation is more than 160 years old. The early experiments of Von Schröder, in 1882, culminated in a mechanical perfusion device in which respiration was artificially maintained through an excised animal lung [16]. This prevented the trauma that was inherent in gas-blood interphase and may be the first use of an extracorporeal membrane apparatus. The development of a practical heart-lung apparatus by Gibbon [18], and its actual clinical application by Dennis [12] in 1950, spurred the development of oxygenators in many directions. The direct blood-gas contact inherent in the function of all bubble, disc, screen, and other filming designs has been shown to produce a variety of deleterious changes in the blood that limit the safe use of such devices to about 5 hours. Newer designs have added some safety to prolonged use of gas-liquid interphase type oxygenators, but they remain unsuitable for prolonged use. The membrane lung, like the natural lung, interposes a diffusion membrane between the blood and gas phases. In any artificial extracorporeal device there are many factors that contribute to blood trauma, which may be either selective or involve all elements.

In general, there are two factors operative in the blood trauma of extracorporeal devices—the pump, and the surface area or surface forces to which the blood is exposed [42]. The trauma is usually manifest by hemolysis, increased fragility of red cells, loss of white cells and platelets by surface aggregation, and denaturation of proteins [13]. This last effect on plasma proteins is the most significant in that it is the most toxic and limits the bubble oxygenator by its progressive effects on the physiology of circulation [33]. In bubblers, a much larger surface area with large surface forces are exposed to blood, and these forces are several times that produced between blood and membrane materials. Thus, the interposition of a membrane between gas and blood greatly reduces these surface forces and the protein changes that result [34].

The changes in protein configuration result in loss of solubility and changes of biologic activity. Lipoproteins may be separated from their fat molecules, which may then form aggregates large enough to obstruct capillaries. Fat embolization has been reported in clinical cases as a possible cause of death after prolonged perfusions with bubble oxygenators. This phenomenon was not found in comparable circumstances when a membrane lung was used [40]. Marked changes in viscosity, turbidity, and coating of red cells also result from bubble oxygenators, a result of the changes produced in the cellular and protein components of the blood [37, 53]. The effect on clotting by the synthetic surfaces varies with the species and with the material. Significant changes in viscosity and coagulation were not found during 6-hour perfusions with a silicone membrane, though larger exposures might be needed to identify these changes [44]. The membrane lungs show a decreasing rate of hemolysis with time, whereas the disc revealed a constant rate. About half of the total hemolysis is due to the circuits exclusive of the oxygenators.

DEVELOPMENT

Currently available commercial models of membrane lungs are based on a long background of experimental trial and human clinical application even before the availability of efficient nontraumatic membranes. Kolff and Berk [26], in 1944, observed that venous blood would brighten during its course through cellophane dialyzing tubing. Cellophane proved to be an impractical membrane when high flows are needed, though Kolff et al. [27] described a coiled polyethylene apparatus that was used successfully in the canine laboratory around 1956. Clowes et al. [9, 10] developed an artificial lung in 1955 that used a finely grooved surface to hold two sheets of ethylcellulose together. This was developed into a multi-layered apparatus with a surface area of 6 square meters, eventually incorporating Teflon sheets because of better permeability. This was the first clinically practical oxygenator and was used by Clowes routinely for open-heart operations. The limitation of materials and the complexity of the apparatus prevented its widespread use. The stationary membrane oxygenator with alternating layers of blood and gas arranged in a pile to form a large surface area remains one of the basic designs for modern oxygenators now available in disposable form at a reasonable cost. Attempts to introduce other designs such as a rotating drum and oscillating envelopes did not pass the critical test of simplicity and efficiency until the present flood of technical as well as material improvements, which allow a variety of designs tested by routine clinical application.

Present membrane oxygenators have effectively provided for normal gas exchange and acid-base balance of the human subject under basal conditions. The human lung is marvelously versatile in its capacity and design. Thus, blood flow may range from 3 to 30 liters with a gas exchange of 200 to 2,400 ml/min. Current oxygenators available commercially offer an oxygen exchange of 200 to 300 ml/min and carbon dioxide transfer of 160 to 250 ml/min. These are obviously basilar conditions, though versatility is added by changes of flow per square meter and by changes of temperature. It is no longer possible to compare oxygenators on the basis of gas exchange per square meter of surface area because design variations have introduced capillary tubes, rotating membranes, and toroidal flow to improve efficiency and reduce the membrane surface area. Seven oxygenators are generally available for clinical use, four of which are disposable or have disposable inserts. These are presented in Table 23-1 with some of their characteristics.

Important differences in resistance to flow and the operating gas pressures in the gas layers may require two pumps instead of one. This is true of the Peirce-GE [42], the Bramson [7], and the Travenol-Modulung [1] lungs. The Lande-Edwards [33], the Sci-Med Kolobow [28], and the Searle [21] can be operated by gravity flow into the oxygenator or by a single arterial pump for the return of blood. Ob-

Table 23-1. Seven oxygenators generally available for clinical use [15, 52, 44]

Name	Design	Membrane	Surface Area (M^2)	Rated Flow	Oxygen Transfer	Carbon Dioxide Transfer	Pumps	Pressure Limits (torr)
Bramson	Sandwich, 20 cells (adult), built-in heat exchange	Silicone	5.3	3 L/min	30 ml/M^2 or 160 ml/min		1	
Lande-Edwards	Sandwich, 20 layers/M^2	Silicone	1 2 3		20–40 ml/min/M^2		1 or 2	0–80 gravity flow
Peirce-GE	Sandwich, 26 layers/M^3	MEM 213, copolymer of dimethyl silicone and polycarbonate	1 3	0–3 L/min	50 ml/min/M^2	40 ml/min/M^2	2	0–300
Searle	Rotating disc inducing secondary flow	Microporous	0.65	0–7 L/min	370 ml/min		1	Gravity flow, low resistance
Travenol-Modulung	Accordion-pleated	Silicone	0.25 0.75 1.5 3.0	250 ml/min 750 ml/min 1,500 ml/min 3,000 ml/min			1	Gravity flow, low resistance
Sci-Med Kolobow	Spiral coil	Silicone	2.5	2.5 L/min	60 ml/min/M^2		1	0–450
Dow	Capillary	Silicone	4.2	2.4 L/min	35 ml/min/M^2	155 ml/min	1 or 2	High resistance

Note: Not all disposable models are listed. A variety of sizes are available for Sci-Med-Kolobow and Dow. The Peirce-GE is not currently available.

viously, a one-pump system simplifies the technical problems of operation over a long period of time. All these devices when properly operated have adequate capabilities, and the safety of each depends on knowing the system and its limitations. Some characteristics of membrane oxygenators in the laboratory may be summarized as follows: destruction of red cells and rate of hemolysis are well within the tolerable levels for hemoglobin and cell ghosts, considered to be approximately 1 mg/kg/min [45]. Peak levels of plasma hemoglobin are seen at 12 to 18 hours and then decrease. Plasma hemoglobin levels rarely rise above 80 mg per 100 ml. Platelets and white cells demonstrate a transient decrease, up to 50 percent, in the first 24 hours, followed by a rise toward normal.

Occasional platelet transfusions are required, varying somewhat with the design of the oxygenator [21, 28]. The function of the remaining platelets may be abnormal as shown by decreased ability to aggregate in collagen, adenosine diphosphate, and epinephrine [43]. More detailed study of platelet activity and changes during extracorporeal membrane circulation reveal conflicting conclusions [6, 12, 40] about the effect of sequestration and of antiplatelet drugs such as aspirin and dipyridamole. Platelet activity is reduced even more. Reappearance of platelets after the bypass to near normal levels has been ascribed to sequestration in the liver. Comparative autopsy studies using the Techna (Searle) membrane and a Bentley bubble oxygenator revealed normal findings in the membrane group. In the bubble group, bloody diarrhea, gross hematuria, hemorrhage, pericardial and peritoneal effusions, hemorrhagic lungs, post-pump respiratory insufficiency, and decerebration were frequent [51]. These findings corresponded to abnormally high serum enzymes and plasma hemoglobin in the bubble group. Platelets were also reduced less at 24 hours in the membrane (54 percent of control) than in the bubble (34 percent of control) group.

Certain technical problems of cannulation and types of bypass have been investigated. The prolonged use of a veno-venous type of flow with an oxygenator in the line may present certain problems of filter lung damage, though prolonged bypass in lambs by several authors [39, 51] has been performed with safety without producing significant histologic damage to the lungs or other organs. This type of bypass would be ideal for pure pulmonary failure without cardiac or circulatory insufficiency. It is easily instituted using femoral and jugular veins. Its disadvantage is that it does not reduce pulmonary artery pressure.

Femoral vein-to-femoral artery bypass has been favored because of the potential "filter" damage to lungs from embolic particles produced by the extracorporeal circuit; this bypass is more appropriate in states of pulmonary embolism, cardiogenic shock, and following cardiac and great vessel injuries. In this technique, there may be a great disparity between oxygen pressure at femoral and aortic arch areas depending on the amount of poorly oxygenated blood arriving from the lungs. Thus, the lower body might be well oxygenated, whereas the upper body would receive poorly oxygenated and acidotic blood from the lungs. The PO_2 level at the aortic arch has been observed to be as low as 20 torr, whereas the lower body was perfused with blood having a PO_2 of 400 torr [35]. This disadvantage of femoral vein-to-femoral artery bypass has been circumvented by cannulation of the proximal aorta from the femoral artery using a thin-walled polyurethane cannula to achieve proximal mixing of membrane lung return with the blood arriving from the lung [38]. Another suitable technique for proximal mixing is the use of an axillary or right subclavian artery for arterial return. Hill et al. [22] favor a combined veno-venous and veno-arterial bypass as the best way of reducing pulmonary artery pressure, improving pulmonary artery saturation, and contributing to arterial saturation and pressure support.

CLINICAL INDICATIONS

The principal indication for extracorporeal membrane lung respiratory assistance is respiratory insufficiency of a reversible nature that cannot be managed by other means. This principle allows a wide latitude of judgment. Initial cases of all series appear to be desperate end-of-the-line attempts to salvage or support patients who obviously could not survive otherwise. Reversibility in any specific situation may be very difficult to ascertain. The exact timing of intercession becomes critical to the problem of reversibility, and this will undoubtedly become clearer as experience increases and complications of long-term anticoagulation and extracorporeal circulation come under better control. It is difficult to justify early or prophylactic use of extracorporeal membrane oxygenation at this stage.

Current indications are a PA_{O_2} of 45 torr on 100% oxygen, using PI_{O_2} of 45 cm H_2O and PEEP of 15 cm H_2O or more [19, 43]. The presence of myocardial or cerebral ischemia at higher arterial oxygen tensions may be reasons for liberalizing the criteria. Hill et al. [22] reported that in a group of 25 patients receiving prolonged respiratory support, if the patients were on a volume-controlled respirator using 100% oxygen and PEEP of 15 cm H_2O, about half had a consistent PA_{O_2} of less than 40 torr and the others ranged from 40 to 60 torr. Many authors report more extreme circumstances before initiating extracorporeal respiratory assistance.

The problem of reversibility is more difficult to define, as is the problem of when to discontinue assisted oxygenation by an extracorporeal membrane. Open lung biopsy under general anesthesia may offer positive information to help in the selection of patients [22]. Diffuse cystic necrosis, diffuse pulmonary hemorrhage, and diffuse nodular intrapulmonary masses in the lung are bad prognostic signs. These all indicate a diffuse pulmonary fibrosis. Reversible pulmonary disease on microscopic examination reveals interalveolar fluid, interstitial edema, alveolar infiltrates, hyaline membranes, nonspecific inflammatory cellular response, and fat emboli.

Contraindications to extracorporeal membrane bypass are (1) active bleeding; (2) irreversible brain damage; (3) progressive systemic disease such as cancer, chronic obstructive pulmonary disease, severe heart failure, or central nervous system disease; (4) if the pulmonary disease has been present for more than 3 weeks [22]. To this list should be added those patients who have diffuse destruction of lung tissue at the time of lung biopsy. Replacement of the lung by giant cysts and fibrosis does not offer a possibility of success in a matter of days.

PATHOPHYSIOLOGY AND RESULTS

The clinical indications for extracorporeal oxygenation fall into three general categories: (1) infant hyaline membrane disease; (2) acute respiratory insufficiency in adults from an infectious agent; and (3) trauma with such sequelae as shock lung, fat embolism, respiratory burn, and pulmonary embolism. Pierce [43] also includes oxygen toxicity and respiratory failure in conjunction with heart failure as possible reasons for the use of membrane oxygenation.

In infants, the principal cause of reversible pulmonary insufficiency is hyaline membrane disease. Although the prognosis for this disease has improved with current techniques of pulmonary care, about 50 percent of cases remain irreversible. The prognosis of this disease can be determined with reasonable accuracy. Stohlman et al. [50] have outlined a linear discriminant for determining prognosis. Though the respiratory distress syndrome of infants is a potentially reversible condition, little success has been obtained in trials of this technique by White et al. [54] and Dorson et al. [14]. The principal cause of death was hemorrhage. However, though these infants were moribund, partial reversibility of the pulmonary lesions and the effectiveness of pulmonary support was demonstrated.

The long-term successes of extracorporeal membrane oxygenation for acute respiratory insufficiency have been in adults. To date, there have been over 130 patients treated for respiratory insufficiency by extracorporeal membrane oxygenation, with 15 known survivors [22]. The conditions that have been treated include a variety of pneumonias and the sequelae of trauma. The results in pneumonia have been disappointing, though these may be related to the advanced stages of other organ dysfunction at the time bypass is instituted. The conditions in the survivors were generally related to trauma with short-term pulmonary insufficiency requiring extracorporeal support. Hill et al. [22] have the most extensive experience in membrane support for pulmonary insufficiency using the Bramson lung. They reported 12 patients with pneumonia, of whom 8 died during bypass; there were no long-term survivors. Awad et al. [1], on the other hand, reported a 5-year-old child with mucoviscidosis and extensive bilateral pneumonia caused by *Staphylococcus aureus* and *Pseudomonas aeruginosa* who survived after a 48-hour membrane support. Rea et al. [47] reported 3 patients, 2 of whom had pneumonia, one a fulminating viral pneumonia, the other an overwhelming infection with *Klebsiella pneumoniae*. Though neither of these patients was a long-term survivor, they both demonstrated marked improvement in lung function and compliance, were removed from membrane assistance, and died because of a technical problem with the membrane and a cerebral hemorrhage.

Chang et al. [8] reported experience with two patients with pulmonary infection, one of whom was a long-term survivor. Joseph et al. [25] performed veno-venous and veno-arterial oxygenation in 5 cases of pulmonary infection, 2 of which were bacterial pneumonia and 3, *Pneumocystis carinii* pneumonia. One patient with *P. carinii* pneumonia perfused with a veno-venous bypass for 5 days was a long-term survivor. Kolobow et al. [29] also had one survivor with pulmonary insufficiency caused by *P. carinii* pneumonia requiring a bypass of 9.5 days. Gannon [17] has added a survivor with influenza A pneumonia. Thus, there are at least 5 out of 35 reported cases surviving long term after overwhelming infections by virus, bacteria, *P. carinii*, or aspiration pneumonia. In addition to these, there are a significant number of patients who were treated by membrane support for these conditions who improved enough to be removed from support only to die later of recurrent respiratory failure, complications of the procedure, or unrelated disease.

Trauma, under which are classified such entities as shock lung, fat emboli, lung contusion, postsurgical states, respiratory burns, and amniotic fluid emboli, forms the other large group of conditions for which extracorporeal membrane oxygenation has been used successfully. Hill et al. [22] had 4 survivors in 13 patients in this group, 3 of whom were classified as having shock lung secondary to trauma, and one as suffering from fat emboli. In a collected group of 27 patients from many authors, there were 6 survivors, including the 4 reported by Hill et al. One of the additional cases was a postoperative atrioventricular canal assisted for 43 hours [48], and the other a multiple trauma assisted for 4.5 days [56].

FACTORS THAT APPEAR TO INFLUENCE SURVIVAL

It is obvious from the case reports that many of the patients were not salvageable, or that therapy was applied too late in the course of their disease. Experience will liberalize the indications for this form of therapy and reduce the number of irreversible conditions that are treated.

Bad prognostic signs include prolonged therapy before extracorporeal membrane oxygenation, hypercapnea in progressive lung failure, severe heart failure, renal shutdown, a diffuse cystic or fibrotic disease of the lungs by biopsy, and a fixed intrapulmonary shunt. Disseminated intravascular coagulopathy is not necessarily a contraindication, because satisfactory reversal of this condition during perfusion has been observed [22]. There is some evidence that patients with a short severe course in general are better candidates than those approaching 2 weeks of therapy. A marked increase in pulmonary vascular resistance in the absence of hypoxemia may signify extensive destruction of pulmonary vasculature. Active bleeding, such as from a peptic ulcer, should be considered a contraindication.

The timing of death in those who were not long-term survivors reveals that approximately 50 percent of all patients die during bypass and another 25 percent die after removal from membrane support [22]. Causes of death are generally progressive lung failure, hemorrhage, cardiac failure or arrest, and central nervous system damage. In Hill's series [22], progressive lung failure from a variety of causes (infection, fistula, fibrosis) was the most common cause of death, with hemorrhage less prominent. In the larger series reported by Quist et al. [47], hemorrhage accounted for over 20 percent of the deaths, and was perhaps the single most common cause along with pulmonary, cardiac, and cerebral damage.

Evaluation of pulmonary function for improvement or deterioration while on extracorporeal perfusion is difficult. Measurements of fixed or variable shunts, alveolar-arterial oxygen gradients ($AaPO_2$), compliance, and the functional residual capacity (FRC) have been used to assess lung function periodically. In addition, the ability of the patient to respond to decreasing membrane support and finally to test periods off the membrane are important methods of deciding the critical questions of when to stop extracorporeal support. During extracorporeal bypass, respiration with positive pressure and positive end expiratory pressure generally must be continued. However, tidal volume and inspiratory oxygen concentration (FI_{O_2}) may be reduced to lower the peak inspiratory pressure below 45 cm H_2O and to reduce oxygen toxicity effects. Zapol [56] states that radiography, functional residual capacity, and compliance are not affected by changes in extracorporeal blood flow or cardiac output, thus making them excellent methods for evaluation of pulmonary function during bypass.

The calculation of pulmonary shunting ($\dot{Q}s/\dot{Q}T$) may have prognostic significance in that if the shunt is reduced by positive end expiratory pressure or by the membrane, it indicates reversibility of the pulmonary insufficiency [22] (Figure 23-1). The shunt may also be followed by periodic measurements during the bypass for improvements in lung function. The fixed shunt fraction is generally very high in all patients before being treated by extracorporeal membrane oxygenation, ranging from 50 to 80 percent. Cannulation and perfusion patterns significantly affect the response of pulmonary hemodynamics and gas exchange during bypass and thus affect prognosis. Veno-venous, veno-arterial, or combined veno-venous and veno-

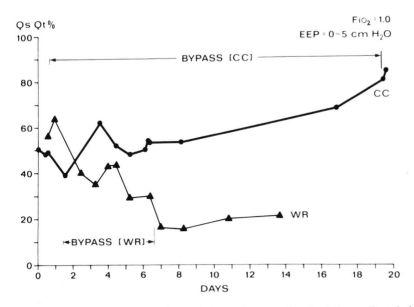

Figure 23-1. Graph showing the changes in intrapulmonary shunting in two patients before, during, and after bypass. Rapid decrease of shunting (patient W. R.) was followed by survival. The progressive increase in intrapulmonary shunting (patient C. C.) was followed by death shortly after bypass. (Reproduced with permission from Hill, J. D., et al. Prognostic factors in the treatment of acute respiratory insufficiency with long-term extracorporeal oxygenation. *Journal of Thoracic and Cardiovascular Surgery* 68, 1974, p. 905. Fig. 4, p. 908.)

arterial modes result in a variety of perfusion patterns of all organs, particularly of the heart and lungs. In those patients in whom membrane oxygenation reversed the disease, the best criterion of improvement was an improvement in arterial oxygen pressure, a decrease in the shunt fraction across the lung, and a decrease in total pulmonary vascular resistance (Figure 23-2). Veno-venous bypass tends to increase pulmonary flow and shunting, whereas a combined pattern of veno-venous and veno-arterial bypass offers the best opportunity for improvement. The pulmonary insufficiency index (PII), based on the construction of effective alveolar-arterial oxygen gradient graphs for each patient, may be used to predict mortality rates and thus to select patients for extracorporeal membrane oxygenation [23]. Although this method is helpful for selecting the high-risk acute patients for extracorporeal membrane oxygenation, it is not helpful after the onset of bypass because the alveolar-arterial gradient is altered by this procedure.

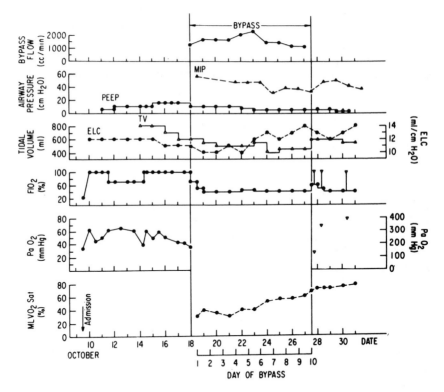

Figure 23-2. Respiratory function before, during, and after membrane bypass for ten days. PEEP = positive end-expiratory pressure; MIP = maximal inspiratory pressure; ELC = effective lung compliance; TV = tidal volume; FI_{O_2} = inspired oxygen concentration; Pa_{O_2} = arterial oxygen tension; MLV_{O_2} = oxygen saturation of venous blood entering the membrane lung. (Reproduced with permission from Kolobow, T., et al., Acute respiratory failure. Survival following ten days' support with a membrane lung. *Journal of Thoracic and Cardiovascular Surgery* 69, 1975, p. 947. Fig. 2, p. 249.)

HEMATOLOGIC PROBLEMS OF EXTRACORPOREAL MEMBRANE OXYGENATION

The management of coagulation during perfusion is critical, as judged by the high incidence of hemorrhage into various compartments of the body and by the high incidence of bleeding as a major cause of death or interruption of extracorporeal flow. Heparin has been universally used as the anticoagulant. Maintenance of the proper heparin level is important for the prevention of clotting in the extracorporeal circuit and hemorrhage in the patient. The traditional glass-tube whole-blood clotting time of Lee and White has serious disadvantages when dealing with continuous heparin administration because of the long time periods involved and the consequent delay in obtaining information that is critical to the conduct of the bypass on a minute-to-minute basis. The activated partial thromboplastin time (APTT) has been used to monitor heparin levels [49, 57], but the accuracy of this when whole-blood clotting times are longer than 20 minutes has been questioned by Ray and Harper [46] because of poor correlation with clotting times.

The activated clotting time (ACT) has been used by Hill and his group [20] as the most sensitive, rapid, and reproducible test of heparin activity. This test can be performed by hand or by an automated machine to record clotting time in seconds even with high levels of anticoagulant activity. It is sensitive to all drugs or factors that alter coagulation, and it can be repeated at frequent intervals with little loss of time or effort. In this test, a metered amount of blood is placed in a glass tube containing diatomaceous earth as an accelerent for the clotting mechanism. Hemochron (International Technedyne, Box 2200, Menlo Park Station, Edison, N.J.) has developed an automatic method whereby the tube is rotated with a magnet stirrer at $38°$ C and records the formation of a clot automatically. There is a close correlation between the activated clotting time and the Lee-White clotting time. Similarly, there is a good correlation between the hand-held activated clotting time apparatus and the Hemochron time. An ACT of 200 to 300 sec is adequate for long-term perfusions, and this level is not associated with excessive ooze in the surgical fields. The activated clotting time can be kept within close range, though the heparin dose will vary from patient to patient and may vary with such variables as body temperature and hemodilution. Heparin is best administered with a continuous infusion pump that allows for exact changes of rate according to the activated clotting time. The whole blood recalcification time (BART) is useful and more linear in its relationship to heparin activity than the activated partial thromboplastin time [43]. Because the half-clearance time for heparin is about 1 to 2 hours, the test for anticoagulation effect should be carried out at least once an hour, or preferably every half hour.

Bleeding problems vary with the control of heparin activity, with the type of bypass, and with the control of platelet activity. Heparin control is best monitored by the activated clotting time at two or three times normal levels. Veno-venous bypass is associated with less blood loss than is veno-arterial bypass. The factors leading to blood loss are increased for combined veno-venous and veno-arterial bypass. Incisional and cannulation site losses are compounded by the presence of a tracheostomy [29] or bleeding into the pleural or gastrointestinal tracts [8, 47]. Blood loss resulting from frequent blood samples may be large and may exceed 200 ml per day. Wound bleeding tends to subside after 2 or 3 days of bypass.

The management of platelets is also important to internal and incisional blood loss. Platelets may be maintained by fresh platelet transfusions, though these are not always necessary. Adequate activity appears to be present if levels are kept above 20,000/ml [29], though some groups prefer to maintain levels of 40,000 to 60,000/ml. Platelet consumption tends to plateau as bypass continues, but may be accelerated at any time that a membrane and tubing are changed. Thus, adding new surface areas is avoided unless required by impairment of gas transfer or leaks. The newer microporous membranes do not differ significantly from the Silastic membranes in their effect on platelets and clotting factors [4, 15].

The management of fluid and blood components during bypass requires frequent monitoring of hematocrit, platelets, fibrinogen, prothrombin time, fibrin split products, and activated clotting time. All cellular and protein fluids except platelets should be passed through microfilters to remove macroaggregates. It is preferable to use saline–washed frozen red cells and albumin because of the improved oxygen-carrying capacity and elimination of hazards such as hepatitis, megaloviruses, and antigenic reactions of foreign white cells, platelets, and plasma.

The hematocrit is maintained above 30 percent and preferably closer to 40 percent. Hemodilution is avoided because of the tendency toward extravascular fluid retention. Excessive hemodilution may be controlled by repeated doses of ethacrynic acid, furosemide, or albumin.

Disseminated intravascular coagulation may be present before, during, or after the extracorporeal membrane oxygenation. This condition may produce diffuse bleeding and organ dysfunction, and may cause death by itself if not reversed; it is also the consequence of shock or hypoxia. It was present in 8 patients reported by Hill et al. [22], in most before extracorporeal membrane oxygenation was started. Four of these patients showed a reversal of disseminated intravascular coagulation during perfusion.

THE CIRCUITRY

The clinical experience points up three basic circuits that have been used successfully, each with theoretical advantages and disadvantages. A review of 44 patients by Lefrak et al. [36] reveals that veno-arterial and veno-venous circuits were used about equally, and all methods can now be done with a one-pump system. Veno-venous (Figure 23-3) or prepulmonary oxygenation has the advantage of allowing the heart to distribute the newly oxygenated blood in a fairly uniform manner, presuming the absence of congestive heart failure. It is especially adaptable for children or infants. Through a cervical and femoral incision, a drainage cannula is usually inserted proximally to the diaphragm. A cannula is also inserted into the distal vein. Pump return is to the internal jugular vein, though the direction of blood flow may be reversed according to cannulation problems. Hill feels that the

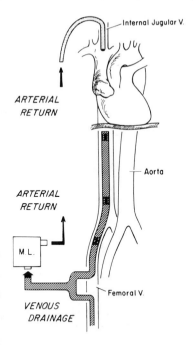

Figure 23-3. A veno-venous circuit for extracorporeal oxygenation using the Kolobow lung. (Reproduced with permission from Zapol, W. M. Extracorporeal perfusion for acute respiratory failure. *Journal of Thoracic and Cardiovascular Surgery* 69:439, 1975. Fig. 1, p. 440.)

veno-venous component of the bypass is important to maintain a proper venous saturation and blood flow for healing.

The pulmonary circuit is the principal source of blood supply for the lung. There is evidence that during veno-arterial bypass (Figure 23-4) pulmonary artery pressure and flow are reduced, and this may have deleterious effects on the primary hope of the procedure, namely, improved lung function. Hill combines veno-venous with veno-arterial flow for improved organ perfusion and for control of pulmonary artery pressure (Figure 23-5). He attempts to maintain a pulmonary artery saturation above 70 percent and a pulmonary artery pressure of 20 to 25 torr. This combined technique offers the advantages of both, namely, a high bypass flow, improvement of aortic arch desaturation, and improved organ perfusion with heart failure. McEnany [38] has described the long femoral artery-to-aortic arch cannula for veno-arterial bypass to obviate aortic arch desaturation, but this will undoubtedly present problems of resistance and problems of passage through small or arteriosclerotic vessels (Figure 23-6). The veno-venous or the combined veno-venous and veno-arterial modes appear to be the preferred techniques now. Cannulation of the right axillary artery for the arterial return has also been used. The axillary artery is a small vessel, and this technique poses inherent dangers to the arm and brachial plexus.

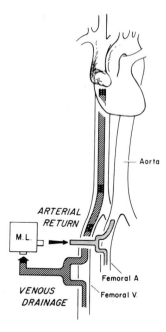

Figure 23–4. Veno-arterial perfusion. (Reproduced with permission from Zapol, W. M. Extracorporeal perfusion for acute respiratory failure. *Journal of Thoracic and Cardiovascular Surgery* 69:439, 1975. Fig. 2, p. 440.)

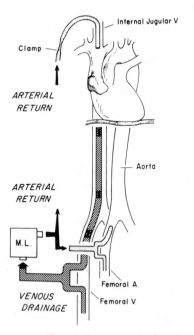

Figure 23–5. Mixed veno-venous and veno-arterial perfusion. (Reproduced with permission from Zapol, W. M. Extracorporeal perfusion for acute respiratory failure. *Journal of Thoracic and Cardiovascular Surgery* 69:439, 1975. Fig. 3, p. 441.)

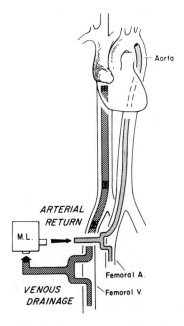

Aorta

ARTERIAL
RETURN

M.L.

Femoral A.

VENOUS
DRAINAGE

Femoral V.

Figure 23-6. Veno-arterial arch perfusion. (Reproduced with permission from Zapol, W. M. Extracorporeal perfusion for acute respiratory failure. *Journal of Thoracic and Cardiovascular Surgery* 69:439, 1975. Fig. 4, p. 441.)

Cannulations should be performed both proximally and distally to the extremities to avoid venous congestion or arterial insufficiency. If not done, pain and discomfort will occur in many patients, even though the limb is not threatened.

Bypass time has varied up to 21 days [22] although most bypasses have required 2 to 4 days. It is of interest that bypass in 9 known survivors varied from 43 hours to 9½ days [8, 29, 45, 56].

PERFUSION EQUIPMENT

The type of perfusion equipment needed varies with the oxygenator. Two-pump, one-pump, and no-pump systems have been used, though the preference at the moment is for a one-pump system servoregulated for ease of control over a long period of time. A closed bag reservoir may be used as the sensing device for automatic control of the pump to activate an on-and-off switch and prevent suction, should the flow suddenly change. More sophisticated weight devices can be used to regulate the speed of the pump automatically. Continuous monitoring of oxygen pressure is most helpful in both the arterial and venous lines. A multilumen pulmonary artery catheter positioned for measurement of wedge and mean pulmonary artery pressures and thermodilution cardiac outputs is necessary for managing and monitoring the various modes of perfusion. Inlet and outlet pressures of the oxygenator are helpful to detect changing resistance that heralds the need for change of oxygenator.

The frequency of oxygenator change may be determined by the changing resistance to flow and decreasing gas transfer calculation. Kolobow [29] used 3 oxygenators in a 10-day perfusion. Zapol et al. [56] change the Kolobow oxygenators if output flow saturation falls below 90 percent. The duration of a single oxygenator will vary with the design, the flow, and the level of heparinization. It is common experience that the inlet and outlet ports and corners are most susceptible to clotting; and that high flows and higher levels of anticoagulation reduce the problems of clot or fibrin and platelet deposition, which in turn will effect the life of the oxygenator. The size of oxygenator or surface area for a particular patient will vary with the size of the patient, and a wide variety of sizes are now available.

Because of the changing designs and the increased efficiency of certain membranes such as the microporous membranes, it is probably no longer feasible to speak of surface area of the conventional silicone membrane, but rather of rated oxygen delivery and flow. Rated blood flow, namely, the maximum flow at which an oxygenating device will maintain an arterial outflow saturation of 95 percent when presented with blood having a saturation of 60 to 75 percent and a hematocrit of 40 to 42 percent, more adequately reflects the capability of any one device irrespective of membrane type of area. Oxygen transfer will vary with the flow within certain limits, but present oxygenators provide adequate excess capacity such that changes of flow are inconsequential or may be compensated for by changes of shim pressure. Thus, most silicone membrane oxygenators will have oxygen transfer capabilities of 25 to 50 ml/min/M^2, depending on the model and flow rates. The microporous membranes have much higher oxygen and carbon dioxide transfer capabilities per square meter, and these are variable depending on the width of the blood layer. Thus, 2.5 M^2 of this type membrane in the Travenol-Teflo system is rated for 6 liters/min flow of blood or equivalent to about 6 M^2 of silicone rubber or copolymer membranes. Partial bypass in adults should have a rated flow of at least 3 L/min or 150 ml of oxygen transfer capabilities. Total pulmonary failure will require twice this capacity.

The need or the feasibility of an ultrafilter in the system for prolonged extracorporeal membrane oxygenation has not been established on a clinical level. There is evidence that microemboli are fewer with membrane oxygenation when used during short-term bypasses in open-heart operations. The need for filters on a long-term basis is not known. The disadvantages of platelet loss and gradient problems because of the marginal anticoagulation would argue against their use. They may add many problems of potential bleeding without adding any advantages. This is particularly true of the veno-venous type of bypass. Newer experimental systems that allow extracorporeal bypass without heparinization would alter this view and probably require some sort of filtration, because a high rate of particle infusion may add damage to already damaged organs.

REFERENCES

1. Awad, J. A., et al. Biologic studies with a membrane oxygenator during prolonged arteriovenous bypass. *Int. Surg.* 59, 1974, p. 548.

2. Baeza, O. R., Wagner, R. B., and Lowery, B. D. Pulmonary hyperinflation: A form of barotrauma during mechanical ventilation. *J. Thorac. Cardiovasc. Surg.* 70, 1975, p. 790.

3. Bartlett, R. H., et al. Mortality prediction in adult respiratory insufficiency. *Chest* 67, 1975, p. 680.

4. Bartlett, R. H., et al. Hematologic responses to prolonged extracorporeal circulation (ECC) with microporous membrane devices. *Trans. Am. Soc. Artif. Intern. Organs* 21, 1975, p. 250.

5. Birnbaum, D., and Eiseman, B. Laboratory evaluation of a new silicone membrane oxygenator. *J. Thorac. Cardiovasc. Surg.* 64, 1972, p. 441.

6. Bloom, S., et al. Platelet destruction during 24 hour membrane lung perfusion. *Trans. Am. Soc. Artif. Intern. Organs* 20A, 1974, p. 299.

7. Bramson, M. L., et al. A new disposable membrane oxygenator with integral heat exchange. *J. Thorac. Cardiovasc. Surg.* 50, 1965, p. 39.

8. Chang, V. P., et al. Acute respiratory failure managed by prolonged partial extracorporeal oxygenation. *Med. J. Aust.* 1, 1974, p. 350.

9. Clowes, G. H. A., Jr., Hopkins, A. L., and Kolobow, T. Oxygen diffusion through plastic films. *Trans. Am. Soc. Artif. Intern. Organs* 1, 1955, p. 23.

10. Clowes, G. H. A., Jr., Hopkins, A. L., and Neville, W. E. An artificial lung dependent upon diffusion of oxygen and carbon dioxide through plastic membranes. *J. Thorac. Cardiovasc. Surg.* 32, 1956, p. 630.

11. deLaval, M., et al. Platelet kinetics during extracorporeal circulation. *Trans. Am. Soc. Artif. Intern. Organs* 18, 1972, p. 355.

12. Dennis, C., et al. Development of a pump-oxygenator to replace the heart and lungs. An apparatus applicable to human patients and application to one case. *Ann. Surg.* 134, 1951, p. 709.

13. Dobell, H. R. C., et al. Biologic evaluation of blood after prolonged recirculation through film and membrane oxygenators. *Ann. Surg.* 161, 1965, p. 617.

14. Dorson, W., et al. Response of distressed infants to partial bypass lung assist. *Trans. Am. Soc. Artif. Intern. Organs* 16, 1970, p. 345.

15. Eiseman, B., et al. A new gas permeable membrane for blood oxygenators. *Surg. Gynecol. Obstet.* 135, 1972, p. 732.

16. Galletti, P. M., and Brecher, G. A. *Heart-Lung Bypass. Principles and Technique of Extracorporeal Circulation.* New York: Grune & Stratton, 1962, p. 61.

17. Gannon, P. Personal communication, 1975.

18. Gibbon, J. H., Jr. Artificial maintenance of circulation during experimental occlusion of pulmonary artery. *Arch. Surg.* 34, 1937, p. 1105.

19. Hill, J. D., et al. Clinical prolonged extracorporeal circulation for respiratory insufficiency: Hematological effects.
Trans. Am. Soc. Artif. Int. Organs 18, 1972, p. 546.

20. Hill, J. D., et al. A simple method of heparin management during prolonged extracorporeal circulation. *Ann. Thorac. Surg.* 17, 1974, p. 129.

21. Hill, J. D., et al. Technique for achieving high gas oxygen rates in membrane oxygenation. *Trans. Am. Soc. Artif. Intern. Organs* 208, 1974, p. 249.

22. Hill, J. D., et al. Prognostic factors in the treatment of acute respiratory insufficiency with long-term extracorporeal oxygenation. *J. Thorac. Cardiovasc. Surg.* 68, 1974, p. 905.

23. Hill, R. N., et al. Adult respiratory distress syndrome: Early predictors of mortality. *Trans. Am. Soc. Artif. Intern. Organs* 21, 1975, p. 199.
24. Holdefer, W. F., and Tracy, W. G. The use of the rated blood flow to describe the oxygenating capability of membrane lungs. *Ann. Thorac. Surg.* 15, 1973, p. 156.
25. Joseph, W. L., et al. Membrane lung support in acute respiratory insufficiency. *Med. Ann. D.C.* 42, 1973, p. 599.
26. Kolff, W. J., and Berk, H. T. J. Artificial kidney: Dialyzer with great area. *Acta Med. Scand.* 117, 1944, p. 121.
27. Kolff, W. J., et al. Disposable membrane oxygenator (heart-lung machine) and its use in experimental surgery. *Cleve. Clin. Q.* 23, 1956, p. 67.
28. Kolobow, T., and Bowman, R. L. Construction and evaluation of an alveolar membrane artificial heart-lung. *Trans. Am. Soc. Artif. Intern. Organs* 9, 1963, p. 238.
29. Kolobow, T., et al. Acute respiratory failure. Survival following 10 days support with a membrane lung. *J. Thorac. Cardiovasc. Surg.* 69, 1975, p. 947.
30. Kolobow, T., et al. Superior blood compatibility of silicone rubber free of silica filler in the membrane lung. *Trans. Am. Soc. Artif. Intern. Organs* 20A, 1974, p. 269.
31. Lamy, M., et al. Effects of extracorporeal membrane oxygenation (ECMO) on pulmonary hemodynamics, gas exchange, and prognosis. *Trans. Am. Soc. Artif. Intern. Organs* 21, 1975, p. 188.
32. Lande, A. J., et al. A new membrane oxygenator dialyzer. *Surg. Clin. North Am.* 47, 1967, p. 1461.
33. Lee, W. H., Jr., et al. Comparison of the effects of membrane and nonmembrane oxygenators on the biochemical and biophysical characteristics of blood. *Surg. Forum* 12, 1961, p. 200.
34. Lee, W. H., Jr., et al. Denaturation of plasma proteins as a cause of morbidity and death after intracardiac operations. *Surgery* 50, 1961, p. 29.
35. Lefemine, A. A., and Harken, D. E. Extracorporeal support of the circulation by means of venoarterial bypass with an oxygenator. *J. Thorac. Cardiovasc. Surg.* 62, 1971, p. 769.
36. Lefrak, E. A., et al. Clinical use of membrane lungs in acute respiratory insufficiency. *Thoraxchirurgie* 21, 1974, p. 494.
37. Lyman, D. J., Muir, W. M., and Lee, I. J. The effect of chemical structure and surface properties of polymers on the coagulation of blood. I. Surface free energy effects. *Trans. Am. Soc. Artif. Intern. Organs* 11, 1965, p. 301.
38. McEnany, M. T., et al. Cannulation of the proximal aorta during chronic membrane lung perfusion. Presented at the 55th Annual Meeting of the American Association for Thoracic Surgery April 14–16, 1975. 70:631 1975.
39. Mielke, C. H., Jr., deLaval, M., and Hill, J. D. Drug influence on platelet loss during extracorporeal circulation. *J. Thorac. Cardiovasc. Surg.* 66, 1973, p. 845.
40. Owens, G., Adams, J. E., and Scott, H. W., Jr. Embolic fat as a measure of adequacy of various oxygenators. *J. Appl. Physiol.* 15, 1960, p. 999.
41. Peirce, E. C. The membrane lung. Its excuse, present status, and promise. *J. Mt. Sinai Hosp.* 34, 1967, p. 437.

42. Peirce, E. C., II. A comparison of the Lande-Edwards, the Peirce and the General Electric–Peirce membrane lungs. *Trans. Am. Soc. Artif. Intern. Organs* 16, 1970, p. 358.

43. Peirce, E. C., II. The role of the artificial lung in the treatment of respiratory insufficiency. A perspective. *Chest* 62, 1972, p. 107S.

44. Peirce, E. C., II, et al. Comparative trauma to blood in the disc oxygenator and membrane lung. *Trans. Am. Soc. Artif. Int. Organs* 15, 1969, p. 33.

45. Quist, A. J., Hansen, D. D., Pontoppidan, H. Parteil perfusion med. membrano Ksygenatorer i be hand lingen ab akut respirations. Uges Kr. Laeger 135; 1808, 1973.

46. Ray, P., and Harper, T. Comparison of activated recalcification and partial thromboplastin tests as controls of heparin therapy. *J. Lab. Clin. Med.* 77, 1971, p. 901.

47. Rea, W. J., et al. Long-term membrane oxygenation in respiratory failure. *Ann. Thorac. Surg.* 15, 1973, p. 170.

48. Schulte, H. D., Birchks, W., and Dudzeak, R. Erste Erfahrungen mit der Bramson-Membran-Lunge. *Thoraxchirurgie* 20, 1972, p. 54.

49. Spector, I., and Corn, M. Control of heparin therapy with activated partial thromboplastin times. *J.A.M.A.* 201, 1967, p. 75.

50. Stohlman, M. T., et al. Prognosis in hyaline-membrane disease. Use of a linear discriminant. *N. Engl. J. Med.* 276, 1967, p. 303.

51. Subramanian, V. A., Wright, W. L., and Berger, R. L. A new efficient disposable membrane oxygenator vs Bentley bubble oxygenator. *Surg. Forum* 25, 1974, p. 132.

52. Ward, B. D., and Hood, A. G. Comparative performance of clinical membrane lungs. *J. Thorac. Cardiovasc. Surg.* 68, 1974, p. 830.

53. Waugh, D. F. Proteins and Their Interactions. In Oncley, J. L. (ed.), *Biophysical Science.* New York: Wiley, 1959, p. 84.

54. White, J. J., et al. Prolonged respiratory support in newborn infants with a membrane oxygenator. *Surgery* 70, 1971, p. 288.

55. Whitely, D. E., et al. 24 hour membrane oxygenation without systemic heparin. *Surg. Forum* 23, 1972, p. 244.

56. Zapol, W. M., et al. Extracorporeal perfusion for acute respiratory failure. Recent experience with a spiral coil membrane lung. *J. Thorac. Cardiovasc. Surg.* 69, 1975, p. 439.

57. Zucker, S., and Cathey, M. Control of heparin therapy: Sensitivity of the activated partial thromboplastin time for monitoring the antithrombotic effects of heparin. *J. Lab. Clin. Med.* 73, 1969, p. 320.

Maurice S. Segal

Glossary of Therapeutics

24

The most commonly employed medications in respiratory care include the following: the bronchodilators (beta adrenergic stimulants and aminophylline), the steroids, the sputalytics (mucolytic aerosols and iodides), and the newer preventive mediator release agents. The tables list the numerous therapeutic drugs available to the physician for managing the problems of bronchodilation, bronchial inflammation, paranasal sinus involvement, and the blocking of (allergic) mediator release substances.

ADRENERGIC BRONCHODILATORS
    Beta adrenergic bronchodilator aerosols   Table 24–1
    Beta adrenergic injectables   Table 24–2
    Alpha adrenergic nasal decongestants   Table 24–3
    Therapeutic aerosols   Table 24–4
AMINOPHYLLINES
    Oral   Table 24–5
    Rectal   Table 24–6
    Injectable   Table 24–7
STEROIDS
    Glucocorticoids   Table 24–8
    Commonly employed steroids   Table 24–9
    Steroid aerosols   Table 24–10
    Nasal steroid aerosols   Table 24–11
MUCOLYTIC AEROSOLS   Table 24–12
IODIDE PREPARATIONS   Table 24–13
SPECIFIC MEDIATOR RELEASE BLOCKING DRUGS   Table 24–14

Table 24-1. Beta Adrenergic Bronchodilator Aerosols

BRONCHODILATORS

Beta adrenergic receptor-stimulating drugs (agonists) are available as pressurized aerosols (freon-powered) and some in solution and oral (see Table 24-5) forms. Some have more bronchoselective (beta 2) and less cardioselective (beta 1) properties, acting by means of the activation of the enzyme adenyl cyclase, which catalyzes the conversion of adenosine triphosphate into adenosine cyclic 3', 5' monophosphate (cyclic AMP), the smooth muscle relaxing substance (SMRS).

The functions of these bronchodilators vary with their structural alterations from the basic isoproterenol hydrochloride formula. They differ as to onset, intensity, and duration of bronchodilation. However, unlike isoproterenol, several (e.g., metaproterenol, salbutamol, terbutaline) may be effective orally, because they are not metabolized by catechol-O-methyl transferase or sulfatase enzymes in the gut. Taken orally, they resemble ephedrine sulfate in their action.

SIDE EFFECTS

The physician is advised to check carefully all the ingredients in the aerosol, other than the principal agent; namely, the excipients, dyes, preservatives, adjuvants, and the inert fluorocarbon propellants. Potential toxicity, idiosyncrasy, and allergic reactions from the agents must be kept in mind. Notable side effects include nervousness, insomnia, tremors, headaches, palpitations, blood pressure changes, tachycardia, arrhythmias, nausea, vomiting, abdominal pains, and paradoxical asthma.

PRECAUTIONS

Individual allergies or idiosyncrasies, cardiovascular disease, hyperthyroidism, stroke, and the like. Usually not more than 2 puffs at 4- to 6-hour intervals is recommended for these aerosols. Consult physician when more is required.

PHARMACODYNAMICS OF AIRWAYS SMOOTH MUSCLE

The bronchoconstricting mediators (e.g., histamine and slow-reacting substance of anaphylaxis, SRS-A) are produced by antigen-antibody (IgE) interaction on sensitive cells. A humoral *first messenger* substance is *endogenously* produced or is liberated by a neuron or mast (generating) cell, or *exogenously* introduced drug. This messenger interacts with its specific (physiologic) receptor on the muscle cell surface, setting off a series of steps by means of an enzyme system; this process ultimately leads either to an increase of the intracellular chemical *second messenger*, cyclic AMP (the SMRS), resulting in bronchodilation, or to a decrease in cyclic AMP, resulting in bronchoconstriction. Specific receptors for the pharmacologic mediators have been postulated as attached to surface enzymes, namely, *adenyl cyclase, phosphodiesterase,* or *prostaglandin synthetase.* Bronchoactive pharmacologic mediators act by stimulating or inhibiting these receptors. Thus humoral bronchodilators (e.g., adrenaline and the beta adrenergic agonists) act by means of their specific receptors and the adenyl cyclase mechanism, producing cyclic AMP and mediating bronchodilation. It has been proposed that the specific receptor for prostaglandins E_1 and E_2 is also attached to adenyl cyclase, which it activates, leading to production of cyclic AMP and bronchodilation. On the other hand, the receptor for $PGF_{2\alpha}$ may be on phosphodiesterase, which it activates, leading to cyclic AMP destruction and bronchoconstriction. Theophylline accomplishes the same result by inhibiting phosphodiesterase, thus effectively altering histamine release by delaying cyclic AMP degradation, leading to bronchodilation.

Trade Name	Company	Content	Delivered Dosages
Aerolone Compound	Lilly	Cyclopentamine hydrochloride	0.5 gm in 100 ml solution
		Isoproterenol hydrochloride	0.25 gm in 100 ml solution
			Fine-mist nebulization, 1 to 2 inhalations q4h prn, or diluted in saline. Air-oxygen or demand valve for 5 to 10 min prn for slow nebulization
Alupent	Boehringer Ingelheim	Metaproterenol sulfate	0.65 mg/puff-dose, metered dosages
Asthma-Meter	Rexall	Epinephrine	0.25 mg/puff-dose, metered dosages
Bronkometer	Breon	Isoetharine (0.61%)	340 µg/puff-dose, metered dosages
		Phenylephrine hydrochloride (0.125%) in 30% alcohol	70 µg/puff-dose, metered dosages
Bronkosol	Breon	Isoetharine (1%)	In solution form, nebulization techniques
		Phenylephrine hydrochloride (0.25%)	
Duo-Medihaler	Riker	Isoproterenol hydrochloride	0.16 mg/puff-dose, metered dosages
		Phenylephrine bitartrate	0.24 mg/puff-dose, metered dosages
Iso-Autohaler	Riker	Isoproterenol hydrochloride	0.16 mg/puff-dose, metered (controlled) single dosage
Isuprel Mistometer	Winthrop	Isoproterenol hydrochloride	125 µg/puff-dose, metered dosages
Isuprel	Winthrop	Isoproterenol hydrochloride	In solution form, 1:100 and 1:200 (1 to 2 puffs q4h of 1:200): Nebulization techniques (hand bulb, continuous, or IPPB)
Luf-Iso	Mallinckrodt	Isoproterenol sulfate	0.075 mg/puff-dose, metered dosages
Medihaler-Epi	Riker	Epinephrine bitartrate	0.16 mg/puff-dose of epinephrine base, metered dosages
Medihaler-Iso	Riker	Isoproterenol sulfate	0.075 mg/puff-dose, metered dosages
Metaprel	Dorsey	Metaproterenol sulfate	0.75 mg/puff-dose, metered dosages
Norisodrine Aerotrol	Abbott	Isoproterenol hydrochloride	0.125 mg/puff-dose, automatic single dosages
Norisodrine sulfate Aerohalor	Abbott	Isoproterenol sulfate	Aerohalor cartridge 10%: 0.45 mg/puff-dose
			Autohalor cartridge 25%: 0.11 mg/puff-dose
			Powder inhaler technique
Vaponefrin Metermatic	Fisons	Racemic epinephrine	0.3 mg/puff-dose, metered dosages
Vaponefrin solution	Fisons	Racemic epinephrine (2.25% epinephrine base)	1:200 solution: 1 or two puffs q4h, prn, nebulization techniques
Vapo-Iso solution	Fisons	Isoproterenol hydrochloride (0.5%)	1:200 solution: 1 or 2 puffs q4h, prn, nebulization techniques

Table 24-1 (continued)

Not available at present in the U.S.A.

Note: Some have more beta 2 bronchoselective properties, less beta 1 cardioselective properties, and longer duration of action.

Trade Name	Company	Content	Delivered Dosages
Albuterol	Schering	Salbutamol	1:200 solution: 1 or 2 puffs q4h, prn, delivered dosages
Bricanyl	Astra	Terbutaline sulfate	250 µg/puff-dose, 1 or 2 puffs q4h prn, metered dosages
Pulmadil	Riker	Rimiterol hydrobromide (suspension)	200 µg/puff-dose, metered dosages or automatic single dosages
Ventolin	Allen & Hanbury's	Salbutamol	100 µg/puff-dose, 1 or 2 puffs q4h prn, metered dosages

Table 24-2. Beta Adrenergic Injectables

Trade or Generic Name	Company	Contents	Forms and Dosages Available
Adrenalin Epinephrine	Parke-Davis (and others) USP	(1) Adrenaline chloride, 1:100 (2) Adrenaline in oil, 1:500 (3) Epinephrine hydrochloride, 1:1000	Ampules for parenteral use (1 and 3) or intramuscular use only (2)
Bricanyl	Astra	Terbutaline sulfate (1 mg/ml)	Ampules, dose 0.3 ml SC
Bronkephrine	Breon	Ethylnorepinephrine hydrochloride, aqueous solution (2 mg/ml)	Ampules, dose 0.3–1.0 ml SC or IM
Isuprel	Winthrop	Isoproterenol hydrochloride, 1:5000	Ampules, 0.2 mg/ml parenterally
Sus-Phrine	Cooper	Epinephrine aqueous suspension, 1:200 (5 mg/ml)	Ampules of slow- and rapid-release gel, dose 0.1–0.3 ml SC

Not available at present in the U.S.A.

Rimiterol	Riker	Rimiterol hydrobromide	Ampules, dose 0.05 to 0.2 µg/kg IV
Salbutamol	Allen & Hanbury's	Salbutamol sulfate	Ampules, dose 0.025 to 0.1 µg/kg IV

Table 24-3. Alpha Adrenergic Nasal Decongestants (Mediate Vasoconstriction)

Caution: Avoid abuse and tolerance. Advise use for 3 days and stop for 3 days.

Trade Name	Company	Contents	Forms and Dosages Available
Afrin	Schering	Oxymetazoline hydrochloride NF	Solution, 0.05% (1:200) Spray, 0.05% (1:200)
4-Way	Bristol-Myers	Phenylephrine hydrochloride 0.25%, naphazoline hydrochloride 0.5%, phenylpropanolamine hydrochloride 0.5%, pyrilamine maleate 0.05%, 0.20%, 0.25%, 0.5%	Atomizer use
Isophrin	Riker	Phenylephrine hydrochloride	Solution, 0.167%, 0.25%, 0.50%, or 1.0% Spray, 0.25%
Neo-Synephrine HCl	Winthrop	Phenylephrine hydrochloride, benzalkonium hydrochloride 0.02%	Solution, 0.125%, 0.5%, or 1.0% Spray, 0.25% or 0.5% Nasal jelly, 0.5%
NTZ	Winthrop	Phenylephrine hydrochloride 0.5%, thenyldiamine hydrochloride 0.1%, benzalkonium hydrochloride 1:5000	Spray
Otrivin	Geigy	Xylometazoline hydrochloride NF 0.05% and 0.1%	Nose drops Spray
Tyzine	Pfizer	Tetrahydrozoline hydrochloride 0.05% and 0.1%	Nose drops Spray

Table 24-4. Therapeutic Aerosols

Family of Agents	Specific Agents
Anticholinergics	Pamine bromide; atropine (synthetic analogues)
Antihistaminics	Pyribenzamine; Benadryl; Chlor-Trimeton (nasal form)
Antimicrobials	Penicillin; streptomycin; amphotericin-B
Bischromones	Cromolyn sodium (Intal; Aarane [micronized form] [lungs] ; Rynacrom [nasal form])
Bronchodilators	
Catecholamines	Norepinephrine (bronchodilation and bronchovasoconstriction)
	Epinephrine: racemic epinephrine (Vaponefrin)
	Isoproterenol: Isuprel; Isoprenaline
	Rimiterol: Pulmadil
Resorcinols	Metaproterenol: orciprenaline (Alupent; Metaprel)
	Terbutaline: Bricanyl
Saligenins	Salbutamol: Ventolin; Albuterol
Under investigation	Prostaglandins: prostaglandins E_1 and E_2
	Saligenin: Salmefamol
	Sulfonanilide: Soterenol
	Quinolone: Quinprenaline
	Papaveroline: Trimetoquinol
Bronchovasoconstrictors	Phenylephrine (Neo-Synephrine)
Detergolytics	Alevaire; Tergemist (sodium 2-ethyl-1-hexyl sulfate and potassium iodide)
Enzymes	Pancreatic dornase (Dornavac)
	Acetylcysteine (Mucomyst)
Steroids	Turbinaire Decadron (nasal form); Respihaler Decadron (lungs)
	Beclomethasone dipropionate (Becotide [lungs] ; Vanceril [lungs] ; Beconase [nasal form]
	Betamethasone valerate (Bextasol, lungs)
	Triamcinolone acetonide (lungs)
Miscellaneous	Water (ultrasonic nebulization, steam)
	Saline (physiologic)
	Propylene glycol (heated)

Table 24-5. Bronchodilators: Theophylline Preparations for Oral Use

Note: Bronchodilation occurs with release of cyclic AMP, the active smooth muscle relaxing substance (SMRS) Theophyllines inhibit the degradation of cyclic AMP by the specific enzyme phosphodiesterase.
*Dosages and duration of therapy to be individualized by the physician.

Trade Name	Company	Content	Forms Available
Aerolate	Fleming	Theophylline (anhydrous) 260 mg (Sr.); 130 mg (Jr.); 65 mg (III); elixir, 160 mg/ml, 10% alcohol	Capsules (3 strengths), elixir
Amesec	Lilly	Aminophylline (anhydrous) 130 mg, ephedrine hydrochloride 25 mg, amobarbitol 25 mg	Enseals, pulvules
Aminodur Dura-Tabs	Cooper	Aminophylline (anhydrous) 300 mg	Tablets (prolonged release)
Asbron G Inlay-Tabs, Elixir	Dorsey	Theophylline (equivalent) 150 mg, guaifenesin 100 mg, phenylpropanolamine hydrochloride 25 mg; elixir, same ingredients/15 ml 15% alcohol	Tablets, elixir
Aminophylline	Various companies	Theophylline (anhydrous) 86%, ethylenediamine 14%; various dosages depending on form	Tablets, suppositories, solutions
Bronchobid Duracap	Meyer	Theophylline 260 mg, pseudoephedrine hydrochloride 50 mg	Capsules (timed action)
Bronchodyl*	Breon	Theophylline (anhydrous) 100 mg or 200 mg	Capsules (micropulverized; 2 strengths)
Brondecon	Warner/Chilcott	Oxtriphylline (choline theophyllinate) 200 mg, guaifenesin 100 mg; elixir, same ingredients/5 ml, 20% alcohol	Tablets, elixir
Bronkotabs	Breon	Theophylline (anhydrous) 100 mg, ephedrine sulfate 24 mg, guaifenesin 100 mg, phenobarbital 8 mg	Tablets (2 strengths)
Bronkolixir	Breon	Theophylline 15 mg, ephedrine sulfate 12 mg, guaifenesin 50 mg, phenobarbital 4 mg/5 ml, 19% v/v alcohol	Elixir
Choledyl	Warner/Chilcott	Oxtriphylline 100 or 200 mg; elixir, 100 mg/5 ml, 20% alcohol	Tablets, elixir

Table 24-5 *(continued)*

Trade Name	Company	Content	Forms Available
Dainite Day	Mallinckrodt	Aminophylline 200 mg, sodium pentobarbital 16 mg, ephedrine hydrochloride 16 mg, aluminum hydroxide 160 mg, Benzocaine 16 mg	Tablets
Dainite Night	Mallinckrodt	Aminophylline 260 mg, phenobarbital 24 mg, sodium pentobarbital 32 mg, aluminum hydroxide 160 mg, Benzocaine 16 mg	Tablets
Dainite KI	Mallinckrodt	Aminophylline 200 mg, ephedrine hydrochloride 16 mg, phenobarbital 16 mg, potassium iodide 325 mg, aluminum hydroxide 160 mg, Benzocaine 16 mg	Tablets
Dilor	Savage	Dyphylline (dihydroxypropyltheophylline) 200 mg or 400 mg; elixir, 160 mg/15 ml; ampules, 250 mg/ml	Tablets (2 strengths), elixir, ampules
Duvovent	Mallinckrodt	Theophylline (anhydrous) 130 mg, ephedrine hydrochloride 24 mg, phenobarbital 8 mg, guaifenesin 100 mg	Tablets
Elixophyllin	Cooper	Theophylline (anhydrous) 200 mg in polyethylene glycol 400	Capsules
Elixophyllin, Pediatric	Cooper	Theophylline (anhydrous) 100 mg/5 ml; no sugar, dye, or alcohol	Suspension
Elixophyllin Elixir	Cooper	Theophylline (anhydrous) 80 mg/15 ml, 20% alcohol	Elixir
Elixophyllin-KI	Cooper	Theophylline (anhydrous) 80 mg, potassium iodide 130 mg/15 ml, 10% alcohol	Elixir (compound)
Emfaseem	Saron	Dyphylline 200 mg, guaifenesin 100 mg; elixir, same ingredients/30 ml	Tablets, liquid
Isuprel Compound	Winthrop	Theophylline 45 mg, isoproterenol hydrochloride 2.5 mg, ephedrine sulfate 12 mg, potassium iodide 150 mg, phenobarbital 6 mg/15 ml, 19% alcohol	Elixir (compound)
Isuprel Mistometer	Winthrop	Isoproterenol hydrochloride 125 g/puff-dose from 15 ml vials of 1:200 or 1:100 solution	Liquid

Product	Manufacturer	Composition	Dosage forms
Lixaminol, Mini-Lix	Ferndale	Lixaminol: Aminophylline (anhydrous) 250 mg/15 ml, 20% alcohol (dye-free and sugar-free) (for adults); Mini-Lix: aminophylline 100 mg/15 ml, 20% alcohol (for children)	Elixir
Lufyllin*	Mallinckrodt	Dyphylline 200 mg; guaifenesin 100 mg; elixir, same ingredients/30 ml, 20% alcohol	Tablets, elixir
Lufyllin GG*	Mallinckrodt	Dyphylline 200 mg, guaifenesin 200 mg; elixir, same ingredients/30 ml, 17% alcohol	Tablets, elixir
Lufyllin EPG*	Mallinckrodt	Dyphylline 100 mg, ephedrine hydrochloride 16 mg, guaifenesin 200 mg, phenobarbital 16 gm; elixir, same ingredients/10 ml, 5.5% alcohol	Tablets, elixir
Marax	Roerig	Theophylline 130 mg, ephedrine sulfate 25 mg, hydroxyzine hydrochloride 10 mg; syrup, same ingredients/20 ml, 5% v/v alcohol (caution: contains a tartrazine dye—may cause hypersensitivity reactions; available in dye-free pints)	Tablets, syrup
Mudrane	Poythress	Aminophylline (anhydrous) 130 mg, ephedrine hydrochloride 16 mg, potassium iodide 195 mg, phenobarbital 21 mg	Tablets
Mudrane GG	Poythress	Aminophylline (anhydrous) 130 mg, ephedrine hydrochloride 16 mg, guaifenesin 100 mg, phenobarbital 21 mg; elixir, theophylline 20 mg, ephedrine hydrochloride 4 mg, phenobarbital 5.4 mg, guaifenesin 26 mg/5 ml, 20% v/v alcohol	Tablets, elixir (pediatric)
Mudrane 2	Poythress	Aminophylline (anhydrous) 130 mg, potassium iodide 195 mg	Tablets
Mudrane GG-2	Poythress	Aminophylline (anhydrous) 130 mg, guaifenesin 100 mg	Tablets
Neothyllin	Lemmon	Dyphylline 200 mg or 400 mg: elixir, dyphylline 160 mg/15 ml, 18% alcohol; injection, dyphylline 500 mg/2 ml	Tablets, elixir, injectable

Table 24-5 (continued)

Trade Name	Company	Content	Forms Available
Quibron	Mead Johnson	Theophylline (anhydrous) 150 mg, guaifenesin 90 mg; elixir, same ingredients/15 ml, 15% alcohol	Capsules, elixir
Quibron Plus	Mead Johnson	Theophylline (anhydrous) 150 mg, ephedrine hydrochloride 25 mg, butabarbital 20 mg, guaifenesin 100 mg; elixir, same ingredients/15 ml, 15% alcohol	Capsules, elixir
Quadrinal	Knoll	Theophylline (anhydrous) (equivalent) 65 mg, ephedrine hydrochloride 24 mg, phenobarbital 24 mg, potassium iodide 320 mg; suspension, same ingredients/10 ml	Tablets, liquid suspension
Slo-Phyllin Gyrocaps	Dooner	Theophylline (anhydrous) 125 mg or 250 mg	Gyrocaps (timed release)
Slo-Phyllin GG	Dooner	Theophylline (anhydrous) 150 mg, guaifenesin 90 mg; syrup, same ingredients/15 ml, non-alcoholic	Capsules, syrup
Slo-Phyllin 80	Dooner	Theophylline (anhydrous) 80 mg/15 ml, non-alcoholic	Syrup
Somophyllin Oral Solution	Fisons	Theophylline base 90 mg/5 ml, nonalcoholic and sugar-free	Solution
Tedral	Warner/Chilcott	Theophylline 130 mg, ephedrine hydrochloride 24 mg, phenobarbital 8 mg; elixir, same ingredients/20 ml, 15% alcohol	Tablets, elixir
Tedral-25	Warner/Chilcott	Theophylline 130 mg, ephedrine hydrochloride 24 mg, butabarbital 25 mg	Tablets
Tedral SA	Warner/Chilcott	Theophylline (anhydrous) 180 mg (immediate release layer 90 mg; sustained release layer 90 mg), ephedrine hydrochloride 48 mg (immediate release layer 16 mg, sustained release layer 32 mg), phenobarbital 25 mg (immediate release layer)	Tablets (layered, sustained action)

Tedral Pediatric Suspension	Warner/Chilcott	Theophylline 65 mg, ephedrine hydrochloride 12 mg, phenobarbital 4 mg/5 ml, nonalcoholic	Liquid suspension (pediatric)
Tedral Expectorant	Warner/Chilcott	Theophylline 130 mg, ephedrine hydrochloride 24 mg, phenobarbital 8 mg, guaifenesin 100 mg	Tablets
Theobid Duracap	Meyer	Theophylline 260 mg	Capsules (timed action)
Theokin	Knoll	Theophylline (anhydrous) (equivalent) 225 mg, potassium iodide 450 mg; elixir, same ingredients/15 ml, 9.5% alcohol	Tablets, elixir
Theo-dur	Key	Theophylline (anhydrous) 100 mg, noscapine 15 mg; or theophylline (anhydrous) 200 mg, noscapine 30 mg	Tablets (timed release; 2 strengths)
Theo-Organidin	Wallace	Theophylline (anhydrous) 120 mg, iodinated glycerol 30 mg/15 ml, 15% alcohol	Elixir
Theophyl	Knoll	Theophylline (anhydrous) 225 mg/30 ml, 5% alcohol	Elixir
Verequad	Knoll	Theophylline (anhydrous) (equivalent) 65 mg, ephedrine hydrochloride 24 mg, phenobarbital 8 mg, guaifenesin 100 mg; suspension, same ingredients/10 ml, nonalcoholic	Tablets, liquid suspension

Table 24-6. Theophylline and Aminophylline for Rectal Use

Trade Name	Company	Contents	Forms and Dosages Available
Wyanoids (aminophylline supposi-tories)	Wyeth	Aminophylline	Suppositories 250 and 500 mg
Fleet Brand Theophylline	Fleet	Theophylline monoethanolamine, 0.30% methyl-paraben and 0.06% propylparaben as preservatives	Single-squeeze, disposable rectal units 250 mg/37 ml and 500 mg/37 ml
Rectalad Aminoph-ylline	Wallace	Aminophylline solution	Single-squeeze disposable small, plastic units, 300 mg/3 ml and 450 mg/5 ml
Somophyllin	Fisons	Aminophylline solution	5 ml syringe and plastic tip for measured dosages 300 mg/5 ml

Table 24-7. Aminophylline and Diphylline Injectables

Trade or Generic Name	Company	Contents	Forms Available
Aminophylline	Searle and others	Theophylline, ethylenediamine	Ampules (250 and 500 mg) 10–20 ml IV
		Theophylline, ethylenediamine	Ampules (250 mg) 2 ml IM
Lufyllin	Mallinckrodt	Diphylline ([7-(2,3-dihydroxypropyl] theophylline)	Ampules 250 mg/ml; 2 ml (500 mg) IM
Neothylline	Lemmon	Diphylline; may contain sodium hydroxide or hydrochloric acid to adjust pH	Ampules (500 mg/2 ml) IM

Table 24-8. Glucocorticoids

Trade Name	Contents	Company	Comparison Equivalent Dosages (mg)	Relative Antiinflammatory Potency	Relative Sodium-Retaining Potency
	Cortisone	USP	25	0.8	0.8
Cortef	Hydrocortisone	Upjohn	20	1	1
	Prednisone	USP	5	4	0.8
	Prednisolone	USP	5	4	0.8
Medrol	Methylprednisolone	Upjohn	4	5	0.5
Aristocort } Kenacort }	Triamcinolone	{ Lederle { Squibb	4	5	0
Haldrone	Paramethasone acetate	Lilly	2	10	0
Celestone	Betamethasone	Schering	0.75	25	0
Deronil	Dexamethasone	Schering	0.75	25	0
Decadron	Dexamethasone	Merck Sharp & Dohme	0.75	25	0

Source: Based on data in Goodman, L. S., and Gilman, A. *The Pharmacologic Basis of Therapeutics* (5th ed.). New York: Macmillan, 1975.

Table 24-9. Commonly Employed Steroids

Caution: Dosages and therapeutic regimens to be individualized.

Trade or Generic Name	Company	Contents	Form and Dosage
H.P. Acthar Gel	Armour	Purified corticotropin, gelatin 16%, phenol 0.5%, cysteine not more than 0.1%	Vials 40, 80 units/ml or 5 ml (only for SC or IM) (rapid and delayed action)
Acthar	Armour	Corticotropin—lyophilized powder (reconstitute in water)	Vials 25, 40 USP units (for SC, IM, IV)
Aristocort	Lederle	Triamcinolone (9 α-fluoro-16 α hydroxyprednisolone)	Tablets 1, 2, 4, 8, 16 mg
Aristocort	Lederle	Triamcinolone diacetate	Syrup 2 mg/5 ml
Aristocort Forte Parenteral	Lederle	Triamcinolone diacetate micronized suspension	Injectable 40 mg/ml IM (for sustained action)
Celestone	Schering	Betamethasone (9 α-fluoro-16 β-methylprednisolone)	Tablets 0.6 mg
Celestone	Schering	Betamethasone 0.6 mg/5 ml, alcohol less than 1%	Syrup 0.6 mg/5 ml
Celestone Soluspan	Schering	Betamethasone sodium phosphate 3 mg *and* betamethasone acetate 3 mg/ml suspension	Injectable suspension 1, 2 ml IM (for rapid and repository action): 6 mg/ml
Cortef	Upjohn	Hydrocortisone (cortisol) (prototype glucocorticoid)	Tablets 5, 10, 20 mg
Solu-Cortef	Upjohn	Hydrocortisone sodium succinate (Mix-O-Vial reconstituted)	Injectable IV or IM in 100–1,000 mg
Cortisone Acetate	Upjohn	Cortisone acetate in sterile aqueous suspension	Injectable suspension for IM only; 25 mg/ml
Cortisone Acetate	Upjohn	Cortisone acetate	Tablets 5, 10, 25 mg
Decadron	Merck Sharp & Dohme	Dexamethasone (major antiinflammatory) (9-fluoro-11β,17,21-trihydroxy-16 α methylpregna-1,4-diene-3,20-dione)	Tablets 0.25, 0.5, 0.75, 1.5, 4 mg
Decadron	Merck Sharp & Dohme	Dexamethasone 0.5 mg, alcohol 5%/5 ml; benzoic acid 0.1% as preservative	Elixir 0.5 mg/5 ml

			Injectable (longer-acting)—*not intravenous*
Decadron-LA*	Merck Sharp & Dohme	Dexamethasone acetate 8 mg/ml	Injectable IM, IV (rapid-short action)
Decadron Phosphate	Merck Sharp & Dohme	Dexamethasone phosphate (equivalent) 4 mg/ml; inactive ingredients	
Deronil	Schering	Dexamethasone	Tablets 0.75 mg
Haldrone	Lilly	Paramethasone acetate (6 α-fluoro-16 α methylprednisolone)	Tablets 1, 2 mg
Kenacort	Squibb	Triamcinolone	Tablets 1, 2, 4, 8 mg
Kenacort	Squibb	Triamcinolone diacetate (anhydrous) 4.85 mg/5 ml	Syrup 5 ml ⇔ 4 mg tablet
Medrol	Upjohn	Methylprednisolone	Tablets 2, 4, 16 mg
Medrol Medules	Upjohn	Methylprednisolone	Medules 2, 4 mg capsules
Solu Medrol	Upjohn	Methylprednisolone sodium succinate	Injectable (IV) 40mg/ml–1,000mg/16 ml
Meticortelone Acetate	Schering	Prednisolone acetate 25 mg/ml (aqueous suspension)	Vials 5 ml multiple-dose (for IM)
Meticortelone Soluble	Schering	Prednisolone 50 mg (equivalent)	Powder 50 mg/vial (for IM or IV)
Meticorten	Schering	Prednisone (17.21-dihydroxy-pregna-1,4-diene-3,11,20-trione)	Tablets 1, 5 mg
Prednisone	Various companies	Prednisone	Tablets 1, 2.5, 5, 10, 20, 50 mg
Prednisolone	Various companies	Prednisolone	Tablets 1, 2.5, 5 mg

Table 24-10. Steroid Aerosols

Caution: Dosages and duration of therapy to be individualized by physician.

Trade Name	Company	Contents	Dosages	Comments
Decadron	Merck Sharp & Dohme	Dexamethasone	4 mg/ml	Solution for nebulizer techniques
Decadron Respihaler	Merck Sharp & Dohme	Dexamethasone sodium phosphate	0.1 mg/puff-dose	Metered dosages
Medrol	Upjohn	Methylprednisolone	40 mg/ml	Solution for nebulization techniques
Becotide Inhaler*	Allen & Hanbury's	Beclomethasone dipropionate	50 µg/dose (2 puffs q6h; 8 puffs = 5 mg prednisone)	Metered dosages (nasal and oral aerosols)
Vanceril Inhaler	Schering	Beclomethasone dipropionate	50 µg/dose (8 puffs = 5 mg prednisone)	Metered dosages
Bextasol Inhaler*	Glaxo	Betamethasone valerate	100 µg/dose (1 puff q6h; 4 puffs = 5 mg prednisone)	Metered dosages (nasal and oral aerosols)
Triamcinolone Inhaler**	Lederle	Triamcinolone Acetonide	0.05 mg/puff-dose (16 puffs/day = 0.8 mg)	Metered dosages

*Not available at present in U.S.A.
**Distribution in U.S.A. pending FDA approval.

Table 24-11. Nasal Steroid Aerosols

Trade Name	Company	Contents	Form and Dosages
Turbinaire Decadron	Merck Sharp & Dohme	Dexamethasone phosphate (equivalent)	Nasal spray 0.1 mg/sniff-dose 2 sprays each nostril 3 to 4 times/day
Beconase Nasal Spray*	Allen & Hanbury's	Beclomethasone dipropionate	Nasal spray 50 µg/sniff-dose 2 sprays each nostril 3 to 4 times/day

*Not available at present in U.S.A.

Table 24-12. Mucolytic Aerosols

Caution: Dosages and duration of therapy to be individualized by physician.

Trade Name	Company	Contents	Dosages	Comments
Dornavac	Merck Sharp & Dohme	Pancreatic dornase	In saline solution, 100,000 units/dose, 3 to 4 times/day up to 7 days/course	Slow nebulization techniques, possible protein sensitization
Mucomyst	Mead Johnson	Acetylcysteine (N-acetyl-L-cysteine)	3–5 ml of 20% solution— aerosol; 6–10 ml of 10% solution—aerosol; both 3 to 4 times/day	Solution for nebulization, intratracheal, or lavage techniques; use with isoproterenol to prevent bronchospasm.

Table 24-13. Iodide Preparations

Trade or Generic Name	Company	Contents	Forms Available
Organidin	Wallace	Iodinated glycerol (organically bound iodine) 50 mg/ml	Tablets, solution, elixir
Iodo-Niacin	Cole	Potassium iodide 135 mg, niacinamide hydroiodide 25 mg	Coated tablets 25 mg
Pima	Fleming	Potassium iodide in black raspberry base	Syrup, 5 gr/5 ml
Sodium Iodide	Lilly	Sodium iodide solution	Ampules 1 gm/10 ml (0.5–1.0 gm for IV)
SSKI	Lyne	Potassium iodide in saturated solution	Dropper (30 gm KI in 21 ml water) solution
SSKI	Upsher-Smith	Potassium Iodide	Dropper (300 mg KI in 0.3 ml water) solution
KI-N	Mallinckrodt	Potassium Iodide	Tablets 10 gr

Table 24-14. Specific Mediator Release Blocking Drugs (inhibits mediator release; no role during acute asthma attacks)

Caution: Dosages and duration of therapy to be individualized by physician.

Trade Name	Company	Contents	Dosages	Comments
Aarane (Inhaler)	Syntex	Cromolyn sodium	20 mg/capsule/dose 4 times/day	Local irritation at times
Intal (Spinhaler)	Fisons	Cromolyn sodium	20 mg/capsule/dose 4 times/day	Local irritation at times
Intal (Rynacrom)*	Fisons	Cromolyn sodium	Nasal use, only as directed	For nasal insufflation
Lomusol*	Fisons	2% w/v sodium cromoglycate	1 spray only as directed	Nasal spray solution

*Not available at present in the U.S.A.

Index

Index

Acetylcholine
acetylcholinesterase and, 282, 283
alpha adrenergic agents and, 360
asthma and, 308
bronchial tone and, 361–362
as neurohumoral transmitter, 281, 282, 283
receptor for, 360
Acid, defined, 102
Acid-base balance. *See also* Hydrogen ion
concentration (pH)
bicarbonate–carbonic acid system and, 102–
103
disturbances, defined, 103–105
neuromuscular blocking agents and, 288
Acidosis
lactic, tissue oxygenation and, 196
metabolic, 103–104, 105
respiratory, 103, 104, 143, 324. *See also*
Respiratory acidosis
Action potential
defined, 281
neurohumoral transmission and, 281–282
Activated clotting time (ACT) in heparin
monitoring, 437
Activated partial thromboplastin time (APTT)
in heparin monitoring, 437
Adenosine 3′, 5′ cyclic monophosphate. *See*
3′, 5′ cyclic adenosine monophosphate
(cyclic AMP)

Adenosine triphosphate (ATP)
hemoglobin affinity for oxygen and, 199
oxidative metabolism and, 193
Adrenergic agents. *See* Alpha adrenergic
agents; Beta adrenergic agents
Adult respiratory distress syndrome (ARDS),
139–140, 321–337
alveoli in, 321–324
edema, 324, 337
gas delivery and exchange and, 322, 323,
324
cardiopulmonary factors in, 325, 328
pulmonary capillary wedge pressure, 140
continuous positive airway pressure in, 328,
337
diagnosis and clinical signs, 324
fat embolism syndrome, 324, 328–331
fluid balance in, 325, 328
infections and, 325
lung pathology in, 324–325, 326, 327
mechanical ventilation in, 325
mediators and, 325
narcotic overdose and, 324, 335–337
neurogenic pulmonary edema, 324, 332–
335
oxygen therapy, 324, 325, 328, 337
positive end expiratory pressure in, 325,
328, 335–336, 337
prognosis, 324, 337

Adult respiratory distress syndrome (ARDS)
— *Continued*
  progression of, 324
  pulmonary edema and, 336
  pulmonary function tests in, 71, 88
  shock and, 324, 332, 335
  shock lung, 331–332, 333
  steroid therapy and, 325
  usefulness of classification, 321
Aerosol(s), 357–367; *See also specific agent,*
    e. g., Beta adrenergic agents, aerosols
  alpha adrenergic, 360
  anticholinergic, 358, 361–364
  antimicrobial, 188, 452
  beta adrenergic, 358–361, 447, 448–450
  classification of, 452
  cromolyn sodium, 358, 365
  defined, 357
  dosage distribution, 358
  infection and, 178
  metabolic fate, 358–359
  mucolytic, 463
  particle size and therapeutic delivery, 357–
    358
  prostaglandins, 358, 364–365
  steroids, 358, 366–367, 452, 462
Aerosol masks in humidity delivery to lungs,
    59, 64–65
Afterburner, 65
Agammaglobulinemia, 153
Agar radial diffusion kits, 155
Air
  alveoli and gas exchange, 321–324
  inspired, temperature and humidity varia-
    tions in, 171, 172
  low resistance, 292–293
Air filters. *See* Filters
Air leaks, pulmonary, in neonates, 342, 347–
    348
Airclean S-99 (Puritan Bennett), 66
Air velocity index (AVI), defined, 78
Airways
  beta adrenergic agents and, 448
  closure measurement, 84–87. *See also*
    Closing volume (CV)
  colonization
    pneumonia and, 187–188
    prevention, 184
  continuous positive pressure. *See* Con-
    tinuous positive airway pressure (CPAP)
  elasticity and ventilation, 94
  fetal formation, 292
  flow-volume loops in dysfunction diagnosis,
    93
  mucociliary apparatus, 113, 114, 115–116,
    172, 400
  mucus secretion
    in chronic bronchitis, 297, 298

  normal, 299
  obstruction
    in asthma, 94
    differential diagnosis, 314
    exercise bronchospasm in, 99, 100
  flow rates and, 89
  inhalation challenge test in, 99
  patency maintenance, in respiratory failure,
    400, 403–405
  pressure, 20
    expiration and equal pressure point
      (EPP), 89–91
    flow and equalization of, 293
    hemodynamics of changes, 230
  pulmonary gas flow and caliber of, 291
  resistance (R_{aw})
    compliance and, 77–78
    conductance and, 78
    high lung volume and, 292–293
    measurement, 78
    oxygen transport and, 193, 194
    of small airways vs. total, 301
    ventilation and, 94
  small airways disease, 106, 291, 301–304.
    See also Small airways disease
Alkalosis
  metabolic, 103–104, 105
  respiratory, 103, 104, 143, 208, 247. *See*
    also Respiratory alkalosis
Allergic bronchopulmonary aspergillosis, 160
Allergies. *See* Hypersensitivity reactions;
    Immune reactions
Alpha adrenergic agents
  bronchovasoconstriction and, 360
  as nasal decongestants, 447, 451
Altitude
  diphosphoglyceride actions and, 207
  hypoxia and, 209
Alveolar-capillary block theory of hypoxia,
    211
Alveoli
  alveolar-arterial oxygen gradient, 83, 215,
    220, 245, 247, 301
  development of, 292
  edema, 324, 337
  filling mechanics, 292
  gas delivery and exchange by, 79, 322,
    323–324
  oxygen toxicity and, 213
  phagocytosis by macrophages, 113, 116
  pressure, defined, 89
  structural and functional interrelationships,
    321–324
  surfactant, hyaline membrane disease and,
    339–340, 341
Alveolitis, extrinsic allergic, 160
Aminophylline. *See also* Theophyllines
  administration methods, 380–382

injection, 381, 458
oral, 380–381, 453–457
rectal, 381–382, 458
circulatory function and, 379
cyclic AMP mechanism and action of, 373, 374–375
dosage, 379–382
drug interactions, 374
toxicity and side-effects, 375–376, 379, 380–381
Amsterdam infant ventilator, 19–20
Anaphylaxis
aggregate vs. cytotrophic, 158
asthma and, 308
described, 157
eosinophilic chemotactic factor of (ECF-A), 161
prostaglandins and, 163
slow-reactive substance of (SRS-A), 308
Anemia
diphosphoglycerate and hemoglobin oxygen affinity and, 204, 205
hemoglobin Seattle and, 206
Anesthesia
for bronchoscopy, 132
complications and, 133
multistage gas regulators in delivery of, 59, 60
Angioedema, 314–315
Antibiotics. See Antimicrobial agents
Antibody, defined, 173. See also Immunologic factors
Antibronchomucotropic agents, defined, 125
Anticholinergic agents
aerosols, 358, 361–364, 452
bronchial tone mediation and, 361–363
ideal agent, described, 364
side-effects, 363
Anticholinesterases, neuromuscular blocking and, 283
Antigen, defined, 173. See also Immunologic factors
Antihistaminic aerosols, 452
Antimicrobial agents
aerosol, 188, 452
classification, 188, 189
criteria for choice of, 188
in meconium aspiration, 346
neuromuscular blocking agents and, 287
prophylactic, 187–188
Antitrypsins
bronchitis and, 297
emphysema and, 295
Apgar score in neonatal assessment, 345
Apnea, 287
monitoring, 26, 38–39
morphine and, 289
neuromuscular blocking agents and, 286–287

in premature neonates, 348–349
Apneustic respiratory control centers, 97
ARDS. See Adult respiratory distress syndrome (ARDS)
Arrhythmias, 142–148
assessment of, 391
atrial, 144–147
beta adrenergic aerosols and, 361
blood gas and acid-base imbalances in, 143
countershock in, 144, 146, 147, 148
digitalis in etiology of, 145
incidence in pulmonary disease, 142
neuromuscular blocking agents and, 286, 287
respiratory alkalosis and, 143, 247
supraventricular, 143–144
ventricular, 146, 147–148
Arthus phenomenon, 159
Artificial gas transport systems, 222–224. See also Artificial lung
Artificial lung, 427, 442
in acute respiratory distress syndrome, 337
available for clinical use, 429, 430–432
background and history, 428, 429
blood trauma and, 428–429
bypass time, 441
cannulation and bypass in use, 431–432
contraindications, 432, 434
hematologic problems, 428–429, 431, 437–438
indications for, 428–429, 432, 433–434
mixed veno-venous and veno-arterial perfusion, 439, 440
perfusion equipment, 441–442
prognostic signs with, 434–436
pulmonary function and, 434–436
veno-aortic arch perfusion, 439, 441
veno-arterial perfusion, 436, 438, 439, 440
veno-venous perfusion, 436, 438–439
ASA triad, 309, 310–311, 317
Aspergillosis, 183
allergic bronchopulmonary, 160
pulmonary infiltration with eosinophilia in, 317
Asphyxia, neonatal, 341, 343–345
hypovolemia in, 344–345
meconium and, 346
persistent fetal circulation and, 350
resuscitation in, 344, 345
Aspiration
of food, 122–123
of pathogens in infections, 184
pulmonary. See Pulmonary aspiration
tracheal, of risk neonates, 346
transtracheal, in sputum collection, 117
Aspirin sensitivity, nasal polyps, and asthma (ASA triad), 309, 310–311, 317

Assessment, 390–394
    daily checklist, 395–398
    diagnostic tests in, 393–394
    family as aid in, 391–392
    past history and present problem in, 390–
        391
    of patient behavior, 391–392
    physical examination data in, 392–393
    priority areas in, 390
    in treatment planning and nursing care, 390
Asthma, 291, 307–319
    airways obstruction and, 94
    ASA triad, 309, 310–311, 317
    asthmatic bronchitis, 309, 310, 317
    blood gas profile in, 308–309, 312, 318
    bronchial tree in
        acetylcholine and parasympathetic system
            and, 361–362
        cyclic AMP and cyclic GMP and, 362–363
    cardiac, 314
    character of, 307
    classification of, 293
    cromolyn sodium in prevention of, 162
    differential diagnosis of, 313–317
    exercise-induced, 309, 311, 317, 359
    extrinsic, 307, 309, 310, 317
    high-risk patients
        profile of, 312, 318
        therapy for, 361
    immunologic factors and, 307, 309–310
        hypersensitivity reactions, 307, 309–310,
            311
        immunoglobulins, 157, 173
    intrinsic, 309–310, 317
    parasympathetic system and, 361–362, 363–
        364
    pharmacologic mediators and, 308
    prostaglandins and, 163
    pulmonary function in, 105, 312, 377–379
        flow-volume loops, 93, 94, 302
        therapy and, 318
    sputum in, 120
        Charcot-Leyden crystals, 121–122, 307
        Curschmann's spirals, 121–122, 307
    therapy, 302, 311, 312. See also specific
        agent
        anticholinergic aerosols, 358, 361–364
        atropine analogues, 360
        beta adrenergic aerosols, 358–361
        cautions with propranolol, 146
        correlation with physical signs, 311–312
        cromolyn sodium, 365–366
        high-risk patients, 361
        immunotherapy, 158
        isoproterenol, 364, 365
        laboratory studies and, 318
        mediator release blocking drugs, 462
        prostaglandins, 364–365

    pulmonary function tests and, 318
    steroids, 311, 318, 366–367
    theophyllines, 373–382
    vagus and experimental antigen-induced, 362
    variant, 309, 311, 313
Asthmatic bronchitis, 309, 310, 317
Atelectasis
    compliance and, 4
    inactivity and, 173
    oxygen toxicity and, 213
Atrial fibrillation
    described, 145, 146–147
    digitalis conversion of atrial flutter to, 146
    treatment, 147
Atrial flutter, 145–146
Atrial premature beats (APB), 144
Atrial tachycardia, 144–145
Atropine for asthma
    aerosols, 362, 363, 364
    analogues, 360
Auscultation in patient assessment, 392–393

B cells, immunologic factors and, 151–152,
    173, 175
Barotrauma, pulmonary, 235–237
Base, defined, 102
Beclomethasone, diproprionate (Becotide) for
    asthma, 366
Belladonna alkaloids (Bellafoline) for asthma,
    363
Bellows spirometer, 51–52
Bendix RSS oxygen delivery system, 61–62
Bennett MA-1 ventilator
    adaptation
        for assisted positive and expiratory pres-
            sure, 240, 241
        for intermittent assisted ventilation, 251
        for intermittent mandatory ventilation,
            249
        for interrupted positive end expiratory
            pressure, 241–243
    alarms, 6
    described, 3, 4–6
    oxygen therapy and nebulization, 4, 5
    sigh volume, 5–6
Bennett monitoring spirometer, 51, 52
Beta adrenergic agents
    aerosols, 358–361, 447
        agents, described, 449–450
        functions, 448
        side-effects and precautions with, 360–361,
            448
    agonist catechol and noncatechol, 358–361
    aminophylline and, 374
    in arrhythmias, 146
    cautions for asthmatics, 146
    cyclic AMP mechanism and, 359
    injectables, 447, 450

receptors for, 360
Betamethasone valerate (Bextasol) for asthma, 366
Bicarbonate
  carbonic acid system and, 102–103
  excretion, metabolic acidosis and alkalosis and, 103–104, 105
Bile flow, positive pressure breathing and, 232–233
Biopsy with fiberoptic bronchoscope, 132
Bischromone aerosols, 452
Blast transformation, defined, 173–174
Blood. See also Anemia; Eosinophils; Hemoglobin; Leukocytes; Transfusion
  abnormalities, hypoxia and, 212
  artificial substitutes for, 222–224
  carbon dioxide. See Blood gases, carbon dioxide
  effects of extracorporeal devices and, 428–429
  gases. See Blood gases
  hematologic problems with artificial lung, 437–438
  hydrogen ion concentration. See Blood hydrogen ion concentration (pH)
  hypovolemia
    in hyaline membrane disease, 341, 343
    in neonatal asphyxia, 344–345
  oxygen. See Blood gases, oxygen
  platelets and extracorporeal circulation, 431, 438
Blood flow, pulmonary. See Perfusion; Ventilation/perfusion (V/Q) ratio
Blood gases
  alveoli and, 321–324
  arrhythmias and, 143
  carbon dioxide
    exercise and, 98, 99
    hemoglobin affinity for oxygen and, 197, 199, 202, 204
    hypoventilation and, 209
    monitoring, 45–46
    partial pressure, 100–101
    respiratory chemoreceptors and, 97
    tension, 98, 99, 100–101, 102, 209, 245, 247
    transport, 101–102
    ventilation and, 101, 102
    voluntary hyperventilation and, 98
    weaning from respirators and, 245, 247
  clinical usefulness of determining, 100–101
  continuous monitoring, 44–46, 47–48
  in diffusion defects, hypoxia and, 211
  measurement
    arterial vs. venous, 100
    tissue gas measurement vs., 48
  oxygen. See also Hemoglobin, oxygen affinity; Hypoxia

alveolar-arterial gradient, 83, 215, 220, 245, 247, 301
arteriovenous differences, 140, 195–196, 204, 205, 206–207
in cardiac output determination, 140
monitoring, 44–45
muscle pH and, 48–49
oxygen toxicity and, 215, 220
partial pressure of, 100–101
pulmonary diffusing capacity measurement, 80
respiratory chemoreceptors and, 97
in small airways disease, 301
tension, 83, 100–101, 193, 247–249
tissue oxygenation and, 195–196, 204, 205, 206–207
transport, 101, 193–203, 208, 211
weaning from respirators and, 245, 247, 248
in patient assessment, 391–392
profile in asthma, 308–309, 312, 318
serial studies, 391
Blood hydrogen ion concentration (pH)
  in asthma, 309
  bicarbonate–carbonic acid system and, 102–103
  hemoglobin oxygen affinity and, 199, 200–201, 202, 204
  monitoring, 45
  neuromuscular blocking agents and, 288
  respiratory chemoreceptors and, 97
  weaning from respirators and, 247
Blood pressure
  central venous pressure (CVP), 138, 139
  direct monitoring, 26
  neuromuscular blocking agents and, 286
  pulmonary. See Pulmonary blood pressure
Body plethysmography
  in airway resistance measurement, 78
  in functional residual capacity determination, 71, 72–73
Bohr integration
  alkalosis and, 208
  carbon dioxide tension calculation with, 80, 247
  described, 143
  in diffusing capacity calculation, 83–84
  hemoglobin oxygen affinity and, 200–201, 202, 203
Bolus technique of closing volume measurement, 84, 85
Bradykinin, asthma and, 308
Breath sounds, normal vs. adventitious, 392–393
Briggs adapter (T-piece)
  artificial humidification of lungs and, 65
  attachment for weaning, 247
Bronchial asthma. See Asthma

Bronchial breath sounds, 392
Bronchial cells in sputum, 121, 123
Bronchial glands, 114
Bronchiectasis, 291, 300
  classification, 300
  pulmonary function in, 107, 293
Bronchiolitis, 315
Bronchitis, 291
  asthmatic, 309, 310, 317
  chronic, 297–300
    classification, 293
    defined, 297
    diagnosis and differential diagnosis, 297–298
    emphysema and, 294, 296
    mucus hypersecretion in, 297
    pulmonary function in, 105, 297, 300
    sputum in, 120
    therapy, 300
  pulmonary function in, 94, 105, 297, 300
Bronchoconstrictors, aerosol, 452
Bronchodilators, 447, 448–450, 452, 453–457, 458. See also specific topic, e.g., Asthma, therapy; Beta adrenergic agents
  aerosol, 447, 448–450, 452
  beta adrenergic, 358–361
    aerosols, 447, 448–450
    cyclic AMP mechanism and, 359
    injectables, 450
  in chronic bronchitis, 300
  cromolyn sodium as, 365
  in emphysema, 295, 296
  mechanism of action, 453
  theophyllines
    injectable, 458
    oral, 453–457
    rectal, 458
Bronchomucotropic agent, defined, 123
Bronchopulmonary dysplasia, neonatal, 342, 348
Bronchoscopy, 129–134
  in bronchiectasis, 300
  flexible fiberoptic
    complications of use, 132, 133, 134
    described, 129–131
    technique of use, 131–132
    premedication and anesthesia for, 131–132
    complications, 133
  rigid bronchoscope, 129, 130
Bronchospasm
  alpha adrenergic agents and, 360
  aminophylline and, 373, 374–375
  cyclic AMP mechanism and, 373, 374–375
  exercise, in airways obstruction testing, 99, 100
  hyperventilation and, 312
  theophyllines and, 373–382
  tubocurarine and, 286

Bronchovesicular breath sounds, 392
Bypass, pulmonary. See Artificial lung

Candida species
  mucocutaneous candidiasis, 155–156, 185
  pulmonary disease and, 183
Cannula(s)
  cannulation for extracorporeal oxygenation, 431, 432, 441
  oxygen, 63
Carbaminos, carbon dioxide transport as, 101
Carbon dioxide
  blood. See Blood gases, carbon dioxide
  excretion, 102, 103, 104
  production calculation, 80, 81
Carbon monoxide
  affinity for hemoglobin, 222, 223
  poisoning
    oxygen therapy for, 221, 222
    therapy problems, 223
  in pulmonary diffusing capacity calculation, 79–80
Carbonic acid
  bicarbonate and pH and, 102–103
  carbon dioxide transport as, 101
Carbonic anhydrase, carbon dioxide transport and, 101
Carboxyhemoglobin, 44, 46
Carcinoid syndrome, 315
Cardiac arrhythmias. See Arrhythmias
Cardiac asthma, 314
Cardiac output
  determination methods, 140
  hypoxia and inadequate, 212
  positive pressure breathing and, 229–232, 232–233
    minimizing effect of, 230–232
  pulmonary embolism and, 137
Cardiopulmonary factors, 137–148. See also Arrhythmias; Blood; Blood pressure; Cardiac output; Pulmonary embolism; Shunt(s)
  adult respiratory distress syndrome and, 325, 328
  aerosol distribution and, 357–358
  beta adrenergic agents and, 361
  cannulation and bypass for extracorporeal oxygenation, 431–432. See also Artificial lung
  cardiac catheterization and, 137
  cor pulmonale, 295, 297, 393
  diphosphoglycerate and hemoglobin oxygen affinity and, 204–205
  exercise-testing, 98–99
  hyaline membrane disease and, 341–342
  hypoxia and, 211–212
  infections and, 170, 173
  left atrial pressure approximation, 138–139

left ventricular function in obstructive lung disease, 140
neonatal pulmonary air leak, 342, 347–348
neuromuscular blocking agents and, 286–287
persistent fetal circulation, 350
phasic alterations and cardiac systole, 137
positive pressure breathing and, 229–233
  cardiac output, 229–232
  portal blood flow, 232–233
  pulmonary vascular resistance, 230
pressure determinations and blood sampling techniques, 137
pulmonary venous hemodynamics, 80, 138–140
radioisotopic perfusion scanning in evaluation of, 95–97
renal blood flow and, 234
right atrial and venous filling pressures, 138
theophyllines and, 377–379
tissue oxygenation and, 195–196, 204, 205, 206–207
vascular resistance and, 138, 230
Cascade oscilloscopes, 39–40
Catecholamines
  aerosols as bronchodilators, 452
  asthma and, 311
  beta adrenergic aerosol agonists, 358–359
Catheter(s)
  for blood gas monitoring, 48
  infection and, 169, 170, 184–185
  oxygen, 63
  in sputum aspiration for collection, 117
Cathode ray oscilloscopes, 39–40, 43
Cavitron PV-10 pediatric ventilator, 18–19
Central airway obstruction, 314
Central venous pressure (CVP) monitoring, 138, 139
Charcot-Leyden crystals in sputum, 121, 122, 307
Chediak-Higashi syndrome, 165
Chelating agents as artificial gas transport system, 223
Chemoreceptors and respiration, 97–98
Chemotaxis, 164
Chemetron Gill 1 Ventilator, 11–12
Chest wall diseases, 106
Chloride shift, 101
Cholinergic drugs for tachycardia, 144
Chronic granulomatous disease in children, 165
Chronic obstructive pulmonary disease (COPD), 291–305. *See also specific condition, e.g., Asthma; Emphysema*
  air velocity index in, 77
  cardiac arrhythmias in, 142
  categorization of, 291
  fetal development and predisposition to, 292

incidence, 291
left ventricular function in, 140
normal lung structure and function and, 291–293
pulmonary function tests in, 105, 302, 303, 304
  closing volume, 87, 89
  flow-volume loops, 92, 302, 304
  functional residual capacity, 71
  regional lung volume, 96–97
  residual volume/total lung capacity ratio, 73
pulmonary pressure in, 140
weaning from ventilators in, 245
Cilia of respiratory tract, 113, 114, 115–116, 172, 400
Cirrhosis, 205
Cladding, defined, 130
Clark, PO_2 electrode, described, 44–45
Closing capacity of lung, defined, 87
Closing volume (CV), 69, 84–88, 89–90
  in calculation of dead space gas, 87
  and closing capacity, 87
  defined, 84
  distribution of, 87, 88
  functional residual capacity and, 87–88, 90
  measurement
    bolus technique in, 84, 85
    resident gas technique in, 84–85, 85–87
  in obstructive pulmonary disease, 87, 89, 303, 304
  position change and, 87
  vital capacity and, 85, 87, 88
Coanda effect in fluidics, 16, 17
Collagen diseases, 153, 154
Colonization
  of airways, 184, 187–188
  defined, 180
  differentiation from infection, 180
Color code for gas cylinders, 61
Coma, airway patency in, 400
Combined (Swiss type) immune deficiency disease, 153
Competitive neuromuscular blocking agents, 282, 283
Complement system, 156–157
  cytolysis and, 158
  soluble antigen-antibody complexes and, 159
Compliance, 69, 76–78
  clinical usefulness of test, 76
  defined, 76
  diagnosis of changes, 4
  frequency dependence of, 76–78
  oxygen toxicity and, 215, 216, 218, 220
  resistance and, 77–78
  static and dynamic, related, 76–77
  static pressure volume curve, 76, 77

Computer(s), 26–27, 27–32
  alarm systems, 32
  analog, 26–27, 28
  analog-to-digital converter, 26–27, 31
  basic operations, 28, 31
  data processing by, 26–27, 29, 31
  defined, 27
  digital, 26–27, 28–31
  Fick method of data calculation, 27
  hardware-implemented algorithms, 31–32
  history, 27–28
  input, 26, 27, 31
  memory and data storage, 27, 28, 29, 31
  multiplexers, 27
  output of data, 28, 30, 32
Congestive heart failure, 139, 204–205
Continuous flow ventilation, 248–249
Continuous positive airway pressure (CPAP)
  in adult respiratory distress syndrome, 328,
    337
  in alveolar collapse, 248
  delivery systems, 19, 238, 239
  described, 239
  in hyaline membrane disease, 342
  jaundice and, 232
  in meconium aspiration, 346
Co-Oximeter, IL Model 182, 46, 47
COPD. See Chronic obstructive pulmonary
    disease (COPD)
Cor pulmonale, 295, 297, 391
Corticosteroids. See Steroid(s)
Coughing
  bronchomucotropic agents and, 125
  mechanics of effective, 91
  in variant asthma, 311, 313
Countershock in arrhythmias, 144, 146, 147,
    148
Counterweighted spirometer, 49, 50
CPAP. See Continuous positive airway pres-
    sure (CPAP)
Cromolyn sodium
  aerosols, 358, 365
  asthma prevention and, 162
  mode of action, 365
  nasal preparations, 365–366
Curschmann's spirals in sputum, 121–122,
    307
CV. See Closing volume (CV)
Cyanotic heart disease, 205
3′, 5′ Cyclic adenosine monophosphate
    (cyclic AMP)
  adenyl cyclase and beta adrenergics and, 360
  bronchospasm control by theophyllines and,
    373, 374–375
  cyclic GMP and, 362–363
  formation, 162–163
Cyclic AMP. See 3′, 5′ Cyclic adenosine mono-
    phosphate (cyclic AMP)

Cylinders, gas, 59
  color coding, 61
  described, 60–61
  duration of gas flow determination, 61
Cystic fibrosis, 297, 316
Cytochromes, respiration and, 192–193
Cytologic studies of sputum, 117–123
Cytolysis, immunologic, 158
Cytomegalovirus, pulmonary disease and, 181,
    183–184

Dead space, 69, 81
  closing volume in calculation of, 87
  defined, 81
  evaluation of, 81
  physiologic vs. anatomic, 81
  tidal volume and, 245, 246–247
Decontamination of equipment, 186, 187,
    188
Decubitus ulcer prevention, 185
Depolarizing neuromuscular blocking agents
  action of, 283
  described, 282–283, 284–285
Detergolytics, aerosol, 450
Devilbiss ultrasonic nebulizer, 23
Diabetes, 205, 206
Diaphragm, electromyography, 98
Differential transformer transducer, 36–37
Diffusing capacity, 69, 79–80, 84
  in chronic bronchitis, 300
  distribution of, 83–84
  hypoxia and, 211–212
  measurement of, 79–80
  oxygen toxicity and, 220
DiGeorge's syndrome, 153
Digital-to-analog converter, 39
Digitalis
  in arrhythmias, 144–145, 146, 147
  toxicity, 145, 146, 147
Dioctylphthalate (DOP) fog test, 66
Diphosphoglycerate (DPG)
  alkalosis and synthesis of, 208
  altitude and, 207
  disease states and, 201, 203–208
  hemoglobin oxygen affinity and, 197, 198,
    199, 201, 202–208
    cardiopulmonary disease and, 204–205
    metabolic disturbances and, 205–206
    modes of action, 203
  hypoxia and, 208
  production in erythrocytes, 203, 204
Diphyllines, injectable, 456
Direct patient monitoring, 26, 27, 36–39
  in apnea, 26, 38–39
  electrocardiogram in, 26, 38
  transducers in, 36–37, 38
Display systems and recorders, 27, 39–44
  galvanometric, 40–42

light beam recorders, 41, 43–44
oscilloscopes, 39–40
potentiometric recorders, 41, 42–43, 44
selecting devices, 44
X-Y recorders, 41, 43, 89
Disseminated intravascular coagulation (DIC), 438
DPG. See Diphosphoglycerate (DPG)
Drager hand-held pump spirometer, 53, 54
Drug abuse
  adult respiratory distress syndrome and narcotic overdose, 324, 335–337
  hypoxia and, 336
  pulmonary aspiration and, 336–337
  pulmonary edema and, 336
Dual neuromuscular block, described, 283
Dysplasia, neonatal bronchopulmonary, 342, 348

Ectopic heartbeats, 144, 147
Edema
  alveolar and interstitial, 213
  pulmonary. See Pulmonary edema
Edrophonium chloride (Tensilon), neuromuscular blocking and, 283
Elastic recoil pressure, defined, 89
Electrocardiogram, monitoring, 26, 38
Electrodes, monitoring
  Clark PO_2, 44–45
  continuous blood gas, 47–48
  pH, 45
  Severinghaus PCO_2, 45–46
Electrolyte(s). See also Acid-base balance
  fluid-electrolyte balance
    in adult respiratory distress syndrome, 325, 328
    nursing care in imbalances, 401, 407
  neurohumoral transmission and, 281, 282
  neuromuscular blocking agents and, 287–288
  secretion, positive pressure breathing and, 235
  tests for, in asthma, 318
Electromyography, 98
Embolism. See Fat embolism syndrome; Pulmonary embolism
Emerson 3MV intermittent mandatory ventilation ventilator, 12–13
Emphysema, 293–297
  centrilobular, 292, 295–296
  classification, 293, 294
  clinical picture, 295, 296
  defined, 293–294
  fiberoptic bronchoscopy in, 130
  incidence, 291
  inheritance pattern, 294–295
  interstitial, in neonates, 342, 347
  panacinar (panlobular), 293, 294

nonhereditary, 295, 296
positive end expiratory pressure in, 235, 328
pulmonary function in, 71, 73, 106, 295, 296
  flow in expiration, 293
  static compliance, 76
  ventilation/perfusion ratio, 296
subcutaneous, 235
therapy, 295
x-ray studies, 296
End expiratory pressure
  negative (NEEP), 19, 239–240, 342
  positive. See Positive end expiratory pressure (PEEP)
  zero (ZEEP), 19
Endotracheal intubation
  arrhythmias and, 142–143
  artificial humidification of lungs and, 65, 403
  infections and, 169, 170, 172
    prevention, 184, 188
  nursing care, 403, 404
    pharyngeal suctioning, 400, 403
    tube care and repositioning, 404
Environment
  control for neonates, 343, 345
  as infection source, 170, 177–179, 186–187
  toxins, respiratory response to, 316
Enzymatic aerosols, 452
Eosinophils
  in asthma, 308, 318
  eosinophilic chemotactic factor of anaphylaxis (ECF-A), 308
  pulmonary infiltration with eosinophilia (PIE), 316–317
  in sputum, 121–122
  tropical eosinophilia, 317
Epoxymethamine bromide (Pamine) in asthma, 363
Equal pressure point (EPP) in expiratory limb of flow-volume loops, 89–91, 94
ERV. See Expiratory reserve volume (ERV)
Escherichia coli pneumonia, 182
Exercise
  in emphysema therapy, 295
  metabolic acidosis and, 311
  oxygen consumption in, 81, 193
  tests
    in airways obstruction, 99, 100
    of cardiopulmonary reserves, 98–99
    techniques, 98–99
Exercise-induced asthma, 309, 311, 317, 359
Expectorant, defined, 123
Expiration
  flow-volume loops in, 89–91, 91–92, 94
  maximal flow, 291, 292
  normal vs. adventitious breath sounds in, 392–393

Expiration—*Continued*
  pathophysiology of obstructions to, 293
  peak expiratory flow, 91
  pressure relationships in, 89–91
    alveolar pressure, 89
    equal pressure point (EPP), 89–91, 94
    at steady lung volume, 89
  tests with forced, 293
Expiratory reserve volume (ERV)
  in adult respiratory distress syndrome, 71
  defined, 70
  determination, 70
Extracorporeal oxygenation. *See* Artificial
    lung
Extrinsic allergic alveolitis, 160–161
Extrinsic asthma, 307, 309, 310, 317
Extubation. *See* Weaning

Fast space ventilation, defined, 83
Fat embolism syndrome, 324, 328–331
  artificial lung for, 433, 434
  causes, 428
  pathophysiology, 329–331
  therapy, 331
FEV. *See* Forced expiratory volume (FEV)
Fiberoptic bronchoscope
  complications of use, 132, 133, 134
  described, 129–131
  technique of use, 131–132
Fick method
  cardiac output determination, 140
  computer data calculation, 27
  tissue oxygenation calculation, 195
Filters
  high-efficiency particulate air (HEPA), 59,
    65–66
  in infection prevention, 186
  ultrafiltration need in artificial lung, 440
Flanders filters Model 9, 66
Fleisch pneumotachograph, 55
Flow-volume loops and pulmonary function,
    69, 88–94
  airways and elasticity and, 89
  in asthma, 93, 94, 302
  in chronic obstructive pulmonary disease,
    302, 304
  determination, 88–89
  equal pressure point (EPP), 89–91, 94
  expiration and inspiration and, 91–92
  gas density and viscosity and, 93, 94
  information from, 91–93
  normal patterns, 92, 302
  peak expiratory flow, 91
  pressure and expiratory flow, 89
  in restrictive diseases, 302
  volume of isoflow, defined, 93, 94
Fluid-electrolyte balance
  in adult respiratory distress syndrome, 325,
    328

  nursing care in imbalances, 401, 407
Fluidics
  Coanda effect, 16, 17
  manipulation of stream attachment, 16–18
  Monaghan 225 Ventilator and, 15–16
  RETEC fluidic IPPB manifold, 16–17
Food aspiration, 122–123, 346
Forced expiratory spirogram, 74–75
Forced expiratory volume (FEV), 76
  in asthma, 312
  defined, 74
  exercise and, 311
  measurement, 74, 75
  normal, 74
  respiratory center depression and, 97
  in restrictive vs. obstructive diseases, 75
  for weaning from respirators, 246
Forced vital capacity (FVC)
  defined, 74
  measurement, 74, 75
Foregger 210 ventilator, 13–15
FRC. *See* Functional residual capacity (FRC)
Free radical theory of oxygen toxicity, 218–
    219
Friedländer pneumonia, 181–182
Functional residual capacity (FRC), 71–73
  in adult respiratory distress syndrome, 71,
    328
  in chronic bronchitis, 300
  closing volume and, 87–88, 90
  defined, 71
  determination
    body plethysmography in, 71, 72–73
    closed-circuit helium dilution method, 71
    open-circuit nitrogen washout method,
     71–72
  in obstructive vs. restrictive diseases, 71
  pleural pressure and, 85
  position change and, 87
  residual volume and, 73
Fungal infections, 176
  classification of antifungal agents, 189
  diagnosis, 177
  pneumonias, 181, 183
Furosemide in hyaline membrane disease,
    343
FVC. *See* Forced vital capacity (FVC)

Gallamine triethiodide (Flaxedel) as neuro-
    muscular blocking agent, 283, 284, 288
Galvanometric recorders, 40–42
Gamma globulins
  agammaglobulinemia, 153
  hypogammaglobulinemia, 152, 154–155,
    185
  intravenous administration, hazards of, 155
Gas(es)
  artificial transport systems for, 222–224
  blood. *See* Blood gases

cylinders, 59, 60–61
delivery systems, 59–66
flow
  density and viscosity and, 93, 94
  duration of, 61
  fluidics, 16–18
  regulation, 59–60
partial pressure, defined, 100
Gas exchange ratio. See Respiratory quotient
  (RQ)
Gear pump spirometers, 53, 54
Gibbs-Donnan effect, 203
Glomerular filtration rate, mechanical ventila-
  tion and, 235
Glucocorticoids in therapy, 459
Glycolysis, respiration and, 192
Gram negative pneumonias, 181, 182
Gram's stain of sputum, 174, 176
Granulomatous disease in children, 165

Hageman factor, 162
Hardware-implemented algorithms (HIA), 31–
  32
Hay fever, 157, 158
Heart block, 144, 145
Heart failure, 139, 204–205
Heart rate monitoring, 26
Heimlich valve for neonatal chest drainage,
  348
Hemodynamics. See Cardiopulmonary factors
Hemoglobin
  carbon monoxide affinity for, 222, 223
  carboxyhemoglobin, 44, 46
  free solutions as artificial gas transport sys-
    tems, 223, 224
  monitoring and analysis devices, 44, 46
  oxygen affinity, 196, 197–203
    as adaptive mechanism, 213
    artificial systems in defects of, 223
    Bohr effect and, 200–201, 202
    carbon dioxide and, 197, 199, 202
    carbon monoxide and, 222, 223
    diphosphoglycerate and, 197, 198, 199,
      201, 202–208
    in fetus, 207
    hydrogen ion and, 197, 199, 200–201,
      202
    hypoxia and, 202, 204, 207–208
    ligands and, 199–200
    molecular changes and, 198, 199
    oxygen binding, 197–200
    structure and, 206
    temperature and, 197, 198, 199
    tissue oxygenation and, 198, 206–207
  Seattle, 206
  structure of, 197, 206
Hemophilus influenzae infections, 181
Hemorrhage
  artificial blood advantages in, 223

artificial lung and, 437, 438
oxygen toxicity and intraalveolar, 213
Henderson-Hasselbalch equation, 102–103
HEPA filters, 59, 65–66, 186
Heparin
  anticoagulation management in artificial
    lung, 437
  for fat embolism syndrome, 331
  for pulmonary embolism, 142
Hereditary angioneurotic edema, 157
Herpesvirus, pulmonary disease and, 181, 183
High-efficiency particulate air (HEPA)
    filters, 59, 65–66, 186
  described, 65
  efficiency standards, 65, 66
  types, 66
Histamine
  antihistaminic aerosols, 452
  asthma and, 308, 311
  immunologic reactions and, 160, 161
  inflammation and, 164
  release, 162
    neuromuscular blocking agents and, 286
Histiocytes. See Macrophages (histiocytes)
Hot wire spirometers, 53–54
Humidification, 171, 172
  delivery of
    aerosol masks in, 59, 64–65
    Amsterdam infant ventilator in, 19, 20
    Bennett MA-1 ventilator in, 6
    Cascade ventilator in, 6, 15
    Foregger 210 ventilator in, 15
    nasal oxygen cannulas and, 63
    Ohio Critical Care Ventilator in, 7
    Puritan nebulizer in, 21
    Searle VVA ventilator in, 10
    Venturi oxygen masks in, 63
  gas flow meters used with humidifiers, 60
  infection and humidifiers, 178–179, 186,187
  in infection prevention, 184
  for intubated patients, 405
  in mucolysis, 126, 127
  nursing care and, 405
Hyaline membrane disease, 339–343
  artificial lung in, 433
  cardiopulmonary factors in, 341–342
  continuous positive airway pressure in, 342
  intermittent positive pressure breathing in,
    342
  lung surfactant and, 339–340, 341
  oxygen therapy in, 341–342
  positive end expiratory pressure in, 342
  prevention of, 339, 343
  prognosis, 343
  pulmonary edema and respiratory failure
    and, 347
  pulmonary rupture in, 342, 347
  risk factors and prediction of, 340–341
  supportive measures in, 343

Hydrogen ion concentration (pH)
  blood. *See* Blood hydrogen ion concentration (pH)
  defined, 102
  monitoring muscle, 48
Hyperbaric oxygen therapy, 222, 223
Hypersensitivity reactions
  Arthus phenomenon, 159
  asthma and, 307, 309–310, 311
  chemical mediators and, 160, 162–163
  cytolysis and, 158
  delayed, 159–160, 173–174
  immediate, 157–158
    anaphylaxis, 157. *See also* Anaphylaxis
    assays in, 157–158
    immunotherapy, 158
    prostaglandins and, 163
  immunoglobulins and, 173
  mixed reactions, 160–161
  soluble antigen-antibody complexes and, 158–159
Hyperventilation
  alkalosis and, 143
  blood carbon dioxide and, 98, 101
  bronchospasm and, 312
  forced expiratory volume and, 311
  hypoxia and, 101–102
Hypogammaglobulinemia
  acquired, 154–155, 185
  physiologic fetal, 152
Hypothalamus, respiration and, 97
Hypoventilation
  absolute vs. relative, 210
  blood carbon dioxide and, 101, 209
  defined, 209
  hypoxia and, 208, 209–210, 212
  pulmonary function profile, 107
Hypovolemia
  in hyaline membrane disease, 341, 343
  neonatal asphyxia and, 344–345
Hypoxia
  alkalosis and, 208
  altitude and, 209
  apnea of prematurity and neonatal, 348
  assessment of, 393–394
  blood abnormalities and, 212
  classification of mechanisms of, 208, 209
  differential diagnosis, 211–212
  diffusion defects and, 208, 211
  diphosphoglycerate and, 208
  drug abuse and, 336
  in emphysema, 295
  hemoglobin oxygen affinity in, 202, 204, 207–208, 211
  hyperventilation and, 101–102
  hypoventilation and, 208, 209–210, 212
  inadequate cardiac output and, 212
  oxygen therapy in acute, 222

  shunting and, 83, 208, 211
  ventilation/perfusion ratio and, 208, 210–211, 212

IL Model 182 Co-Oximeter, 46, 47
Immune deficiency disease, combined, 153
Immune reactions, 157–161
  cytolysis, 158
  delayed hypersensitivity, 159–160
  immediate hypersensitivity, 157–158, 163. *See also* Anaphylaxis
  mixed reactions, 160–161
  soluble antigen-antibody complexes, 158–159
Immunization against respiratory pathogens, 185
Immunoglobulins, 151, 152
  antibody–antigen reactions in immunotherapy, 158
  asthma and, 157, 173, 307, 309, 311
  classification, 173
  in combined immune deficiencies, 153
  defective synthesis, 153–154
  deficiencies and infections, 174, 175
  described, 152
  in fetus and neonate, 152
  hypersensitivity reactions, 173
  hypogammaglobulinemia, 152, 154–155, 185
  in immediate hypersensitivity, 157–158
  immunity to infections and, 165
  synthesis, 152
Immunologic factors, 151–167. *See also* Hypersensitivity reactions
  abnormalities and dysfunctions, 174, 175
  in asthma, 307, 309–310
    hypersensitivity reactions, 307, 309–310, 311
    immunoglobulins, 157, 173, 307, 309, 311
  B cells and, 151–152, 173, 175
  cell-mediated vs. humoral, 151, 152–153
  chemical mediators and, 160, 161–163
  chronic bronchitis and, 297
  combined immune deficiency disease, 153
  complement system and, 156–157, 158, 159
  defective immunoglobulin synthesis, 153–154
  development in fetus and neonate, 151, 152
  hypogammaglobulinemia, 152, 154–155, 185
  immune reactions, 157–161. *See also* Immune reactions
  immunization, 185
  immunoglobulins, 151, 152. *See also* Immunoglobulins
  immunotherapy, 158
  infections and, 151–152, 165–167, 170, 173–174, 175, 186–187

inflammation and, 163–164
mucocutaneous candidiasis and, 155–156
T cells and, 151–152, 173–174, 175
thymus and, 151, 152–153
treatment of defects, 185
Wiskott-Aldrich syndrome and, 155
Immunosuppressive agents
  infection susceptibility and, 167, 174
  lung transplant rejection and, 421
Immunotherapy of hypersensitivity reactions,
  158
IMV. See Intermittent mandatory ventilation
  (IMV)
Inactivity, complications of, 170, 172–173,
  185
Incentive spirometers, 49, 56–57
Infant respiratory distress syndrome (IRDS)
  continuous positive airway pressure in, 238
  hyaline membrane disease and, 347. See
    also Hyaline membrane disease
  intermittent mandatory ventilation in, 249
  meconium aspiration and, 345–346
  pressure for inflation of premature lung and,
    341
  type II, in neonates, 349–350
Infection(s). See also specific condition, e.g.,
  Bronchitis
  adult respiratory distress syndrome and, 325
  breaching natural barrier and, 169, 170, 171
  classification of antimicrobial agents for,
    188, 189
  clinical aspects, 180–184
  colonization vs., 180
  constitutional factors and predisposition to,
    169, 170, 172–174, 185
  defensive anatomy of respiratory tract and,
    169, 170–172
  drugs and susceptibility to, 169, 172, 174
    366
  environmental sources of, 165, 170, 177–
    179
    control of, 186–187
  equipment and, 188
    decontamination of, 186, 187
  factors in response to, 165, 166–167
  hyperbaric oxygen therapy and anaerobic,
    222
  immunologic factors and, 151–152, 165–
    167, 170, 173–174, 175, 186–187
    B cells, 151–152, 173, 175
    T cells, 151–152, 173–174, 175
  intravenous and intraarterial lines and, 167,
    170, 184–185
  intrinsic vs. extrinsic asthma and, 309
  pathogens in, classification of, 174, 176,
    177
  patient-to-patient transmission of, 186
  personnel in transmission of, 178, 186, 188

prevention of, 184–188
  in hypogammaglobulinemia, 155
  nursing care and, 406–408
  prophylactic antibiotics and, 187–188
  respiratory insufficiency and artificial lung
    in, 433–434
  reverse isolation in, 186–187
  risks in pulmonary disease, 169, 170
  sputum staining and cytologic studies in,
    174, 176, 177
  tracheostomy and, 169, 170, 172, 260, 261
    prevention, 184, 188
  treatment of underlying conditions, 185
Inflammation, 163–164. See also Infection(s)
Inhalation challenge test in airways obstruction, 99
Inspection in patient assessment, 392
Inspiration
  flow-volume loops and, 91–92
  maximal force for weaning from ventilators,
    245, 246
  normal vs. adventitious breath sounds in,
    392–393
Intermittent assisted ventilation (IAV) in
  weaning, 251, 252
Intermittent mandatory ventilation (IMV)
  Bennett monitoring bellows spirometer
    with, 52
  described, 249
  for infant respiratory distress syndrome,
    249
  in weaning, 250–251, 252
Intermittent positive pressure breathing (IPPB)
  decision for, 232
  in hyaline membrane disease, 342
  in meconium aspiration, 346
  pulmonary vascular resistance and, 230
  renal response to, 233–235
Intravenous or intraarterial catheterization,
  infections and, 169, 170, 184–185
Intrinsic asthma, 309–310, 317
Intubation. See Endotracheal intubation;
  Tracheostomy
Iodides, therapeutic preparations, 463
IPPB. See Intermittent positive pressure
  breathing (IPPB)
Isoetharine aerosols, 358
Isoniazid in tuberculosis, 187, 189
Isoproterenol
  areosol
    bronchodilating action of, 359–360, 365
    side-effects of, 358, 361
  in asthma, 364, 365
  inhalation, arrhythmias and, 142, 143

Jones Pulmonar, 51

Kartagener's syndrome, 297

Kidney
  function assessment, 393
  mechanical ventilation and
    blood flow, 234
    urine composition and flow, 233, 234,
      235
  positive pressure breathing and, 235–236
Kinins
  defined, 162
  immunologic reactions and, 160, 161, 162
  inflammation and, 164
Klebsiella pneumoniae pneumonia, 181–182
Krale Pleur-Evac, 235, 236
Krebs (tricarboxylic acid) cycle, 192
Krogh's equation, 79

Lactic acid metabolism, exercise and, 98, 99
Lecithin-sphingomyelin ratio, hyaline mem-
    brane disease and, 341
Leprosy, 165–166
LES disposable pneumotachograph, 55–56
Leukocytes
  in acquired hypogammaglobulinemia, 155
  B cells, 151–152, 173, 175
  cell-mediated immune mechanisms and, 152
  combined immune deficiency disease and,
    153
  phagocytosis in infections, 164, 165, 173,
    174, 175
  in sputum, 121, 123
  T cells, 151–152, 173–174, 175, 184
  transfusion for deficiencies, 186
Lidocaine for arrhythmias, 147–148
Ligands
  defined, 199
  hemoglobin oxygen affinity and, 199–200
Light beam recorders, 41, 43–44
Liver, positive pressure breathing and, 232–
  233
Locked lung syndrome, 361
Löffler's syndrome, 316
Lungs. *See also specific topic, e.g.,* Pulmonary
    function tests
  clearance mechanisms, 116
    alveolar phagocytosis, 113, 116
    mucus transport, 115–116
  normal structure and function, 291–293
Lung scans, 69, 95–97, 142
Lung transplantation, 417–423
  allografts, 419–420, 421, 422–423
  autotransplants, 418–419, 420, 421–422
  failure causes, 418–419, 420
  function after, 417, 420
  histologic response to, 421–422
  history of, 417–418, 422
  incidence, 417
  moral and ethical decisions in, 419
  orthotopic heart–bilateral lung transplanta-
    tion, 423

rejection problems. 417, 419, 421, 423
  survival, 417, 418, 419, 421, 422
Lymphocytes. *See* Leukocytes

MA-1 ventilator. *See* Bennett MA-1 ventilator
Macrophages (histiocytes)
  phagocytosis by alveolar, 113, 116
  in sputum, 119, 121, 122
Magnetic mass spectrometer(s), 27, 33–35
  criteria for, 34–35
  flexibility of system, 33
  gas analysis by, 33
  mechanism of operation, 33–34, 35
Marion Laboratories Spirostat, 53
Mask(s)
  aerosol, in humidity delivery to lungs, 59,
    64–65
  oxygen, 59, 62–64
    fitting, 63–64
    partial rebreathing, 63
    Venturi type, 59, 62–63
Mass spectrometer, 48
Mast cells in sputum, 121
Maximal breathing capacity (MBC)
  in air velocity index calculation, 78
  defined, 75
  measurement, 75–76
  for weaning from respirators, 245, 246
Maximal flow–static elastic recoil curve, 69,
  94
Maximal midexpiratory flow (MMF), 75
  defined, 74
  flow-volume loops and, 91
  measurement, 74
  normal, 291, 292
  in small airways disease, 304
Maximal voluntary ventilation (MVV). *See*
    Maximal breathing capacity (MBC)
MBC. *See* Maximal breathing capacity (MBC)
Mechanical ventilators, 3–20. *See also specific*
    ventilator
  in adult respiratory distress syndrome, 325
  bronchoscopy during use of, 132
  complications, artificial lung and, 427–428
  fluidics, 16–18. *See also* Fluidics
  in infection transmission, 178, 179, 188
  in meconium aspiration, 346
  minute ventilation and, 74
  nursing care during use, 404
  positive pressure breathing in, 229–243. *See*
    also Positive end expiratory pressure
    (PEEP)
  pressure-cycled, 3
  psychological needs in, 404
  pulmonary barotrauma and, 235–237
  renal response to, 233–235
  tidal volume measurement in, 74
  time-cycled, 3–4

volume-cycled, 3, 4–6. *See also* Volume-
cycled ventilators
weaning from, 245–252. *See also* Weaning
Meconium aspiration, 345–346
Mediators
adult respiratory distress syndrome and, 325
asthmatic reaction and pharmacologic, 308
release blocking drugs, 464
Medulla, respiration and, 97, 210, 277
Membrane lung. *See* Artificial lung
Membrane potential, neurohumoral transmission and, 281
Memory cell, defined, 173
Metabolic acidosis
in adult respiratory distress syndrome, 324
asthma and exercise, 311
causes, 103–104
Metabolic alkalosis, 103–104, 105
Metachronal beating, defined, 115–116
Methscopolamine bromide for asthma, 363,
364
Methylxanthines. *See* Aminophylline; Theophyllines
Minicomputers. *See* Computer(s)
Minute ventilation (VE)
defined, 74
measurement, 74
in oxygen consumption calculation, 80
oxygen toxicity and, 220
for weaning from respirators, 245, 246
Minute volume, monitoring, 3
Mitochondria, respiration in, 193
MMF. *See* Maximal midexpiratory flow
(MMF)
Monaghan 225 ventilator
described, 15–16
fluidics, 16, 18
Monaghan M 700 Spirometer, 53–54
Monitor(s), 25–56
advantages and disadvantages, 25–26
basic five-bed monitoring system, 26–27
for blood gases and pH, 27, 44–49
computers and, 26–27, 27–32. *See also*
Computer(s)
defined, 25
direct patient, 26, 27, 36–39
in apnea, 26, 38–39
electrocardiograph, 26, 38
transducers in, 36–37, 38
display systems and recorders, 27, 39–44.
See also Display systems and recorders
magnetic mass spectrometers, 27, 33–35
for muscle pH, 48–49
spirometers as, 27, 49–57. *See also*
Spirometer(s)
Morphine as neuromuscular blocking agent,
289
Motor end-plate, 280–281
Motor unit, 279–281

Mouth occlusion pressure (MOP), 98
MSA fluidic IPPB manifold, 17–18
Mucocutaneous candidiasis, 155–156, 185
Mucoid sputum, described, 118, 120
Mucolytic agents
actions, 125–127
aerosol, 463
defined, 125
humidification and, 127
Mucopurulent sputum, 118
Mucosa, respiratory
mucociliary system, 113, 114, 115–116,
172, 400
mucous blanket, 114, 115–116
mucus. *See* Mucus
structure, 114, 115
Mucus
composition and structure, 114, 117
mucous blanket, 114, 115–116
propulsion of, 115–116
secretion
in chronic bronchitis, 297, 298
normal, 299
Multifocal atrial tachycardia (MAT), 145
Multistage gas pressure regulators, 59, 60
Muscle pH, monitoring, 48–49
Mycoplasma pneumonia, 182
Myasthenia gravis, 287

Naloxene hydrochloride (Narcan) as morphine antagonist, 289
Narco Vitalor, 50, 51
Narcotics. *See also* Drug abuse
adult respiratory distress syndrome and overdose, 324, 335–337
antagonists, 289
Nasal decongestants, alpha adrenergic, 447,
451
Nasal oxygen cannulas and catheters, 63
Nasal polyps, aspirin sensitivity, and asthma
(ASA triad), 309, 310–311, 317
Nasal steroid aerosols, 462
Nebulization
importance, 20
nebulizers
described, 4, 20–23
as infection source, 178–179
ultrasonic, 22–23
particle size and, 357–358
NEEP. *See* Negative end expiratory pressure
(NEEP)
Negative end expiratory pressure (NEEP)
for neonates, 19, 342
systems for delivery, 19, 239–240
Neonates, 339–350. *See also* Pediatric
ventilators
amniocentesis and pulmonary disease risk
calculation, 340–341
Apgar score in assessment, 345

Neonates—*Continued*
  apnea of prematurity, 348–349
  asphyxia, 341, 343–345
  bronchopulmonary dysplasia, 342, 348
  feeding aspiration, 346
  hyaline membrane disease, 339–343, 347,
      433. *See also* Hyaline membrane disease
  hypovolemia and hypervolemia in, 341, 343
  immunologic factor development in, 151,
      152
  inflation pressures for premature lung, 341
  interstitial emphysema, 342, 347
  meconium aspiration, 345–346
  mortality of premature, 343
  negative end expiratory pressure for, 19,
      342
  neuromuscular blocking agents and, 288
  persistent fetal circulation, 350
  pneumomediastinum in, 342, 347–348
  pneumothorax in, 342, 347–348
  prematurity prevention, 339, 341, 343
  pulmonary air leak, 342, 347–348
  recurrent pneumonia, 342
  resuscitation, 344, 345
  sudden infant death syndrome, 349
  tracheal aspiration of risk, 346
  type II respiratory distress syndrome, 349–
      350
Neoplasms, immune defects and, 170, 174
Neostigmine methylsulfate (Prostigmin),
      neuromuscular blocking and, 283, 287
Nerves. *See* Neurological factors; Neuromus-
      cular factors
Neurohumoral transmission, described, 281–
      282
Neurological factors. *See also* Neuromuscular
      factors
  in adult respiratory distress syndrome, 324,
      325
  parasympathetic system and asthma, 361–
      362, 363–364
  in patient assessment, 391–393
Neuromuscular blocking agent(s), 282–290
  classification, 282–283
  clinical standards, 289–290
  competitive
    action of, 283
    described, 282, 283
  depolarizing
    action of, 283
    described, 282–283, 284–285
  drug interactions of, 287–288
  dual block, 283
  effects on neonates, 288
  effects in pregnancy, 288
  glaucoma and, 288
  ideal block, 285, 289–290
  individual responses to, 283, 285

  morphine as, 289
  purpose of use, 285
  side-effects, 285–286
Neuromuscular factors, 277–290
  blocking agents, 282–290. *See also* Neuro-
      muscular blocking agent(s)
  breathing control, 277–282
    central nervous system and reflex, 277–
      279
    drug control sites, 279
    muscles, 277
  motor end-plate, 280–281
  motor unit, 279–281
  neuromuscular junction, 279–282
Neuromuscular junction
  described, 279–281
  neuromuscular transmission at, 281–282
Neutrophils. *See* Leukocytes
Nocardia pneumonia, 181, 183
Noncatecholamines, beta adrenergic aerosol
      agonists, 359, 360
Nonrebreathing oxygen mask, 63
Norepinephrine as neurohumoral transmitter,
      281
Nursing care, 389–412
  assessment, 390–394, 395–398. *See also*
      Assessment
  communication and, 405, 406
  daily checklist, 395–398
  endotracheal tube, 403–404
    pharyngeal suctioning, 400, 403
    tube care and repositioning, 404
  evaluation of plan, 412
  fluid-electrolyte imbalance, 401, 407
  life style and disease chronicity, 389, 390–
      391
  main constants in, 412
  nutritional problems or deficiencies, 402,
      407–409
  patient problems, 394, 399, 400
    defined, 394
    psychological factors and, 389, 403, 405,
      406, 411–412
  planned interventions in, 394, 400, 401–
      403
  in respiratory failure, 400, 401, 403–407
    humidification, 405
    infection prevention, 406–407
    mechanical ventilation, 406
    oxygenation, 403, 405
    patent airway, 400, 403–405
  in sleep deprivation, 402–403, 409–410
  teamwork in, 389
  of tracheostomy, 404–405
Nutritional deficiencies, nursing care in, 402,
      407–409

Obesity, pulmonary function and, 107

Obstructions, extrathoracic, 93
Obstructive pulmonary disease. *See* Chronic
    obstructive pulmonary disease (COPD)
Ohio Critical Care Ventilator
  adaptation for assisted positive end expira-
      tory pressure, 240, 241
  described, 3, 6-7
Ohio Vortex Respiration Monitor, 56
Open-circuit nitrogen washout in functional
    residual capacity, determination, 71-72
Opiates, neuromuscular blocking and, 289
Optoelectric turbine spirometer, 52, 53
Oropharyngeal airway implementation, 400
Oropharyngeal oxygen catheters, 63
Oscilloscopes
  cascade, 39-40
  cathode ray, 40
  light beam recorders and, 43
Owens-Illinois Hydro-Sphere Nebulizer, 20,
    21-22
Oxygen. *See also* Oxygen therapy; Oxygen
    toxicity
  adaptive mechanisms and tolerance limits,
      213
  blood. *See* Blood gases, oxygen
  consumption
    calculation of, 80, 81
    defined, 80
    exercise and, 81, 98, 99, 193
    minimizing in hyaline membrane disease,
        343
    normal, 81
    at rest, 193
  negative feedback and photosynthesis, 213
  tension curve from atmosphere to tissues,
      193, 194
  transport, 101, 193, 194
    artificial systems for, 222-224
Oxygen therapy, 59, 61-64
  in adult respiratory distress syndrome, 324,
      325, 328, 337
  in apnea of prematurity, 349
  Bendix model RSS in, 61-62
  cannulas and catheters in, 63
  clinical recommendations on, 219-220,
      221-222
  in fat embolism syndrome, 331
  in hyaline membrane disease, 341-
      342
  hyperbaric, 222, 223
  masks in, 59, 62-64
    fitting, 63-64
    partial rebreathing, 63
    Venturi type, 59, 62-63
  in meconium aspiration, 346
  in neonatal pneumothorax and pneumo-
      mediastinum, 348
  tolerance limits in, 212-213

Oxygen toxicity, 212-222
  acute, 213-214
  adult respiratory distress syndrome therapy
      and, 325
  chronic, 213, 214
  clinical aspects, 219-222
  enzymes and coenzymes and, 218-219
  evolutionary adaptations to, 192
  exudative and proliferative phases, 213-214
  free radical theory of, 218-219
  hyperbaric oxygen therapy and, 222
  oxygen level and duration of exposure and,
      219-220, 221
  pathology, 213-215
  pulmonary function tests in, 215-218, 220
  symptom masking in, 220
  time course of, 214
Oxyhemoglobin dissociation curve, 198-199,
    200. *See also* Hemoglobin, oxygen
    affinity
  diphosphoglycerate and, 204, 205
  hypoxemia and, 143
  monitoring and analysis of, 44
  unloading and shape of, 206-207

Palpation in patient assessment, 392
Pancuronium bromide (Pavulon) in neuro-
    muscular blocking
  action of, 283, 284
  in pregnancy, 288
  side-effects, 286
Papanicolaou stains of sputum, 118, 119
Paper electrophoresis of gamma globulins, 154
Paralysis, neuromuscular blocking and, 285-
    286
Parenchymal (infiltrative) disease, 106
Paroxysmal atrial tachycardia (PAT), 144-145
Partial pressure of gases, described, 100
Partial rebreathing oxygen mask, 63
Particulate matter, removal from tracheo-
    bronchial tree, 113, 114, 115-116, 171-
    172, 400
Peak expiratory flow rate (PFR)
  defined, 75, 91
  measurement, 75
  normal, 91
Pediatric ventilators
  Amsterdam infant ventilator, 19-20
  Cavitron PV-10, 18-19
  positive pressure, 342
PEEP. *See* Positive end expiratory pressure
    (PEEP)
Percussion in patient assessment, 392
Perfluorocarbons as artificial blood, 223-224
Perfluorotributylamine as artificial blood, 224
Perfusion. *See also* Artificial lung; Ventilation/
    perfusion (V/Q) ratio

Perfusion—*Continued*
  distribution of regional, 96
    compartmental method analysis of, 83–84
    in small airways disease, 301
    oxygen extraction and, 196
    in pulmonary embolism diagnosis, 142
Persistent fetal circulation, 350
Personnel in infection transmission, 178, 186, 188
PFR. *See* Peak expiratory flow rate (PFR)
pH. *See* Blood hydrogen ion concentration (pH); Hydrogen ion concentration (pH)
Phagocytosis
  defined, 165
  in inflammation and infection, 164, 165, 174, 175
Pharyngeal suctioning, 400, 403
Photosynthesis, 192, 213
Platelets, artificial lung and, 431, 438
Plethysmography, body
  in airways resistance measurement, 78
  in functional residual capacity determination, 71, 72–73
Pleural disease, pulmonary function in, 106
Pleural friction rub, 392–393
Pneumococcal pneumonia, 180–181
Pneumocystis carinii pneumonia, 181, 183, 184
Pneumomediastinum
  described, 231
  neonatal, 342, 347–348
  positive pressure breathing and, 235
Pneumonia(s)
  artificial lung in, 423–424
  asthmatic bronchitis and, 310
  hypersensitivity, 160–161
  infectiousness of, 179
  lipid aspiration in, 124
  pathogens and clinical signs of, 180–182, 183–184
  radiologic patterns in, 180, 181
  recurrent, in neonates, 342
  upper airway colonization in, 187–188
Pneumopericardium, neonatal, 348
Pneumotachographs, 49, 55–56
  Fleisch, 55
  LES disposable, 55–56
Pneumotaxic centers, respiration and, 97
Pneumothorax
  compliance and, 4
  described, 231
  neonatal, 342, 347–348
  positive pressure breathing and, 235, 236
Pons, respiration and, 97
Portal blood flow, positive pressure breathing and, 232–233
Positive end expiratory pressure (PEEP), 229–243

  in adult respiratory distress syndrome, 325, 328, 335–336, 337
  decision for, 232
  in emphysema, 328
  in fat embolism syndrome, 331
  hemodynamic effects, 229–233
    cardiac output, 229–232, 232–233
    portal blood flow, 232–233
    pulmonary vascular resistance, 230
  in hyaline membrane disease, 342
  interrupted
    in minimizing effects of continuous, 232
    ventilator adaptation for, 241–243
  jaundice and liver function and, 232, 233
  methods of delivering, 237–238
    Amsterdam infant ventilator, 19
    Bennett MA-1 ventilator, 4, 5, 6
    Cavitron PV-10 pediatric ventilator, 18–19
    Emerson 3MV ventilator, 13
    Foregger 210 ventilator, 13–14
    Monaghan 225 ventilator, 15
    Ohio Critical Care Ventilator, 7
    Siemens Servo Ventilator 900, 9
  optimal level, 232
  patient assisted, 240–241
  pulmonary barotrauma and, 235–237
  renal response to, 233–235
  weaning from, 248, 252
Positive pressure breathing. *See* Positive end expiratory pressure (PEEP)
Potentiometric recorders, 41, 42–43, 44
Potter's syndrome, 348
Premature supraventricular ectopic beats, 144
Preset gas pressure regulators, 59, 60
Pressure
  defined, 59
  gas pressure regulators, 59–60
Pressure-cycled ventilators, 3
Pressure pulse, components of, 137
Procainamide in arrhythmias, 147–148
Propranolol in arrhythmias, 146
Prostaglandin(s) (PG)
  actions and chemistry, 163, 365
  aerosol, 358, 364–365
  asthma and, 308
  bronchodilator duration effects, 365
  described, 364–365
Proteases, emphysema and, 294–295
Pseudomonas pneumonia, 182
Psychological factors
  anxiety reactions, 389, 403, 411–412
  assessment of patient responses, 391–392
  beta adrenergic aerosol abuse, 360
  depression, 403, 411–412
  differential diagnosis of psychogenic illness, 316
  neuromuscular blocking, 285–286

in respiratory failure, 405, 406
in sleep deprivation, 410
Pulmonary air leak in neonates, 342, 347–348
Pulmonary aspiration
   differential diagnosis, 315
   in drug abuse, 336–337
   food, 122–123, 346
   of lipids, pneumonias and, 122
   meconium, 345–346
Pulmonary blood pressure
   arterial, 26, 138
   factors in increased, 138
   monitoring
      in artificial lung, 441
      direct, 26
   in obstructive lung disease, 140
   pulmonary capillary wedge pressure
      (PCWP), 138–140
      in acute respiratory failure, 139–140
      in adult respiratory distress syndrome, 325
      determination methods, 138–139
      monitoring, 26
      normal and abnormal, 139
   pulmonary embolism and, 141
   vascular resistance and, 138, 230
Pulmonary bypass. See Artificial lung
Pulmonary edema
   acute respiratory distress syndrome and, 336
      in hyaline membrane disease, 347
      narcotic addiction and, 336
   neurogenic, 324, 332–335
   pressure relationships in, 139, 324
Pulmonary embolism, 140–142
   diagnosis, 95, 142
   differential diagnosis, 314
   hemodynamic effects, 141
   heparin anticoagulation in, 142
   presenting symptoms, 141–142
   pulmonary function profile in, 107
   pulmonary infarction and, 141, 142
   radioisotopic scanning in, 95
   thrombosis and, 140–141, 173
Pulmonary function tests, 69–107, 391. See
   also specific topic, e.g., Asthma,
   pulmonary function in; Compliance;
   Residual volume (RV)
   air velocity index, 78
   alveolar-arterial oxygen tension gradient, 83
   categories, 69
   closing volume (CV), 69, 84–88, 89, 90
   compartmental method analysis, 83–84
   compliance, 69, 76–78
   criteria, for weaning from respirators, 245–
      247
   dead space evaluation, 69, 81
   diffusing capacity, 69, 79–80, 83–84
   exercise testing, 98–99
   expiratory reserve volume (ERV), 70

flow measurements, 69, 74–76
flow-volume loops, 69, 88–94
functional residual capacity (FRC), 71–73
lung volumes and capacities, 69–76
maximal flow–static elastic recoil curve
   (MFSERC), 69, 94
minute ventilation (VE), 74
need for, 69
normal, 291, 292–293
oxygen consumption and carbon dioxide
   production calculation, 69, 80–81
perfusion, 83–84
radioisotope scanning and, 69, 95–97
residual volume (RV), 73–74
respiratory center and chemoreceptor
   evaluation, 69, 97–98
shunt fraction, 69, 81–83
tidal volume, (TV), 74
total lung capacity (TLC), 73
ventilation, 83–84. See also Ventilation;
   Ventilation/perfusion (V/Q) ratio
vital capacity (VC), 70
Pulmonary infarction
   diagnosis, 142
   pulmonary embolism and, 141, 142
Pulmonary infiltration with eosinophilia (PIE),
   316–317
Puritan nebulizer, 20–21
Purulent sputum, 118–119, 120

QS. See Shunt fraction (QS)
Quinidine for atrial flutter, 146

Radioallergosorbent test (RAST) for immuno-
   globulins, 157–158, 307
Radioimmuneadsorbent test (RIST), 157
Radioisotopic lung scans, 69, 95–97, 142
Radiology
   in adult respiratory distress syndrome, 324,
      325
   in emphysema, 296
   patterns in pneumonias, 180, 181
Rales, 390
Recorders. See Display systems and recorders
Reducing valves, 59
Regional lung volume measurement, 96–97
Renin-angiotensin-aldosterone system, 235
Reservoir tube in lung humidification, 65
Resident gas technique of closing volume
   measurement, 84–85, 85–87
Residual volume (RV), 73–74
   and closing capacity, 87
   defined, 73
   functional residual capacity and, 73
   measurement, 73
   in small airways disease, 304
   total lung capacity/residual volume ratio,
      73–74

Resistance
to air flow at high lung volume, 292–293
airways. *See* Airways, resistance (R_{aw})
compliance and, time constant, 77–78
vascular, 138, 230
Resorcinols as bronchodilators, 452
Respiration. *See also* Pulmonary function
tests; Ventilation *and specific topic, e.g.,*
Respiratory rate; Ventilation/perfusion
(V/Q) ratio
biosynthetic pathways, 192–193
control, 97–98, 210, 277–282
central nervous system and reflex, 277–
279
drug control sites, 279
rhythm, 97
neuromuscular factors in, 277–290
Respiratory acidosis, 103
adult respiratory distress syndrome and, 324
arrhythmias and, 143
diagnosis, 104
Respiratory alkalosis, 103, 104
in acute respiratory failure, 247
arrhythmias and, 143, 247
Bohr effect and, 208
diagnosis, 104
diphosphoglycerate and, 208
Respiratory control centers, 97–98, 210, 277
Respiratory distress syndrome. *See* Adult
respiratory distress syndrome (ARDS);
Infant respiratory distress syndrome
(IRDS)
Respiratory failure. *See also specific topic,
e.g.,* Adult respiratory distress syndrome
(ARDS)
acute, 247
alveolar collapse in, 248
nursing care in, 400, 401, 403–407
humidification, 405
infection prevention, 406–407
mechanical ventilation, 406
oxygenation, 403, 405
patent airway, 400, 403–405
psychological factors and, 405, 406
oxygen therapy problems in, 221
pulmonary capillary wedge pressure in, 139–
140
Respiratory insufficiency, artificial lung for,
433–434
Respiratory muscle detraining, 248
Respiratory quotient (RQ), 69
calculation of, 81
defined, 81
exercise and, 98
normal, 100–101
Respiratory rate
in Amsterdam infant ventilator, 19–20
direct monitoring, 26

in Searle VVA ventilator, 10
Restrictive diseases, pulmonary function
profile in, 73–74, 92–93, 106, 302
Resuscitation
of neonates, 344, 345
in ventricular fibrillation, 148
RETEC fluidic IPPB manifold, 16–17
Reticular activating system (RAS), respira-
tion and, 97
Reticuloendothelial cells in sputum, 119–121
Ronchi, 392
RQ. *See* Respiratory quotient (RQ)
RSS (Bendix) oxygen delivery system, 61–62
RV. *See* Residual volume (RV)

Salbutamol as bronchodilator, 359, 360
Saligenins as bronchodilators, 452
Scar emphysema, 296
Schick test, 154
Scopolamine for asthma, 363
Searle VVA (Volume Ventilator Adult)
ventilator, 9–11
alarms, 11
humidifier, 10
oxygen delivery, 9–10
respiratory rate control, 10
spirometer, 10
Senile emphysema, 296
Serotonin
asthma and, 308
immunologic reactions and, 161–162
inflammation and, 164
Serum sickness, 159
Severinghaus PCO_2 electrode, 45–46
Shake test for surfactant, 340
Shock, adult respiratory distress syndrome
and, 324, 332, 335
Shock lung, 331–332, 333, 431, 432
Shunt(s). *See also* Shunt fraction (Qs)
in adult respiratory distress syndrome, 328
calculation on artificial lung, 433–434
hypoxia and, 83, 208, 211–212
in persistent fetal circulation, 350
pulmonary blood flow and, 138
Shunt fraction (Qs), 69, 81–83
anatomic vs. physiologic, 82
described, 81
expression and estimation, 81–83
weaning from respirators and, 245
Siemens Servo Ventilator 900, 7–9
inspiration and expiration, 8, 9
oxygen delivery, 7–8
pressure gradients, 7–8, 9
Sinus tachycardia, 143–144
Skin tests in immunologic deficiencies, 155
Sleep
nursing care in problems, 402–403, 410–411
stages, described, 409–410

Slow-reactive substance of anaphylaxis (SRS-A), asthma and, 308
Slow space ventilation, defined, 83
Small airways disease, 291, 301–304
  in asthma, 318
  diagnosis, 301–302
  morphologic studies in, 302
  pulmonary function tests in, 106, 301, 302, 303, 304
  symptoms, 302, 304
Spectrometer(s)
  IL model 182 Co-Oximeter, 46, 47
  magnetic mass, 27, 33–35
  respiratory mass, 48
Spirometer(s), 27, 49–57
  bellows, 49, 51–52
  in closing volume determination, 85–87
  described, 69
  in expiratory reserve volume determination, 70
  forced expiratory volume, 74–75
  in functional residual capacity determination, 71–73
  gear pump, 49, 53, 54
  hot wire, 49, 53–54
  incentive, 49, 56–57
  optoelectronic turbine, 52, 53
  pneumotachograph, 49, 55–56
  radiospirometer, 95–97
  in residual volume determination, 73–74
  in tidal volume determination, 74
  vane, 49, 56
  in vital capacity determination, 70
  water-seal, 49–50
  wedge, 10, 49, 50–51
Sputum, 113–127
  bedside appraisal, 118
  bronchomucotropic agents and, 123
  classification, 118, 120
  collection procedures, 116–118
  cytologic studies, 115, 116, 118–119
    cellular and noncellular elements, 119–122, 307
    fixation and staining, 118–119
    in infections, 174, 176, 177
  defined, 117
  examination time, 118–119
  examination of unstained, 118–119
  expectorants and, 123
  gross examination, 118
  mucoid, 118–119, 120
  mucolytic agents and, 125–127
    humidification and, 125–127
  mucopurulent, 118
  "normal," 120
  physical properties in stable bronchial disease, 118, 120
  quantity produced, 117
  stains, 176

Staphylococcal pneumonia, 181
Starling equation of pressure relations, 324
Stead-Wells spirometer, 49–50
Stenosis, tracheal. See Tracheal stenosis, post-intubation
Steroid(s), 459–462
  in adult respiratory distress syndrome, 325
  aerosol, 358, 366–367, 452, 462
  in asthma, 311, 318
    aerosol, 366–367
    oral, 366
  commonly employed, 460–461
  in emphysema, 295
  glucocorticoids, 459
  infection susceptibility and, 167, 174, 184
  in meconium aspiration, 346
Streptococcal pneumonia, 180–181
Succinylcholine chloride (Anectine) in neuromuscular blocking
  acid-base balance and, 288
  action, 282–283, 284–285
  in pregnancy, 288
  side-effects, 286–287
Suctioning, pharyngeal, 400, 403
Sudden infant death syndrome (SIDS), 349
Sulfonamides, 189
Superoxides, free radical theory of oxygen toxicity and, 218–219
Surfactant, hyaline membrane disease and, 339–340, 341

T cells, immunologic factors and, 151–152, 173–174, 175, 185
Temperature
  body
    monitoring, 26
    neuromuscular blocking agents and, 287
  controlled environment for neonates, 343, 345
  hemoglobin oxygen affinity and, 197, 198, 199, 204
  respiratory tract and variations in, 171, 172
Terbutaline, bronchodilating action of, 359, 360
Theophyllines. See also Aminophylline
  administration methods, 380, 382
    injection, 458
    oral, 349, 453–457
    rectal, 458
  for apnea of prematurity, 349
  circulatory function and, 379
  cyclic AMP mechanism and, 373, 374–375
  dosage, 380–382
  drug interactions, 374
  metabolism, 373–374
  pharmokinetics, 376–377
  pulmonary function and, 377–379
  tolerance to, 374

Theophyllines—*Continued*
  toxicity and side-effects, 375–376, 379, 380
Thoracoscope, fiberoptic bronchoscope use as,
    132
Thrombosis
  inactivity and, 173
  prevention, 185
  pulmonary embolism and, 140–141, 173
Thymic cysplasia, 153
Thymus, immunologic factors and, 151, 152–
    153
Tidal volume (TV)
  dead space related to, 245, 246–247
  defined, 74
  measurement, 74
  mechanical ventilators and, 3, 20, 74
    weaning and, 245, 246–247
  pulmonary barotrauma and, 235, 237
  variations in, 74
Time-cycled ventilators
  Amsterdam Infant Ventilator, 19–20
  Cavitron PV-10 Pediatric Ventilator, 18–19
  cycling in, 4
  described, 3–4
TLC. *See* Total lung capacity (TLC)
Total lung capacity (TLC)
  calculation, 73
  defined, 73
  residual volume/total lung capacity ratio,
    73–74
  in restrictive vs. obstructive pulmonary
    diseases, 73–74
  in small airways disease, 304
Total parenteral nutrition (TPN), infection
    and, 170, 184–185
Toxicity. *See* Oxygen toxicity
Toxins, respiratory response to, 316
T-piece (Briggs) adapter
  artificial humidification of lungs and, 65
  attachment for weaning, 247
Trachea
  anatomy, 253–254
  stenosis. *See* Tracheal stenosis, postintuba-
    tion
  tracheoesophageal fistulas, 260
Tracheal aspiration of high-risk neonates, 346
Tracheal stenosis, postintubation, 404
  clinical course, 262–264
  cricoid cartilage and, 253, 261
  cuffed tubes and, 255, 256, 257, 260, 261–
    262, 271
  fiberoptic bronchoscopy in, 130
  incidence, 255
  in infants and children, 272–273
  injury, healing and scarring patterns, 255,
    256, 257, 258, 260
  laminagrams in, 256, 263
  prevention, 271–272

primary disease and, 254
  pulmonary function tests in, 263
  restenosis, 271
  surgical therapy, 257, 259, 264–271
    cervical stenosis, 264–266
    laryngeal release technique, 267, 268–269
    low tracheal, 266–270
    results, 270–271
    subglottic, 266
    tracheal segment replacement, 267, 270
Tracheostomy
  artificial humidification of lungs and, 64,
    65, 403
  equipment and technique in stenosis pre-
    vention, 271–272
  indications and technique, 404
  in infants and children, 272–273
  infection and, 169, 170, 172, 260, 261
    prevention, 184, 188
  nursing care, 404–405
  tracheal stenosis and. *See* Tracheal stenosis,
    postintubation
  tracheoesophageal fistulas and, 260
  weaning from respirators and, 247, 248
Transducers
  in direct patient monitoring, 36–37, 38
  selection of, 44
Transfer factor in T cell deficiency, 185
Transfusion
  in hyaline membrane disease, 343
  in leukocyte defects, 186
  placental, 345
  platelet, 431, 438
  problems and hazards, 223
Tropical eosinophilia, 317
Tuberculin reactions, 160
Tuberculosis
  chemotherapy, 187, 189
  diagnosis in hospital, 183
  preliminary investigation, 182–183
  prophylaxis, 187
  reactivation, 182
Tubing, infection and, 186, 187
Tubocurarine chloride in neuromuscular
    blocking
  acid-base balance and, 288
  action, 282, 283–284
  in pregnancy, 288
  side-effects, 286
Turbine spirometer, 52, 53
TV. *See* Tidal volume (TV)
Type II respiratory distress syndrome in neo-
    nates, 349–350

Ultrasonic nebulizers, 22–23
Unbonded stain gauge transducer, 37, 38
Urinary catheters, infection and, 169, 170,
    184, 185, 188

Urine composition and flow, mechanical ventilation and, 233, 234, 235

Vanceril for asthma, 366
Vane spirometers, 56
Variable gas pressure regulators, 59, 60
Variant asthma, 309, 311, 313
Varicella virus, pulmonary disease and, 181, 183–184
Vasopressin, 233–234
VC. See Vital capacity (VC)
VE. See Minute ventilation (VE)
Ventilation. See also Hyperventilation; Hypoventilation; Ventilation/perfusion (V/Q) ratio
  carbon dioxide tension and, 101, 102
  distribution of, 96
    analysis, 83–84
    diffusing capacity and, 79
    nonuniform, 76–77, 301
    in small airways disease, 301
  exercise and, 98
  lung surface area for, 357
  maximum elasticity vs. airways resistance and, 94
  neuromuscular factors and, 277–290
  oxygen content of air and, 97
  oxygen toxicity and, 215
  slow vs. fast space, analysis of, 83, 84
Ventilation/perfusion (V/Q) ratio, 84
  diffusing capacity and, 79, 83–84
  in emphysema, 295, 296
  end capillary oxygen saturation and, 83
  exercise and, 98, 99
  hypoventilation and, 208, 210–211
  hypoxia and, 208, 210–211, 212
  position and, 87
  radioisotopic perfusion scanning, 69, 95–97
  in small airways disease, 301
Ventilators. See Mechanical ventilators
Ventricular premature beats (VPBs), 147
Ventricular tachycardia, 147–148
Venturi oxygen mask delivery system, 59, 62–63
Vital capacity (VC)
  in air velocity index calculation, 78
  closing volume and, 85, 87, 88
  defined, 70
  equal pressure point, 90, 94
  oxygen toxicity and, 215, 216, 220
  peak expiratory flow and, 91
  ratio of expiratory to inspiratory flow at, 92
  in restrictive pulmonary disease, 74
  tests of, 70
  weaning from respirators and, 245, 246
Volume of isoflow, defined, 93, 94

Volume-cycled ventilators, 3
  adaptation of
    for assisted positive end expiratory pressure, 240–241
    for intermittent assisted ventilation, 251
    for intermittent mandatory ventilation, 249
  advantages of, 3
  Bennett MA-1, 3, 4–6. See also Bennett MA-1 ventilator
  Chemetron Gill 1, 11–12
  described, 3
  Emerson 3MV intermittent mandatory ventilator, 12–13
  Foregger 210 ventilator, 13–15
  Monaghan 225 ventilator, 15–16
  Ohio Critical Care Ventilator, 3, 6–7, 240, 241
  Searle VVA (Volume Ventilator Adult) ventilator, 9–11
  Siemens Servo Ventilator 900, 7–9
V/Q ratio. See Ventilation/perfusion (V/Q) ratio

Water-seal spirometers, 49–50
Weaning
  arterial oxygen tension and, 247–248
  challenge of, 252
  intermittent assisted ventilation in, 251, 252
  intermittent mandatory ventilation in, 249–251, 252
  McPherson construction for continuous flow ventilation and, 248–249
  from positive end expiratory pressure, 248, 252
  pulmonary function test criteria for, 245–247
  respiratory muscle detraining and, 248
  team approach in, 245
  timing correlated with medical status, 248
  T-piece adapter in, 247
  tracheostomy patient, 247, 248
Wedge spirometers, 50, 51
Wiskott-Aldrich syndrome, 155, 160
Wounds, surgical, infection and, 169, 170, 172
Wright vane respirometer, 56
Wright's peak flow meter, 75

X-Y recorder
  in closing volume determination, 85–87
  described, 41, 43
  in flow-volume loop determination, 89

Yokohama asthma, 316

Zero end expiratory pressure (ZEEP) for infants, 19